Barcelona Publishers

Guidelines for Music Therapy Practice in Adult Medical Care

EDITED BY

JOY ALLEN

Guidelines for Music Therapy Practice
in
Adult Medical Care

Edited by Joy Allen

Print ISBN: 978-1-937440-50-3
E-ISBN: 978-1-937440-51-0

To obtain chapters separately in epub or Mobi formats, please visit:
www.barcelonapublishers.com

Distributed throughout the world by:
Barcelona Publishers
4 White Brook Road
Gilsum NH 03448
Tel: 603-357-0236 Fax: 603-357-2073
Website: www.barcelonapublishers.com
SAN 298-6299

Cover illustration and design: © 2013 Frank McShane

Copy-editor: Jack Burnett

Dedication

To

Benjamin, Ellie, & Madeleine Allen

We are no longer waiting for the storm to pass,
but, together, learning to dance in the rain.

Acknowledgments

My utmost gratitude goes to Dr. Kenneth Bruscia for conceptualizing this series. Dr. Bruscia's visionary leadership, clinical expertise, and research expertise have undoubtedly advanced the field of music therapy and my work as a music therapy clinician and researcher. His continual belief in my abilities and unending support have allowed me to grow is so many ways, personally and professionally.

Thank you to my fellow editors within this series for sharing in the vast array of emotions experienced during this process. Knowing others were a part of this incredible journey provided me with continual comfort, reassurance, and guidance.

I thank and appreciate the authors who contributed to this volume. Each author agreed to share his or her expertise while working together to advance the clinical and research knowledge of music therapy with adult medical patients.

I am indebted to my Temple University family, most especially Dr. Darlene Brooks, who has supported my growth since the beginning of my educational pursuits in music therapy and Dr. Cheryl Dileo, who fostered my love of medical music therapy and a biopsychosocial approach with medical patients.

I am grateful to my music therapy students. Their passion, dedication, and commitment to learning about self, music therapy, and the needs of medical patients provides inspiration and motivation to my work as a clinician, researcher and educator.

Lastly, I would like to express my sincerest and deepest gratitude to Benjamin, Ellie, and Madeleine Allen. They blindly joined me on this adventure and provided unwavering excitement, laughter, patience and support. I love you to the moon and back!

Permissions

Table of Contents

Contributors

Joy Allen, PhD, MT-BC is Assistant Professor of Music Therapy at Loyola University, New Orleans. She has extensive experience working with medical patients, primarily focusing on psychological health, pain management, and the family system. She is particularly passionate about working with individuals and families living with chronic illness, including cancer. Dr. Allen has presented on her clinical work and research at several peer reviewed regional, national, and international conferences.

Dr. Nicki S. Cohen is Professor of Music Therapy and Coordinator of Vocal Studies at Texas Woman's University. She received her PhD in Music Education from the University of Kansas, an MA in Vocal Performance from the University of Denver, and a BS in Music Education from Duquesne University. She is a board certified music therapist and a Fellow of the Association for Music and Imagery. Dr. Cohen has published in music therapy and related journals, most specifically about the applications of singing instruction for patients with neurogenic communication disorders. She also has published chapters in music therapy textbooks. Cohen is a regular presenter at music therapy and associated professional conferences.

Amy Clements-Cortés, PhD, MTA, MT-BC, FAMI is a music therapy instructor and clinical supervisor at the University of Windsor and Wilfrid Laurier University; and Senior Music Therapist/Practice Advisor at Baycrest Centre, Toronto, Canada. Dr. Clements-Cortés has worked extensively with geriatrics, adult mental health, complex continuing care, palliative care, oncology, and survivors of the Holocaust. Her work has been presented around the world and published in peer reviewed journals. She also runs a music studio *Notes By Amy* and has produced several recordings. Visit www.notesbyamy.com for more details. Dr. Clements-Cortés is currently the President of the Canadian Association for Music Therapy, and Clinical Commissioner for the World Federation of Music Therapy.

Dr. Barbara Daveson studied music therapy at the University of Queensland, health service management at the University of Manchester, and earned a PhD from University of Melbourne. She has worked clinically in acute care, oncology, palliative care (in hospice, specialist inpatient, day hospice and home-based environments) and neuro-rehabilitation in Australia and the UK. She is currently Research Fellow for the BuildCARE project at the Cicely Saunders Institute at King's College in London.

Simon Gilbertson is Associate Professor and Head of Studies of the 5-year integrated MA in Music Therapy, Grieg Academy, University of Bergen, Norway. Since qualifying in 1993 he has worked as a clinician, researcher and educator in England, Germany and Ireland and has experience with children and adults with cancer, individuals with unique developmental biographies, and neurological illness/trauma. He authored 'Music therapy and traumatic brain injury: A light on a dark night' with David Aldridge and is an Associate Editor of the Nordic Journal of Music Therapy. His current research interests include neurorehabilitation, the Arts, and central, peripheral and social nervous systems.

Annie Heiderscheit, Ph.D., MT-BC, LMFT, Fellow in the Association of Music and Imagery. She is an assistant professor and director of the master's in music therapy at Augsburg College, assistant professor at the University of Minnesota Center for Spirituality and Healing, and clinical music therapist at University of Minnesota Amplatz Children's Hospital. She is also a member of an interdisciplinary research team at the University of Minnesota. Dr. Heiderscheit is president of the World Federation of Music Therapy and frequently speaks and lectures nationally and internationally. She has authored several book chapters and articles based on her research and clinical work with mechanically ventilated patients, eating disorder and chemically dependent clients.

Douglas Keith, PhD, MT-BC, studied music therapy at the University of Georgia, the University of Applied Sciences in Heidelberg, Germany, and Temple University. As a clinician, he has worked with adults with psychiatric disorders, children with developmental disabilities, senior adults with dementia, and adults with HIV/AIDS. His dissertation examined ways that people make meaning of improvised music. Subsequent research has examined technology in music therapy education, music listening for premature infants, and the effects of music on breast milk production by mothers of premature infants. Douglas is currently Associate Professor of Music Therapy at Georgia College in Milledgeville, Georgia.

Christine Pollard Leist, PhD, MT-BC is an Assistant Professor in the Appalachian State University Music Therapy Program in Boone, NC. She holds the BM in music therapy from Florida State University, the MM in music therapy from the University of Miami, and the PhD from Michigan State University. Her clinical experience includes work with adult and older adult populations in a variety of settings and supervision of practicum students across a wide variety of ages and populations. As a member of the American Music Therapy Association, she has been involved in leadership roles at the state, regional, and national levels.

Dr. Wendy Magee studied music therapy at the University of Melbourne and earned a PhD in music at the University of Sheffield, UK. She is a Fellow in Neurologic Music Therapy, and has over 20 years experience working with neurological conditions including traumatic brain injury, stroke, Parkinson's Disease, Multiple Sclerosis, Huntington's Disease, low awareness states, and Locked-in Syndrome. She is a widely published author. Presently Dr. Magee is Associate Professor of Music Therapy at Temple University.

Dr. Jeanette Tamplin is a registered music therapist and researcher specialising in neurorehabilitation for people who have sustained a traumatic brain injury, stroke, spinal cord injury or other neurological disorder. Her clinical and research interests include the therapeutic effects of singing, speech and language rehabilitation, respiratory training, therapeutic songwriting, and coping and adjustment following traumatic injury or illness. Jeanette has published in international and interdisciplinary refereed journals and has contributed chapters to several edited books on music therapy, as well as co-authoring a text with Dr Felicity Baker: 'Music Therapy Methods in Neurorehabilitation: A Clinician's Manual' in 2006 (Jessica Kingsley Publishers).

Dr. Victoria Policastro Vega is an accomplished music therapy clinician, educator, and lecturer. She received her bachelor in music education from West Virginia University, her masters from Loyola University, and her doctorate at Temple University both in music therapy. AMTA activities include; South-Central Regional vice-president and president, Clinical Training and Education Committees, Education and Training Advisory Board, Judicial Review Board, Continuing Education Committee, Assembly of Delegates, Council Coordinator of Professional Practices and AMTA Executive Committee. Dr. Vega is currently the Associate Dean of the College of Music and Fine Arts at Loyola University New Orleans.

Preface

An Evolving Perspective

Kenneth E. Bruscia

Music therapy has grown dramatically in the last 20 years—in theory, practice, and research. New training programs have been founded in many countries, and global networks have been formed through federations, conferences, journals, and online media. The technological revolution has made it possible for professionals and students around the world to communicate their thoughts and discoveries about music therapy in the flash of one simple click. New generations of music therapists have begun to explore the endless horizons of music therapy in different cultures, while the more experienced generations have had the time and resources to reflect upon what has been evolving in the field. Theory, practice, and research can no longer be defined or delimited in terms of a single culture, treatment philosophy, method, training program, or individual.

The traditional modus operandi of music therapists has always been to find or develop the most appropriate methodological approach to meet the unique health needs and resources of each individual client, population, and treatment milieu. This aim has not changed. What has changed, however, is the growing awareness that understanding what these needs and resources are is not as simple as we had previously imagined. Once the strait jackets of a particular theoretical orientation or a single method are removed, and once cultural and individual differences are fully acknowledged, most of the older guideposts disappear, and therapists today are faced with the daunting task of apprehending each client's resources and needs within the full richness and complexity of his or her own unique world.

The primary mission of this series is to provide new, diverse, and more up-to-date guideposts for clinical practice. This mission is based on the belief that music therapy students and professionals have an ethical responsibility to be knowledgeable of *all* approaches to clinical practice that have been found effective for clients within different contexts.

The implications are threefold. First, this series advances the notion that no potentially effective practice should be excluded from the study of music therapy for reasons of personal, organizational, or institutional bias. Gone are the days that music therapists can assert that *only* their own approaches belong within the definitional boundaries of music therapy. Gone are the days when music therapists can assert that music therapy is only improvisational, or that music therapy is only behavioral, or that improvisational or behavioral approaches can be used with every clientele in all contexts. This narrow-mindedness is no longer acceptable. Music therapy is not just what you do, or just what I do—it is what we all do within the boundaries of ethical practice—and within the context of a discipline that also includes theory and research. Moreover, ethical practice can no longer exclude what others do with significant clinical effect.

Second, this series underlines the premise that music therapy is first and foremost a discipline of practice. As such, the practice of music therapy cannot be based solely on theory and research, it must also be informed by what practitioners have learned over the years about what works and what does not work in actual clinical settings. Very often these clinical details and anecdotes cannot be subjected to the rigors of research, yet they have significant practical value. Thus, notwithstanding the contributions of theory and research, clinical practice must be based on the accumulated insights of practitioners who have the experience, expertise, and ethical values needed to serve as our models. In short, music therapy is not merely evidence based or theoretically informed, it is even more essentially clinically based.

Third, this series reinforces the notion that like in other scholarly health care disciplines, music therapists must begin to write about their own clinical work within the context of what others have done in the same area of practice. In the early days, music therapists developed their own ways of working with a particular clientele or method independently of one another, and without the benefit of a world-wide communication network—there were no journals, books, or websites that could provide the wealth of practical information available today. This had a rather bizarre outcome that to some extent still continues today. Not being aware of what had already been done in the field, music therapists often considered and presented themselves as pioneers—touting that their own particular method of working as if it were entirely new—when in fact other music therapists had already been doing the same thing for quite some time. This sometimes made attending a conference a deja-vu experience, where it seemed as if we were proudly re-inventing the wheel and then giving the wheel our own new brand. Mary from Podunk would give a presentation announcing that she had discovered how to use the cello in therapy, when unknown to her, Juliette Alvin had already been doing it for years. Then to further complicate the matter, therapists in Podunk would call it Mary's method, and people in England would call it Alvin's method, even if the methods were practically identical. Of course, this was not the case for the many true pioneers of music therapy who actually invented or created a specific approach or model. But the problem remains: how can one distinguish between ignorant vanity and a truly new contribution to the field? Today there is no excuse for not knowing what others have done, and even less justification for not being interested. All we have to do is a computer search of the rapidly developing literature, and we can find others who are working in the same area of practice. And then our responsibility is quite simple: we have to contextualize what we have discovered about clinical practice in terms of the current state of knowledge in the field. Just like researchers who are expected to review the literature on their research question, modern practitioners are expected to know what they are doing within the context of their discipline.

The specific objectives of the series is to provide practical guidelines for implementing receptive, improvisational, re-creative, and compositional methods of music therapy with major client populations, supported by a comprehensive and critical review of existing literature. These methods are thoroughly defined and discussed in every chapter of the series. The major client populations were identified and categorized by diagnosis and age. As a result, four main areas of practice were identified: developmental health, mental health, pediatric care, and adult medical care. Primary diagnosis was used to distinguish between populations with mental health versus medical needs, and age was used to distinguish between the needs of children, adolescents, and adults.

Authors were carefully selected according to two criteria. First, they had to have extensive clinical experience in the area of practice about which they were writing; and second, they had to acknowledge and recognize significant clinical work done by others in the same area. Their charge then was not to merely write about what they did and believed, but to present a comprehensive picture of a particular area of practice to which they themselves had contributed significantly. Obviously, some areas of practice are more developed than others and in some instances the authors could only rely upon their own experiences. Music therapy is practiced in so many areas that this unevenness in development is to be expected for some time, and also is bound to be evident in the present series.

Given the aims and issues addressed so far in this Preface, it should come as no surprise that unlike many edited books in music therapy that support the "pioneer" syndrome, every chapter in every volume of this series follows the same outline. Authors were not free to determine what would and would not be covered in their respective chapters. A uniform outline was fashioned to ensure not only that the same basic topics would be addressed for each area of practice, but also to ensure that all relevant literature on each area was included. The basic outline is as follows:

1) Diagnostic Information
2) Needs and Resources
3) Assessment and Referral
4) Multi-cultural Issues
5) Overview of Music Therapy Methods
6) Guidelines for Receptive Music Therapy
    a. Method A:
        i. Overview: Definition, indications, goals, contraindications
        ii. Preparation of Session and Environment
        iii. What to Observe
        iv. Procedures for Conducting Session
        v. Possible Adaptations
    b. Method B:
    c. Etc..
7) Guidelines for Improvisational Music Therapy
8) Guidelines for Re-creative Music Therapy
9) Guidelines for Compositional Music Therapy
10) Working with Caregivers
11) Research Evidence
    a. Receptive Music Therapy
    b. Improvisational Music Therapy
    c. Compositional Music Therapy
    d. Re-creative Music Therapy
12) Summary and Conclusions
13) References
14) Resources (Optional)

One of the consequences of following the same outline is that there are bound to be repetitions in the information presented. The editors and authors have done their best to reduce *unnecessary* redundancies, while recognizing that some redundancies are important to keep. For example, many redundancies *between* chapters were left because each chapter will be made available separately in electronic formats, apart from the other chapters. Thus, each chapter had to be a complete presentation in itself, without requiring the reader to consult another chapter that the reader may not have.

Redundancies *within* chapters are another matter. These kinds of repetitions can be quite revealing. Several clinical questions are pertinent. For example, why is it that with a particular population, contraindications or "what to observe" are the same across certain methods but not others, or why are they the same for one population but not others? In some cases, a redundancy can reveal something about the population—that regardless of method, there are certain fundamental considerations that must be made when working with them. In other cases, a redundancy can reveal something about methods and how, though very different, may make the same demands on the client. And lastly, some redundancies can reveal blind-spots in the practitioner, that is when the music therapist can only see certain aspects of the client or clinical situation, regardless of the many complexities or variations present. For this reason, readers are urged to interrogate each redundancy. What does it reveal about the client, method, or therapist?

Another consequence of following the same outline is the opposite problem—disagreements. The authors in these four volumes were sometimes definite about using specific terminology and definitions for music therapy phenomena, even if doing so created disagreements and inconsistencies with other authors or the editors. Sometimes there was good reason, other times there was not. Sometimes it was the "Mary-Podunk" problem of wanting to name and thereby own a particular method or procedure that the author believed that she or he developed; other times it reflected deep theoretical divisions in the field itself; and other times it merely revealed aspects of music therapy that still need further conceptual clarity.

It is important to be aware of these disagreements and inconsistencies, not only to better comprehend what the authors have written, but also to understand the theoretical and practical issues confronting present-day music therapy. Three important differences of opinion became obvious in the planning, writing, and editing of these four volumes—differences that could not always be resolved within the context of the editorial process.

First, there are inconsistencies in how basic terms such as model, approach, method, protocol, procedure, and technique are used and defined. What one calls a model, others call an approach, and what one calls method, others call a technique. In this series, the basic premise was that there are four main "methods" of music therapy: listening (or receptive) experiences, improvisational experiences, re-creative experiences, and compositional experiences, each with their own set of procedural variations. This premise was not shared by all authors.

Second, there are disagreements in how to differentiate these methods. When does improvising become listening, and when does composing a song become improvising? Isn't listening a part of all musical activity, and doesn't listening require activity? So then why and how do we differentiate between receptive and active? An even more important dilemma for music therapy is: Should a method be defined by what the client "experiences" or by what the therapist "does?" If the therapist improvises for the client, is the method improvisational or receptive? Again this dilemma remains unresolved in these volumes.

Finally, there are considerable controversies over what practices a particular "model" (or method, or approach) does and does not include. For example, there is substantive confusion over what practices are legitimately considered part of the "Bonny Method of Guided Imagery and Music (BMGIM)," and which are not, and whether this "method" should be called BMGIM or simply "Guided Imagery and Music" (GIM). Then there is the onslaught of terms for the various "whatevers" that also involve music and imagery. Can anyone explain the procedural differences between the terms "Guided Imagery", "Directed Music Imagery," "Music and Imagery," "Music-imaging," and "Music-assisted imagery?" And do these names actually reflect those procedural differences? This is an example of an area of practice that begs for greater conceptual clarity.

These are not idle or "so what?" questions. How can we communicate about practice if we ignore differences between a model and a method, and if we invent idiosyncratic names for every method and technique? How can we train music therapists in the "discipline" of music therapy if there is no shared vocabulary or common language? How can we develop sensible "protocols" of practice to test through research if we do not understand the basic properties of the music experience that we hope to study, and if we are unclear in specifying what the client experiences and what the therapist does? And, how can we ever imagine an organized body of theory if practitioners and researchers do not use language intentionally and consistently?

It is hoped that this first attempt to present procedural, populational guidelines for practice will highlight the myriad implications of how we talk and write about music therapy. We need to be more aware of our discourses, not only from a philosophical or theoretical perspective (as in feminist and sociocultural streams of thought), but also from a practical point of view. Hopefully, the language problems encountered in this series will lead to a discourse analysis that will spawn more serious efforts to clarify and unify our diverse vocabularies about practice.

One final issue needs to be addressed. This series was envisioned as a teaching tool. Its purpose is to inform students as well as professionals about areas of practice that may not have been studied or experienced previously. The hidden yet obvious assumption is that the way to learn how to practice music therapy is by studying it in reference to each client population rather than by method. This relates directly to the redundancy problem. If the reader scans across "receptive" methods used across different client populations, many redundancies will be found, and the same kinds of repetitions will be found in re-creative, improvisational, and compositional methods. This poses an important pedagogical question: Would it be more economical and effective to first learn how to design music experiences (or use different methods of music therapy), and then learn how to implement or adapt them for different clients? Or is it more economical and effective to first learn about the characteristics and needs of each population, and then learn to design methods within that specific context? Put another way, is it easier and more effective to generalize or extrapolate from method to clients or from clients to method? Should we be training specialists in working with each population, or generalists who master the methods of music therapy? The vote is still out on this because unfortunately these pedagogical issues have not been recognized or discussed widely in the field.

Notwithstanding the decided emphasis given to clinical practice in this series, theory and research are still very much needed in music therapy—and in music therapy education as well. It is hoped that these volumes will stimulate the field to address the myriad research questions and theoretical issues raised by an organized and comprehensive presentation of what we know in practice. Further, it is hoped that this presentation will soon become outdated, and that revised, new, and increasingly more effective methods of practice will be conceived and tested.

GUIDELINES FOR MUSIC THERAPY PRACTICE IN ADULT MEDICAL CARE

Chapter 1

Introduction

Joy L. Allen

Aims

This volume seeks to present the current state of knowledge of medical music therapy practice with adults living with or experiencing a variety of medical conditions. The information presented is based on clinical expertise, along with a comprehensive and critical review of all relevant clinical and research writings. Practical guidelines for implementing music therapy methods with major medical conditions and/or experiences are provided for students and professionals in hope of increasing the knowledge of all viable approaches to clinical practice in medical music therapy with adults.

Medical Music Therapy

Medical crises do not discriminate based on race, disability, ethnicity, age, or socioeconomic status. It is quite likely that every individual will experience a medical crisis during his lifetime. Hopefully, this crisis will be temporary in nature; however, for many, this crisis will have lasting implications on all areas of their functioning and being. Important questions that emerge are: "What separates the area of medical music therapy from other medical interventions?" "From other forms of therapy?" "From other areas of music therapy practice?" Or, in summary, "What is medical music therapy?"

Bruscia (1998) defines medical music therapy as "all applications of music or music therapy where the primary focus is on helping the client to improve, restore, or maintain physical health" (p. 193). The goals may be directed toward change in the biomedical condition; to modify the cognitive, emotional, social, or spiritual factors that contribute to the biomedical condition; or to provide support to the client during the course of illness, medical treatment, or stages of recovery. According to Bruscia, medical music therapy does not include every approach provided to medical patients. Instead, medical music therapy includes only practices that "ultimately seek a change in the client's physical health" (p. 193). Thus it is distinguished from psychotherapy, as psychotherapy seeks psychosocial changes in the client regardless of changes in the client's physical health.

Dileo (1999) argues against distinguishing the practice of medical music therapy based on goals and outcomes. Her argument is supported through research into the mind/body/spirit connection. Accordingly, Dileo defines medical music therapy as music interventions implemented by a board-certified music therapist to meet the complex and diverse needs of medical patients. Medical music therapy always involves a therapeutic process, a music therapist, and a therapeutic relationship established within and through the music. Medical music therapy approaches may address physiological, emotional, social, spiritual, and/or cognitive and behavioral needs. With regard to medical treatment, music therapy may serve as the primary mode, in a supportive role, or in equal partnership with medical treatment.

The American Music Therapy Association has collected data on the demographics and employment of professional music therapists since 1990. Most recent data indicate that 13% of music therapists provide services in medical settings (AMTA, 2011). Furthermore, 16% of survey responders report working with medical, surgical, and/or neurological populations. Job growth in health care settings continues to grow, as several new jobs were created in hospitals, hospices, outpatient medical clinics, oncology settings, wellness programs, rehabilitation facilities, and palliative care units (AMTA, 2011). In addition to employing music therapy with medical patients, approximately 78 medical facilities serve as national association–approved internship sites for music therapy students (AMTA, 2013). Research in medical music therapy has dramatically increased over the previous decades and includes case studies, qualitative studies, descriptive studies, quantitative studies, randomized control studies, meta-analysis, and Cochrane Reviews.

Music therapists work with a wide variety of patients and medical conditions. These include working with patients in various medical units, during diverse procedures, with various medical diseases and disorders, and in addressing physical as well as emotional, social, cognitive, and/or spiritual needs. The effects of music therapy interventions with adult medical patients have been explored with the following populations/conditions: oncology, pain management, surgical patients, HIV/AIDS patients, cardiac patients, burn patients, transplant patients, orthopedics, neurology, intensive care units, ventilator-dependent patients, obstetrics, hospice, palliative care, and support groups. However, music therapists are not exclusive in the use of music experiences with medical patients, and it is necessary to distinguish medical music therapy from other complementary practices using the power of music within medical settings.

Music medicine is the use of music by medical professionals in research and clinical practice (Dileo, 1999). The purpose of music medicine interventions is to reduce the stress of the medical condition, hospitalization, and/or medical procedures, while optimizing physiological functioning such as heart rate, blood pressure, and respiratory rate. Typically, the music experiences in music medicine interventions are prerecorded and not individualized. Furthermore, the therapeutic relationship is not established through the music, and there is not a process of assessment, treatment, and evaluation with regard to establishing and evaluating the music experience (Dileo, 1999). Examples of music medicine as well as the effectiveness of music medicine experiences are prolific in the research literature. A range of music medicine interventions exists and includes such experiences as music piped into waiting areas to decrease anxiety and improve ambiance, the use of music listening experiences during medical procedures such as radiation, surgery, or CAT scans, etc.

Music thanatology is a field whose practitioners provide music comfort, using harp and voice, at the bedside of patients near the end of life (Music-Thanatology Association, 2008). Live music is used to respond to the physiological needs of the actively dying person as well as to serve the emotional and spiritual needs of loved ones. Educational and training requirements are not provided; instead, certification is based on meeting personal, musical, clinical, and medical competencies outlined.

Music practitioners are musicians who work to create a healing environment for the medically ill or dying. The goal of their work is environmental aesthetics vs. the individual needs of the medical patients (Music for Healing and Transition Program, n.d.). Furthermore, music practitioners do not make any attempts to actively engage the patient in the music. Training to become a certified music practitioner is provided through a series of workshops presented in conjunction with the Music for Healing and Transition Program.

"Musicians on Call" is an organization that brings live and recorded music to the bedside of patients in health care facilities. In an addition to professional musician volunteers servicing health care facilities throughout the United States, "Musicians on Call" provides hospitals with music listening libraries for patient use (Musicians on Call, n.d.).

Volunteer musicians are medical facility volunteers who offer to use their musical gifts to improve the overall hospitalized experience. These volunteers may agree to play music in lobbies or open areas, or for specialized events. Some volunteers assigned to patient visitation may spontaneously break into song during a visit with a patient. Volunteer musicians are generally amateur musicians who volunteer their time to improve the aesthetics of medical settings as well as to improve the quality of life of medical patients.

RESEARCH

Faced with financial and other related constraints, which continue to this day, Professor Archibald Cochrane suggested that health care resources be focused on those interventions proven to be effective by way of randomized control trials (Cochrane, 1972). The Institute of Medicine (IOM) defines "evidence-based practice" as a combination of the following three factors: (1) best research evidence, (2) best clinical experience, and (3) consistency with patient values (IOM, 2001). It affirms the right of every individual to receive high-quality care while ensuring that health care decisions are based on the best available, current, and relevant evidence. Limitations on funding and reimbursement demand that music therapists justify services as effective. Furthermore, as clinicians, it is our duty and responsibility to communicate the effectiveness of our work to others, including patients, families, treatment team members, administrators, students, and related individuals.

Within the field of music therapy, Wigram and Gold (2012) proposed three types of evidence:

- Direct evidence: provided through the clinician's assessment, treatment, and evaluation of therapeutic change or maintenance of health
- Related evidence: from literature (including case studies) of clinicians working in similar or related fields
- Research evidence: from both qualitative and quantitative methodologies

Wigram and Gold further created an evidence hierarchy, emphasizing that all levels of evidence are important in the development of evidence-based practice, research, and theory. Expert opinion forms the foundation of this hierarchy, proceeded by, in hierarchal order: qualitative studies, case reports/case studies, case series, case control studies, randomized control studies, review, and systemic review. As you will see throughout this volume, medical music therapy has made great strides in moving up the evidence hierarchy. Several examples of direct evidence, related evidence, and research evidence are provided. The reader is encouraged to review the evidence within each population/condition of medical music therapy, becoming aware of where our strengths and weaknesses lie. An overview of reviews and systemic reviews within medical music therapy as a whole is provided below.

Standley (2000) completed a meta-analysis with regard to researching the effectiveness of music experiences with various medical settings and populations. Primary dependent variables from 92 studies revealed that music within medical/dental care had positive benefits within the following goal areas: reduction of pain; reduction of anxiety and stress; reduction in chemotherapy-related nausea; increase in motor ability and joint ability; shortened labor; increase in capacity and strength in respiration ability; reduction in fear or trauma; assistance in acceptance of death or disability; assistance in symptom management; stimulation or elicitation of responses from those with cognitive dysfunction or those in isolation; improvement in short-and long-term memory; increase in awareness, self-control, and monitoring of physiological responses; reduction in depression/isolation; and increase in feelings of well-being.

Dileo and Bradt (2005) completed a meta-analysis of 183 music-based studies with medical patients. Studies were separated into music medicine experiences vs. music therapy interventions. Results indicated that music therapy interventions were more effective than music medicine interventions. Furthermore, results indicated that music therapy interventions significantly improved medical patients' well-being and life satisfaction and increased oxygen saturation rates. Results also indicated that music therapy interventions were effective in increasing perceived level of control and enhancing mood and were effective in decreasing the following: depression; distress behaviors; hospital stays; pain medication; and physiological measures including heart rate, respiratory rate, blood pressure, and mean arterial pressure. The authors conclude by encouraging future research with emphases on research collaborations to coordinate approaches, methodologies, and outcomes within and between the disciplines of music therapy and music medicine.

Several Cochrane Reviews have examined music interventions on various medical populations/settings/conditions. Cepeda, Carr, Lau, and Alvarez (2006) investigated the effects of music listening on acute, chronic, or cancer pain intensity, pain relief, and analgesic requirements. Fifty-one (51) randomized control trials involving 1,867 subjects and 1,796 different control variables met inclusion criteria. Results indicated that music listening reduced pain intensity and medication request; however, the magnitude of these results is limited due to the wide variety of control variables. Protocol has been submitted for an updated Cochrane Review of music for pain relief (Bradshaw, Brown, Cepeda, & Leon Pace, 2011).

Dileo and Bradt (2009) examined the effects of music interventions on stress and anxiety reduction in coronary heart disease patients. Results from 23 randomized control trials involving 1,461 participants indicated that music listening may have a positive effect on blood pressure, heart rate, respiratory rate, anxiety, and pain. However, the quality of the evidence is not strong and the clinical significance is unclear. The authors noted that 21 of the 23 studies examined involved listening to prerecorded music and did not involve consultation with a trained music therapist. The authors call for more research investigating the effects of music interventions offered by medical music therapists.

Bradt, Dileo, and Grocke (2010) completed a Cochrane Review of music interventions for mechanically ventilated patients. Specifically, they investigated the effects of music experiences on anxiety and physiological responses in mechanically ventilated patients. Results indicated that music listening might have a beneficial effect on heart rate, respiratory rate, and measures of anxiety; however, due to sample size limitations, the evidence was weak. Of the eight studies that met inclusion criteria, music listening was the main variable, and only one study included interventions by a trained music therapist. The authors call for more research investigating the effects of music interventions by trained music therapists.

Bradt, Dileo, Grocke, and Magill (2011) completed a Cochrane Review of music interventions for improving psychological and physical outcomes in cancer patients. Inclusion criteria were met for 17 studies implementing prerecorded music and 13 studies using active music therapy interventions. Results indicated that music experiences might have a beneficial effect on anxiety, pain, mood, and the quality of life of individuals with cancer. However, due to small sample sizes as well as the large variety of outcomes, it was not possible to compare the effectiveness of music medicine interventions with those of music therapy interventions.

In addition to Cochrane Reviews on music-based interventions in medical settings, systematic reviews have been completed of music therapy with specific clinical populations within the field of music therapy. Bradt and Dileo (2010) examined the effects of music therapy on psychological, physiological, and social responses in end-of-life care. Only five studies met inclusion criteria, leading to insufficient evidence. The authors conclude that there may be a benefit of music therapy on the quality of life of people in end-of-life care, but more research is needed.

The effects of music therapy on gait, upper extremity function, communication, mood and emotions, social skills, pain, behavioral outcomes, activities of daily living and adverse events for people with acquired brain injury were examined by Bradt, Magee, Dileo, Wheeler, and McGilloway (2010).

Results of the systematic review indicated that rhythmic auditory stimulation may be beneficial for improving gait, but insufficient data exist on all other measures. The authors call for more randomized control trials to support the effectiveness of Rhythmic Auditory Stimulation as well as research into music therapy interventions targeting movement, cognition, speech, sensory perceptions, and emotions in patients with acquired brain injuries.

Many limitations are present within medical music therapy research studies. These include small sample sizes, wide ranges of dependent variables, inconsistent reporting of music interventions used and the rationale behind selection of said interventions, various experience levels of clinicians, and the vast range of populations and clinical needs with which music therapists work. In an effort to address medical music therapy research limitations, Robb, Burns, and Carpenter (2011) identified and described key reporting guidelines for medical music therapy researchers. An overview of reporting criteria is outlined below.

- Provide a rationale for the music selected, including how the qualities and delivery of the music are expected to impact targeted outcomes.
- Provide the precise details of the music intervention and, when applicable, descriptions of procedures for tailoring interventions to individual patients.
    - Specify who chose the music.
    - Provide references for sheet music or sound recordings; when using improvised or original music, describe the overall structure.
    - Specify the music delivery method.
    - Specify music and/or nonmusic materials.
    - Describe the music therapy technique under investigation.
- Report the number of sessions, session duration, and session frequency, including any practice sessions.
- Specify how many interventionists delivered study conditions, as well as related qualifications and credentials.
- Describe the strategies used to ensure that treatment and/or control conditions were delivered as intended.
    - Include any manualized protocols, intervention monitoring, and/or interventionist training.
- Describe the treatment setting, including location, privacy level, and ambient sound.
- Specify whether interventions were delivered to individuals or groups, including the size of the group.

WHY MUSIC THERAPY?

Medical crises, whether temporary or chronic, can lead to physical, emotional, social, cognitive, and spiritual changes. During and after treatment, individuals may be challenged to balance their own notions of healthy self with their actual experiences of new or different physical, spiritual, emotional, or social capabilities. Music therapy is a form of therapy that allows individuals to identify, explore, and develop new ways of coping, experiencing, relating, and living in a safe and supportive environment. This process aims to connect the mind and body.

As outlined above and throughout this volume, research indicates that medical music therapy is effective on many levels—physiological, psychological, spiritual, behavioral, and social. Few, if any, side effects have been documented, and there are limited contraindications. Music therapy is noninvasive and flexible enough to meet the individual needs of a wide variety of conditions and populations. Research indicates that music therapy is associated with high levels of patient satisfaction (Bradt & Dileo, 2005) and is cost-effective treatment within medical settings (Standley & Walworth, 2005; Walworth, 2005).

In addition to the aforementioned practical considerations, it is striking to take into account the similarities and complementary nature of music and life, and music and health. According to Aldridge (1993), music itself can be a metaphor for life. Music, like life, is synonymous with movement. To live, one must continue to evolve, change, adapt, or, in some cases, maintain a certain level of functioning so as not to lose a needed gain. If our perpetual movement slows or comes to a halt, we are in danger of dying either figuratively or literally. What makes music so great, so interesting, and so appealing is the inherent movement, whether it is between the fundamental elements, within one element, or a shift in one's perception or reaction to the music. When music becomes overly repetitive or fails to develop, we lose interest or we tune out.

We are constantly improvising to meet the internal and external demands of our daily lives (Aldridge, 1996). If we stop improvising, creating, or engaging, we are no longer coping, responding, or, in some cases, living. Music allows for movement—more exploration is possible, and this exploration can come from several different "angles" until a new path is discovered. Sometimes that movement may be in leaps and bounds; sometimes it may be a steady plateau after a small loss or gain. It may be a simple heartbeat or a biopsychosocial balance leading to personal growth. We are all moving physiologically, behaviorally, psychologically, spiritually, and socially. Music therapy interventions provide patients with the opportunity to reconnect with their bodies in a multidimensional way. The music allows for an auditory experience as well as opportunities for kinesthetic, visual, and/or emotional experiences. By using music to address health, we essentially recognize the multidimensional aspects of self as well as the need for multidimensional techniques to access, explore, re-create, and/or create a new way of being.

We are musical beings. From conception on, we are all exposed to and respond to music, whether physiologically (heart rate, respiratory rate), behaviorally (dancing, tapping our toes), emotionally (feelings, memories), socially (interacting with others), or spiritually (connection with a higher power). In our modern culture, we often use a mechanical metaphor for life—when we are ill, we go to a physician to get fixed, often through mechanical application of medical protocol (vs. dialogue on the complex relationship between physical and mental aspects of health). However, I would argue that life and health, like music, are composed of many layers and relationships. Start with rhythm—it is the basis of our existence, as seen with our heartbeat. Next, add melody—our identity, our voice, followed by harmonic structure, form. This is followed by the interplay between the two—our social existence. Next we can add dynamics, layering, progressions, all leading to continued development of interrelationships and emotions. This is followed by aesthetic experience and transcendent qualities of music, or our spiritual connection. When we are born, we are rather simple musically, and as we age and develop, so does the complexity of the music. As adults, if our music doesn't flow, continue to unfold, continue to develop, we are no longer healthy and need to recompose, transpose, simplify, or return to an underlying form so that we can continue to respond to life's challenges. Life and health are not always simple, nor can they be fixed with a single prescription or type of intervention. Music may simply serve as a tool to access, a tool to re-create, a tool to redefine, a tool to express, or a tool for life.

Approaches to Music Therapy

Within medical music therapy, several factors influence the clinical choices that therapists make on a daily basis. The type of patients served is one such factor. This includes the homogeneity or plethora of diagnoses, primary presenting need areas, age, current functioning level, background and culture, and client goals or motivations. It is necessary for medical music therapists to select approaches that are consistent with best practices for the presenting health needs and conditions.

Policies and/or attitudes of employers also influence clinical approaches within medical music therapy. Health care facilities have established policies and treatment priorities that place limits on the types of services available to patients. In turn, this guides the selection of treatment approaches provided by a facility. In addition to workplace policies, the health care and insurance industries have considerable influence over the type and duration of treatment that a patient may receive for a medical condition. Funding and reimbursement of music therapy services is not uniform across populations, conditions, states, insurance providers, or countries. The availability of funds to cover treatment can greatly influence clinical approaches and services provided.

In addition to the needs of clients and the settings in which services are provided, the clinical and educational background of the music therapist has an influence on approaches to music therapy in adult medical care. Families, teachers, friends, and social circumstances influence a therapist. As the field of music therapy expands, so too do the educational opportunities available to students or practicing therapists. Several undergraduate and graduate music therapy training programs are espoused within a particular therapeutic approach or theory. In some cases, we may embrace the beliefs of our mentors; in other cases, we may reject the attitudes or opinions or approaches that our mentors share. As we continue to work, we gain additional experiences in implementing techniques with a variety of clientele. These experiences help us to form our identity as a therapist and may or may not force us to modify or change our previously conceived opinions or beliefs. Our strengths, limitations, values, and beliefs certainly influence our clinical orientation.

As therapists and the field of medical music therapy grow and develop, it becomes increasingly important to continue to stay abreast of current knowledge and trends within the field of medicine while continually examining how closely a selected approach matches our personal philosophy of health and helping those in need. Of utmost importance is our ethical responsibility to balance the needs of our clients within the policies and regulations of our employers and our personal strengths and limitations.

Given the variety of influencing factors on the therapeutic decision-making process, it is not surprising to find diverse theoretical orientations framing the work of medical music therapists. Influences can be found that reflect psychological philosophies, theories, or models, as well as approaches that reflect biomedical models.

Approaches Based on Psychological Theories or Models

Cognitive-behavioral approaches aim to alter cognitive perceptions essential to therapeutic success. They are effective in alleviating client distress in a short period of time. Interventions are designed for the here-and-now as well as to meet the immediate needs of medical patients in crises. Cognitive-behavioral approaches can be used to address the physiological, emotional, cognitive, and/or behavioral needs areas of adult medical patients (Standley, Johnson, Robb, Brownell, & Kim, 2004). Due to the short nature of inpatient medical stays, cognitive-behavioral approaches are widely used in acute medical situations.

Psychodynamic music therapy is based on the concept that events in the past have an impact on the present and that unconscious material drives current behavior. Psychodynamic approaches are used to help patients develop insights into unconscious drives, motives, and conflicts that negatively impact present functioning. Implementing psychodynamic techniques requires extensive and advanced training in psychodynamic music therapy, strong musical skills, and commitment and capacity for insight on the part of the client (Isenberg-Grzeda, Goldberg, & Dvorkin, 1994).

Within medical music therapy, psychodynamic approaches are aimed at addressing the emotional, social, and/or spiritual needs of clients. It is best used in outpatient settings or in long-term rehabilitation settings wherein the therapist and client will have the necessary resources and time to work through issues preventing emotional and/or spiritual healing.

The Bonny Method of Guided Imagery and Music is based upon humanistic and transpersonal theories that aim to increase self-awareness and understanding (Burns & Woolrich, 2004). It is a form of therapy that allows one to imagine, explore, and more fully experience possible life choices in a safe and supportive environment. Advanced training at the graduate level is necessary, and information on specific training programs can be found through the Association for Music and Imagery.

Working with individuals who have a chronic illness is one of the primary applications for Guided Imagery and Music (Bruscia, 2000). Short (2002) suggests that guided imagery and music with medical patients includes ventilation of emotions, insight into problem relations or negative patterns of behaviors, symbolic transformation of body parts, and increased feelings of physical and mental health, in addition to emotional reactions related to self-concept.

Approaches Based on Biomedical Models

Neurological music therapy focuses on utilizing musical stimuli for a variety of neurological disorders. It is defined as "the therapeutic application of music to cognitive, sensory, and motor dysfunctions due to neurological disease of the human nervous system" (Thaut, 1999, p. 221). It consists of standardized clinical techniques for sensory and motor training, speech/language training, and cognitive training in neurological rehabilitation, neuropediatric therapy, neurogeriatric therapy, and neurodevelopmental therapy (Clair & Pasiali, 2004). Clinical training in neurological music therapy is at the postbachelor's level through the Institute for Neurological Music Therapy.

Biopsychosocial theory acknowledges that disease and illness not only manifest themselves in terms of pathophysiology, but also may simultaneously affect many different levels of functioning, from cellular to organ systems, to person, to family, to society (Engel, 1977). It provides for a broader understanding of disease process as encompassing multiple levels of functioning. The biopsychosocial approach seeks to minimize the impact of disease on the physical and emotional development and functioning of the patient and family, as well as to achieve a dynamic balance between disease management and quality of life for the patient and family.

Music Therapy Methods

Evidence from research literature and clinical practice indicates that all four methods of music therapy outlined by Bruscia (1989) are used within medical music therapy. A method is defined as "a particular type of music experience used for assessment, treatment, and/or evaluation" (Bruscia, 1998, p. 114). Each of the four methods will be defined and outlined within the context of the medical care of adults.

Receptive methods involve the client listening to music and responding to the experience either silently, verbally, or through another modality such as art or movement (Bruscia, 1998). With medical patients, changes in physiological measures such as heart rate, respiratory rate, and blood pressure can be considered a response to a music listening experience. The music within receptive methods may be live or pre-recorded and focused on any of the elements within the music and/or song lyrics as facilitators of change. With adult medical patients, receptive methods are implemented to address physical, emotional, cognitive/behavioral, social, and/or spiritual needs.

Bruscia (1998) defines improvisational methods as experiences whereby the client spontaneously creates a melody, rhythm, song, or instrumental piece by singing or playing instruments. The therapist supports the client within this experience by providing appropriate levels of structure to facilitate or guide the client's creation. This may include providing selection of instruments, potential themes, and/or the musical support necessary to meet the needs of the patient during the improvisational experience. With adult medical patients, improvisational methods are implemented to address physical, emotional, social, and/or spiritual needs.

Re-creative methods encompass the client learning or performing precomposed vocal or instrumental music or reproduction of any kind of musical form (Bruscia, 1998). With adult medical patients, variations of re-creative methods are implemented to address physical, social, and/or cognitive/behavioral need areas.

Compositional methods are those experiences in which the therapist provides the necessary structure to facilitate songwriting, lyric writing, or the writing of instrumental pieces by the client (Bruscia, 1998). With adult medical patients, compositional methods may be implemented to meet their emotional, social, and/or spiritual needs.

LEVELS OF PRACTICE

A uniform approach to levels of practice within medical music therapy has yet to be adopted or implemented. Instead, music therapists within the field of medical music therapy categorize the depth of specific interventions on levels developed by Wheeler (1983), Bruscia (1998), and Dileo (1999). Each of these classifications will be described, including typical goals and overall significance within the patient's overall treatment.

Wheeler's psychotherapeutic classification of music therapy practice (1983) was originally based on the various need levels of psychiatric patients but can and has been adapted within medical music therapy. Three categories emerged to categorize the continuum of procedures—supportive, re-educative, and reconstructive. Within the supportive level, music therapy experiences are activity-based and success-oriented. Goals are achieved as a direct result of participation, and the therapeutic focus is on the here-and-now. Potential goal areas, relevant to the field of music therapy, may include social support, reality orientation, diversion from neurotic concerns, healthy use of leisure time, developing skills in dealing with emotions, and decreased anxiety and/or pain perception. At the supportive level, interventions are structured so that the client can practice patterns of behavior and responses, and the role of the music therapist is to establish a positive yet directive role. Music therapy interventions may include structured movement to music, singing, relaxation techniques, and compositional activities. Medical patients who may need a supportive level of care include those dealing with temporary medical crises, those dealing with severe anxiety, and those relearning skills secondary to an acquired medical trauma.

At the re-educative level, activity level is still important; however, there is a greater emphasis on interpersonal relationships and the expression and processing of emotions. Interventions at this level are focused on accessing and exploring personal thoughts, feelings, and interpersonal reactions. Music therapists working at this level need skill in choosing music for sessions that evokes emotions, images, memories, and reactions as well as solid verbal processing skills (Wheeler, 1983). Interventions used may include various forms of improvisation and the use of songs, including song communication, song discussion, songwriting, and song improvisation. At the re-educative level, the therapeutic process revolves around helping patients to cope emotionally with their diagnosis in order to maintain medical stability. Medical patients who may need interventions at this level include those dealing with complex lifestyle changes secondary to a chronic disease or an acquired injury.

According to Wheeler (1983), music experiences at the reconstructive level are used to uncover, relive, or resolve subconscious conflicts. Music is a critical component in accessing and expressing repressed materials, and advanced models of music therapy are required. Interventions include Guided Imagery and Music, vocal psychotherapy, Analytical Music Therapy, and psychodynamic music therapy practices with individuals living with chronic illnesses. Medical patients who may need interventions at this level include those who are medically stable but struggling with integrating aspects of their pre-illness self.

Bruscia (1989, 1998) defines the areas of medical music therapy as well as levels of practice within medical music therapy. According to Bruscia, medical music therapy includes "all applications of music or music therapy where the primary focus is on helping the client to improve, restore, or maintain physical health" (1998, p. 159). This includes music therapy approaches that focus on biomedical illness as well as those focused on psychosocial or ecological issues that impact biomedical illnesses. Levels of practice within the area of medical music therapy include auxiliary, augmentative, intensive, and primary.

Music experiences at the auxiliary level include therapeutic uses of music and music therapy consultations. This may include music experiences using prerecorded music for aesthetic purposes, to decrease distress, to increase relaxation, or for procedural support. At this level, the experience does not depend on a process of assessment, treatment, and/or evaluation by a trained music therapist. Examples of the auxiliary level may include music medicine experiences such as listening libraries, prerecorded music relaxation scripts, and music piped into various medical settings (Bruscia, 1998).

Within augmentative practices, music is primarily within a supportive client–therapist relationship. The therapeutic focus is on using music interventions for procedural support or improving quality of life within medical settings. Within augmentative medical music therapy practices, the therapeutic relationship is brief or time limited, often times comprised of a single session. Examples may include music therapy interventions to decrease perception of acute pain, to alleviate pre-surgical anxiety, or to reduce stress, fear, and related physiological responses during medical procedures such as lumbar punctures, chemotherapy, and bone marrow biopsies. Additionally examples may include music therapy at end of life that is focused on active stages of dying or limited to single session interventions (Bruscia, 1998).

Bruscia (1998) defines intensive practices as those experiences where the music is used as the primary agent of change within a supportive client–therapist relationship over an extended period of time or those experiences where the music and the client–therapist relationship are equal and used over an extended period of time to address the biomedical and/or psychosocial needs of patients overcoming or managing medical problems. Potential goals of medical music therapy within intensive practice may be found within cancer care, chronic pain, palliative care, HIV/AIDS, and chronic medical conditions.

Medical practices at the primary level occur when the music therapy interventions lead to significant and lasting changes in the client's health condition or when the goals and interventions extend beyond the medical condition to include other areas of practice. It is reconstructive in nature. Examples of music therapy at this level include case examples within HIV/AIDS and cancer (Bruscia, 1998).

Dileo (1999) presented a beginning model for delineating the levels of practice within medical music therapy. This model is based on the clinical needs of the patient, the degree of expertise and training of the therapist, the depth of the intended goal, and the function of the music therapy intervention within the overall medical care of the patient. Three levels of music therapy are found within this model—supportive, specific, and comprehensive.

At the supportive level, the needs of the client are temporary in nature, and the therapeutic need is focused on behavioral or physiological responses. Beginning therapists are qualified to implement techniques at this level with the focus on supporting medical interventions (Dileo, 1999). Examples may include music therapy interventions aimed at procedural support, procedural and acute pain management, and anxiety or fear responses. Specific methods may include music-based relaxation strategies, supportive music listening experiences, and re-creative techniques.

At the specific level, the need of the client is more insight-oriented, with the goal of accessing and exploring specific reactions and/or experiences to gain awareness as well as to confront challenging situations. Music therapy interventions at this level are of importance equal to that of medical interventions. Therapists must have advanced clinical and educational experiences and training (Dileo, 1999). Techniques may include the use of songs, improvisational experiences, and imagery techniques.

Music therapy at the comprehensive level is focused on resolution and takes over as the primary need of the client, with medical interventions becoming secondary in importance. At this level, therapists must have specialized training in advanced music therapy models as well as significant clinical experience in meeting the diverse needs of medical patients (Dileo, 1999). Examples of music therapy techniques at this level may include Guided Imagery and Music as well as entrainment.

Despite the lack of uniformity within levels of music therapy practice, areas of overlap between the aforementioned levels can be found. For example, it can be argued that Wheeler's supportive level is similar to Bruscia's augmentative practice and Dileo's supportive level. Regardless of preferred classification system, it is important for the therapist to align with or define her own levels of practice, taking into account the needs of the client, therapeutic intent, role of the music therapist, potential techniques, depth and breadth of the clinical process, and the level of experience and training needed.

Organization of the Book

The reader is encouraged to read "An Evolving Perspective" found at the beginning of every volume within this series. This preface provides the reader with essential information on the organization of chapters as well as the educational intent behind said organization.

This volume can be used in several ways. Music therapists and music therapy students may read specific sections within each or select chapters. The organization of this series allows readers to easily find information on diagnostic criteria, referral and assessment, treatment methods and techniques, and clinical and research evidence supporting selected treatment methods and techniques. This allows the reader to develop, enhance, and/or expand educational and clinical knowledge across specific areas of practice. Educators may assign specific sections within each or select chapters to teach according to personal and/or program learning philosophies. Specifically, educators are free to choose between population- or method-specific models of learning.

Music therapists and music therapy students may choose to read entire chapters, based on an area or population of interest. Likewise, some may choose to read a group of chapters with similar areas of concern. For example, four chapters specifically deal with neurological conditions (stroke, traumatic brain injury, neurodegenerative diseases, and neurocommunication disorders). Given the overlap in needs areas within the field of neurology, it might be beneficial for these chapters to be read in conjunction with one another. Similarly, if an individual is being seen on a palliative care unit secondary to advanced cancer, it might be beneficial to read the chapter on cancer care and the chapter on palliative care/hospice. An index that includes medical conditions and methods discussed in this volume is presented at the end to help the reader access those areas of greatest interest or need.

It is not possible to document every potential diagnosis and condition that adult medical patients may face. Likewise, this volume does not address every major diagnosis, unit, or situation found in various medical settings. However, information can be gained from reading the entire volume, as methods addressed in one chapter may very well be applicable to other disorders, conditions, and/or needs of adult medical patients that may or may not have been discussed in this volume.

Because medical crises are universal to all populations, the reader is encouraged to consult other volumes within this series. It is quite plausible that medical music therapists will treat adults with underlying psychological or developmental conditions in acute care hospitals, clinics, and rehabilitation facilities. Likewise, older adults constitute 60%–70% of acute care admissions and are prone to significant physical, cognitive, and social deterioration and decomposition after even minor medical stressors (Department of Health, 2011; Sager at al., 1996). It is imperative that the therapist be aware of the potential complications and needs facing individuals in these situations, select appropriate assessment tools, and adapt methods accordingly to meet the needs of some of the most vulnerable patients in medical settings.

Concluding Remarks

As I have reached a stopping point in the editing of this volume, it is time to reflect upon the two-year decision-making process and related challenges that the authors and I, as editor, have faced. At the beginning, it was which conditions/populations to include. This was difficult, as it would be impossible to cover every possible diagnosis, condition, or situation faced by individuals and music therapists in medical settings. As disease trajectories continue to change and the treatment of conditions change, so will the populations or conditions with which medical music therapist's work.

Challenges were also faced in defining terms and treatment approaches. Just as several definitions of music therapy exist, so do several definitions of diseases and related needs areas. Various governments and health care insurers define and classify medical conditions differently. As authors in this volume represent several countries throughout the world, efforts were made to use universal definitions or include a selection of definitions. It is important for music therapists to be aware of respective health care policies and the impact on practice and treatment trends.

Assessment methods and techniques faced several challenges. As you will discover, standardized music therapy assessments are hard to find. Instead, many rely on a combination of clinical expertise and methods/tools used by other health care professionals. Some chapters provide the reader with specific examples; other chapters describe specific assessment tools typically used. It is up to the practicing music therapist to choose the tool that best meets the needs of the situation within facility guidelines.

Perhaps of all the sections, the method sections were most difficult. Discussions took place over whether particular techniques were truly one method over another, a combination of methods, or interpretational differences between the author and editor. As not all music therapists ascribe to the methods presented by Bruscia, this was bound to happen. A great effort was made to classify techniques by definitions provided as well as the author's rationale behind any questionable placements. Additional issues revolved around advanced training and supervision requirements. A great effort was made to expose the reader to a variety of techniques. The reader is informed of those techniques that require advanced training and supervision for safe implementation. Readers are encouraged to seek additional training and supervision to expand the abilities and resources they are able to offer their patients.

An additional challenge within the methods section was documenting what we do as music therapists. Our clinical expertise allows us to meet the immediate needs of clients in a variety of situations. It becomes a challenge when we are forced to define what we do vs. describe what we do and why we do it. This is particularly true when asked to provide enough details in our definitions and descriptions to enable others to learn from our experiences as well as compare methods in one chapter to methods described in another.

The dilemma of whether a method was evidence-based came into play. The research within medical music therapy has grown by leaps and bounds but continued growth in this area is needed. However, we must continue to share our clinical experiences in order for this to happen. Some authors had to be encouraged to share techniques regularly implemented despite the lack of research evidence supporting effectiveness.

While it is impossible to cover every condition or situation that music therapists might incur in their work within medical settings, it is hoped that music therapists will be able to use the underlying principles contained in this volume to shape their practice. This work is not a final product and will never be. However, it is an important step in providing current knowledge on the practice of medical music therapy. Just as humans and music continue to grow and evolve, so will the field of music therapy and the music therapists working with adults with medical needs.

References

Aldridge, D. (1993). The music of the body. Music therapy in medical settings. *Advances in Mind-body Medicine, 9,* 17–35.

Aldridge, G. (1996). A walk through Paris: The development of melodic expression in music therapy with a breast cancer patient. *The Arts in Psychotherapy, 23,* 207–223.

American Music Therapy Association. (2011). *Snapshot of the music therapy profession. AMTA 2011 member survey and workforce analysis.* Silver Spring, MD: American Music Therapy Association.

American Music Therapy Association. (2013). *National roster internship site.* Silver Spring, MD: American Music Therapy Association. Retrieved from: musictherapy.org

Bradt, J., & Dileo, C. (2010). Music therapy for end-of-life care. *Cochrane Database of Systematic Reviews, Issue 1.* Article no.: CD007169.

Bradt, J., Dileo, C., & Grocke, D. (2010). Music interventions for mechanically ventilated patients. *Cochrane Database of Systematic Reviews, Issue 12.* Article no.: CD006902.

Bradt, J., Dileo, C., Grocke, D., & Magill, L. (2011). Music interventions for improving psychological and physical outcomes in cancer patients. *Cochrane Database of Systematic Reviews, Issue 8.* Article no.: CD006911.

Bradt, J., Magee, W., Dileo, C., Wheeler, B., & McGilloway, E. (2010). Music therapy for acquired brain injury. *Cochrane Database of Systemic Reviews, Issue 7.* Article no.: CD006787.

Bruscia, K. (1989). *Defining music therapy.* Gilsum, NH: Barcelona Publishers.

Bruscia, K. (1998). *Defining music therapy* (2nd ed.). Gilsum, NH: Barcelona Publishers.

Bruscia, K. (2000). A manual for level one training in Guided Imagery and Music. Unpublished.

Burns, D., & Woolrich, J. (2004). The Bonny Method of Guided Imagery and Music. In A. Darrow (Ed.), *Introduction to approaches in music therapy* (pp. 53–62). Silver Spring, MD: American Music Therapy Association.

Cepeda, M., Carr, D., Lau, J., & Alvarez, H. (2006). Music for pain relief. *Cochrane Database of Systemic Reviews, Issue 2,* Article no.: CD004843

Clair, A., & Pasiali, V. (2004). Neurologic Music Therapy. In A. Darrow (Ed.), *Introduction to approaches in music therapy* (pp. 143-157). Silver Spring, MD: American Music Therapy Association.

Department of Health. (2011). *A & E quality indicators: May 2011.* London: DH. Retrieved from www.dh.gov.uk/health/2011/10/qualityindicators

Dileo, C. (1999). Introduction to *Music Therapy and Medicine*: Definitions, theoretical orientations and levels of practice. In C. Dileo (Ed.), *Music therapy & medicine: Theoretical and clinical applications* (pp. 3–10). Silver Spring, MD: American Music Therapy Association.

Dileo, C., & Bradt, J. (2005). *Medical music therapy: A meta-analysis & agenda for future research.* Cherry Hill, NJ: Jeffrey Books.

Engel, G. (1977). The need for a new medical model: A challenge for biomedicine. *Science, 13,* 18–33.

Institute of Medicine. (2001). *Crossing the quality chasm: A new health system for the 21st century.* Washington, DC: National Academy Press.

Isenberg-Grzeda, C., Goldberg, F., & Dvorkin, J. (2004). Psychodynamic approach to music therapy. In A. Darrow (Ed.), *Introduction to approaches in music therapy* (pp. 79–102). Silver Spring, MD: American Music Therapy Association.

Music for Healing and Transition Program. (n.d.). *Mission Statement.* Retrieved from www.mhtp.org

Musicians on Call. (n.d.). *About musicians on call.* Retrieved from http://www.musiciansoncall.org/site/PageNavigator/About/About_MOC

Music-Thanatology Association International. (2008). *What is music-thanatology?* Retrieved from http://www.mtai.org/index.php/what_is

Robb, S., Burns, D., & Carpenter, J. (2011). Reporting guidelines for music-based interventions. *Music and Medicine, 3,* 271–279.

Sackett, D. (1996). Evidence-based medicine—What it is and what it isn't. *British Medical Journal, 312,* 71–72.

Sager, M., Franke, T., Inouye, S., Landefeld, C., Morgan, T., Rudberg, M., Siebens, H., & Winograd, C. (1996). Functional outcomes of acute medical illness and hospitalization in older persons. *Archives of Internal Medicine, 156*(6), 645–652.

Short, A. (2002). Guided imagery and music (GIM) in medical care. In K. Bruscia & D. Grocke (Eds.), *Guided imagery and music: The Bonny Method and beyond* (pp. 151–170). Gilsum, NH: Barcelona Publishers.

Standley, J. (2000). Music research in medical treatment. In J. Standley (Ed.), *Effectiveness of music therapy procedures: Documentation of research and clinical practice* (3rd ed.; pp. 1–64). Silver Spring, MD: American Music Therapy Association.

Standley, J., Johnson, C., Robb, S., Brownell, M., & Kim, S. (2004). Behavioral approach to music therapy. In A. Darrow (Ed.), *Introduction to approaches in music therapy* (pp. 103–124). Silver Spring, MD: American Music Therapy Association.

Standley, J., & Walworth, D. (2005). Cost/benefit analysis of the total program. In J. Standley, D. Gregory, J. Whipple, D. Walworth, J. Nguyen, J. Jared, K. Adams, D. Procelli, & A. Cevasco (Eds.), *Medical music therapy: A model program for clinical practice, education, training, and research* (pp. 31–40). Silver Spring, MD: American Music Therapy Association.

Thaut, M. (1999). Music therapy in neurological rehabilitation. In W. Davis, K. Gfeller, & M. Thaut (Eds.), *An introduction to music therapy: Theory and practice* (2nd ed.; pp. 221–247). Dubuque, IA: McGraw-Hill.

Walworth, D. (2005). Procedural support music therapy in the healthcare setting: A cost-effectiveness analysis. *Journal of Pediatric Nursing, 20*(4), 276–384.

Wheeler, B. (1983). A psychotherapeutic classification of music therapy practices: A continuum of procedures. *Music Therapy Perspectives, 1,* 8–12.

Wigram, T., & Gold, C. (2012). The religion of evidenced-based practice: Helpful or harmful to health and well-being? In R. Macdonald, G. Kreutz, & L. Mitchell (Eds.), *Music, health, & well-being.* Oxford: Oxford Scholarship Online. DOI: 10.1093/acprof:oso/9780199586974.001.0001.

Chapter 2

Surgical and Procedural Support for Adults

Annie Heiderscheit

Diagnostic Information

In the medical environment, surgery and procedures are tools for diagnosing or treating disease and illness. Surgery is the branch of medicine that deals with the diagnosis and treatment of injury and illness through manual and instrumental means (*Webster's New World Medical Dictionary,* 2008). Medical procedures are categorized by the level of invasiveness and are termed noninvasive, minimally invasive, or invasive. Noninvasive procedures refer to those that utilize external imaging, such as x-rays, magnetic resonance imaging (MRI), computerized axial tomography (CAT) scans, and positron emission tomography (PET) scans. A minimally invasive procedure refers to a procedure that is less invasive than open surgery used for the same purpose. In a minimally invasive procedure, there is minimal damage to biological tissue and the damage that does occur is typically from the insertion of the instrument. Medical procedures that are invasive refer to medical procedures that invade the body, by a device that punctures the skin or an instrument that is inserted into the body (NIH, 2012; *Webster's New World Medical Dictionary,* 2008).

There is a wide array of noninvasive, surgical, invasive, and minimally invasive procedures performed in medical care. These can range from open-heart surgery to cardiac catheterization, labor and delivery, radiation, gynecological exams, burn debridement, wound care, mechanical ventilation, biopsy, dialysis, and a host of others. Patients who experience high levels of anxiety can encounter the negative physiological symptoms, such as increased blood pressure and heart rate, elevated blood cortisol levels, and decreased immune response, which can result in slower wound healing and an increased risk of infection (Scott, 2004). Additionally, patients undergoing medical procedures may have negative experiences or symptoms as a result of their reactions or feelings about the experience or as a result of the invasiveness of the procedure itself. Patients may have fear about undergoing the procedure and experience stress, anxiety, pain and/or discomfort during the procedure.

Music therapy for surgical and procedural support can occur prior to, during, or following the surgery or procedure. Music therapy is a versatile approach with flexible methods that can address the various needs, symptoms, and feelings that patients experience in the perioperative and procedure process. This can range from managing stress and anxiety due to anticipation of the procedure to distracting the patient from fears or pain, facilitating relaxation to manage discomfort or anxiety, or managing symptoms such as nausea. The intensity of these feelings, symptoms, and issues can vary depending on the invasiveness of the procedure, previous experiences of the patient, and the patient's ability to cope.

Needs and Resources

Patients may undergo many different procedures during the course of their hospitalization or treatment. The level of invasiveness varies tremendously from one procedure to the next, and a patient's response may vary from one procedure to the next as well as from one patient to the next. Therefore, it is important to approach each patient based on their circumstances and situation, and to individualize their care. It is important to be observant of body language, facial expression, muscle tension, how they may be positioned, and vital signs, in addition to what a patient may say. It is important to pay attention to details, as all of these are sources of information about the patient and provide indications of the patient's needs.

Patients may not always know or be able to communicate clearly what they need, due to their condition or situation. They may also feel too overwhelmed to even recognize what they need in the moment. This can require the music therapist to assess their needs and introduce the intervention that is potentially the most effective. It is important to ask if the patient does consent to the intervention.

Patients can have a wide range of needs that arise during procedures. Physical needs can include dealing with pain and discomfort, nausea, and increased respiratory or heart rate due to stress or anxiety. Emotional needs may include anxiety, fear, or depression prior to or during the process. Some patients may have spiritual needs to be addressed in this process as well. They may want to feel more connected to God or their Higher Power during this time. In order to best meet these needs, it is helpful to meet with the patient in advance to assess these needs.

Patients who have had previous experiences in undergoing procedures may have a clear understanding regarding how they tend to respond in these situations, or they may have a greater level of comfort due to their familiarity with the process. While this may be very helpful to the music therapist in anticipating their needs, the music therapist still has to be prepared to respond to needs arising in the moment. Previous experiences of the patients with a particular procedure do not guarantee that they will experience it again in the same way.

It is also important to understand what the patient can and cannot do during the procedure. If the patient needs to be still and not move, they will not be able to actively play music. Additionally, it is important to know what access the staff doing the procedure needs to have to the patient. This helps to ensure that an instrument will not be obstructing the procedure and provide insight into how to situate for the procedure to best meet the patient's needs.

During the course of the intervention or therapeutic process, the patient's needs may change. This may necessitate shifting or changing the intervention accordingly. For example, a patient may begin a session by needing active music-making to provide distraction from discomfort. After a period of actively making music, he or she may tire and need to move to an intervention in which they engage in a receptive method. Therefore, it is important to continuously observe the patient's level of engagement and body language to best access their needs and changes therein.

Musical characteristics for this clinical population will vary in many ways. Adults undergoing surgical and medical procedures range in age from late teens/early 20s to older adults well into their 80s. Music preferences for patients in these age ranges will vary greatly, and assessing these preferences will be key to meeting the patient's needs. It is important to be aware that the musical needs of the patient may vary during the procedure, thus requiring the music therapist to be flexible while engaging the patient in the music experience. There will be times when the patient needs very soothing and calming music (based on their preferences) to help them relax, and then in the midst of the same procedure they may need music that serves as a means of distraction.

It is helpful to have a variety of instruments for playing live music for patients during a procedure. This ensures that the patient can make a choice regarding what they would like to hear from moment to moment. When patients are engaged in actively making music, it is important to have a variety of instruments that can be easily played with minimal effort, as the patient may not be able to move a great deal due to the procedure. Sound can also be a consideration, so it is important to have instruments that can also be played quietly and softly in order to not disrupt the staff conducting the procedure or other patients in surrounding rooms.

In the medical environment, there are precautions to follow. Instruments need to be cleaned prior to and after procedures. Ensure that the instruments you will be utilizing with a patient can be cleaned with the wipes utilized by the hospital to sterilize equipment. This may require checking with the manufacturer. Hospital gowns, gloves, and masks will often be required. Observe signs outside patient or procedure rooms, as these will indicate the necessary precautions. Procedures often occur in smaller rooms, so it is important to work with the patient care team to determine how to best situate care providers in the space to provide the best possible patient care.

Referral and Assessment

Music therapy referrals are often a multipronged process involving patient self-referrals, treatment team referrals, and/or music therapist–based referrals. During their scheduling, patients may be given information in advance regarding services available to them before, during, and after the procedure. In this instance, they have the opportunity to self-refer for music therapy. On the other hand, a nurse meeting with the patient to discuss the procedure may suggest or make a referral for music therapy services. As the need for procedures can arise quickly in the medical setting, the music therapist may be paged when the nurse or physician recognizes that music therapy services may be helpful to the patient. Last, music therapists may suggest the service to the patient or the treatment team for certain medical procedures or symptom presentations.

Once a patient has been referred for services, the music therapist should assess music preferences and how music will be used during the medical procedure. It is important to determine if the patient is restricted to music listening or if they may be engaged in simple or subtle playing or singing. A sample music assessment tool (MAT) developed by Chlan and Heiderscheit (2009) is included in Appendix A. This tool can assist in assessing the music preferences of the patient.

There are many considerations when utilizing music and music therapy in the surgical or procedural process. This requires understanding the procedure and what logistically will occur, as well as the needs of the patient and staff. These factors all impact the process and need to be reviewed so that the procedure can be conducted successfully and smoothly. It is important to consider the following when determining what method to employ with a patient.

- An understanding of the process surrounding the procedure:
    - What precautions need to be taken for this procedure?
    - Does the patient have any experience in undergoing procedures?
    - If so, what has been helpful in the past?
- What are the patient's needs?
    - Has the patient expressed any fears or concerns regarding the procedure?
    - Could these needs change during the process or course of the procedure?
- Does the patient have a clear understanding of the procedure (what will take place and how it will occur)?
    - Does the patient want to understand what will take place in the procedure?
- How does the patient tend to respond when feeling stressed, anxious, or overwhelmed?
- What are the patient's music preferences?

- What is required of the patient during the procedure?
    - Is the patient able to move, or does he or she need to be still?
- What are the space considerations and needs of other staff during the procedure?
    - Will family members be present during the procedure?
- Does the procedure staff understand the role of the music therapist?
    - Does the procedure staff understand the role that music can plan during the procedure?

OVERVIEW OF METHODS AND PROCEDURES

The following methods and procedures are most commonly used for surgical and procedural support. These have not been sequenced to reflect relative significance, effectiveness, or complexity.

Receptive Music Therapy

- Music Listening: Facilitating opportunity for patient to listen to preferred music, which may be recorded or performed live
- Directed Imagery and Music: Combines the use of music with guided imagery, usually prerecorded music.

Improvisational Music Therapy

- Meditative Drumming: A subtle and soothing manner of drumming by the patient, supported by the therapist

Re-creative Music Therapy

- Singing: Patient sings or hums preferred music with or without the support of the music therapist

Compositional Music Therapy

- Songwriting: The therapist assists the patient in composing songs with particular words or messages

GUIDELINES FOR RECEPTIVE MUSIC THERAPY

Music Listening

Overview. Listening to patient-preferred music can be initiated prior to the procedure, and then continue through the procedure as well as any recovery time following the procedure. It is appropriate for procedures that require the patient to be still, or when patients are hesitant to engage in more active approaches. The goals for this likely include managing stress, anxiety, and discomfort surrounding the procedure or surgery. Using music listening during a procedure requires a complete understanding of the medical environment, the procedure, and the acute patient needs in this setting. It is contraindicated whenever patients report that they do not want to listen to music.

Preparation. The music therapist should conduct a thorough assessment of the patient's music preferences in order to have music available for the time of the procedure (see Appendix A). The music therapist can either work to put together the music for the patient or work with the patient to put together playlists for the patient to utilize via their own portable device. If portable devices are permitted at the hospital or clinic, this will need to be addressed with the infection control. The music therapist will need to determine the device the music will be administered through (iPod, iPad, MP3 device, or portable CD player). I recommend using a personal device rather than providing music through ambient means. The use of noise-canceling headphones and a portable device allows the patient to listen and helps to block out noise and allow control of the music device.

The environment for the procedure is pre-determined by the hospital or clinic and is therefore beyond the control of both the patient and music therapist. Since this method allows the patient to self-administer the music, there will be no need for the music therapist to prepare the space. It is vital to inform and educate the procedure team about the music listening protocol. This helps to ensure that the team is supportive and that there are no barriers to the implementation of the protocol for the patient.

What to observe. Since the music therapist will not be with the patient during the procedure, it is important to ensure that the music equipment is loaded with music preferred by the patient and that the patient can operate the equipment easily. This will include understanding whether the patient will be able to utilize their hands during the procedure to change or adjust the music. The patient will be closely observed by the procedure team throughout the procedure and while listening to music. It may be helpful to talk with the patient and team following the procedure to evaluate the effectiveness of the music listening protocol.

Procedures. This method is designed as a patient-directed protocol, so the patient can self-direct their use of music. It may be helpful for the music therapist to take time prior to the procedure to make sure the equipment is functioning properly, so that the patient does not need to be concerned with this task.

Adaptations. The music therapist may meet with the patient and provide instructions about how to best use music listening during surgery. At this time, it can be decided whether the patient or music therapist will select the music. The music therapist may encourage the patient to develop his or her own playlists or collection of music to utilize for surgery, or gather the information needed to create a music listening program for the patient. If patients are bringing their own music into the procedure, it is still vital that the procedure team has agreed to this practice and that all infection control policies and issues are addressed.

Song discussion may also serve as a valuable tool for patients who may have thoughts and fears they want or need to express. Patients who also want to connect spiritually prior to a procedure may find it helpful to do so through listening to songs that connect them to God or their Higher Power. Gardstrom and Hiller (2010) provide some considerations when selecting songs for discussion. Overall, it is important to keep in mind the needs of the patient and their music preferences when selecting a song or songs for the sessions.

Recorded Imagery and Music Relaxation

Overview. The therapist creates a recording of imagery suggestions and pre-recorded music, designed to help the patient focus and relax prior to and throughout the procedure. The music may be taken from a recording that the patient is familiar with and utilizes currently, or one that is selected from a collection that is made available to the patient by the music therapist. The music therapist does not create the music for the recording. In most cases, the therapist uses a standard relaxation induction that has been prepared beforehand.

This method is appropriate for a patient undergoing a procedure when they have a difficult time managing their anxiety or when they are not able to self-initiate an imagery experience. The goals for this intervention may range from providing a distraction from the procedure to managing anxiety, stress, and discomfort. The method is contraindicated if it conflicts with a patient's religious beliefs or if the patient does not enjoy imaging.

Preparation. It is beneficial to have the patient practice using the recording to allow them to determine what will work best for them. This can be done at home or in the presence of the therapist. In the latter situation, the therapist can immediately address any issues or struggles that may arise and make the necessary adjustments.

It is important that the listening device the patient uses during the procedure has been approved by the procedure team and that it has also been reviewed and approved by infection control. It will need to be determined who will clean the device prior to the procedure. It may be the music therapist who oversees this task or a member of the procedure team.

The environment will be the procedure space provided, which will be predetermined and over which the patient or music therapist will not have control. Since this method allows the patient to self-administer the music, there will be no need for the music therapist to prepare the space. It is vital to inform and educate the procedure team about the music listening protocol. This helps to ensure that the team is supportive and that there are no barriers to the implementation of the protocol for the patient.

What to observe. The music therapist will not be with the patient during the procedure, so it is important to ensure that the music equipment is loaded with the appropriate music, and that the patient can operate the equipment easily. The patient must be able to change or adjust the music throughout the procedure. The patient will be closely observed by the procedure team while listening to the recording. It may be helpful to talk with the patient and team following the procedure to evaluate the effectiveness of the intervention.

Procedures. This method is designed as a patient-directed and -controlled intervention, so the patient can self-direct the design of the recorded imagery and music, and the listening process. The music therapist should take time prior to the procedure to make sure the equipment is functioning properly, so that the patient does not need to be concerned with this task. The music therapist may meet with the patient and provide instructions on how to use and control the listening device.

Adaptations. This method can be varied in many ways, depending upon the situation and patient need. In some instances, the therapist may attend the procedure and actually voice the relaxation suggestions while the patient listens to recorded music selected by the patient. This gives optimal flexibility to responding to what the patient is experiencing moment to moment. There may also be instances when the therapist will want to create special music for the recording, based on the patient's preferences. Finally, the patient may also choose to record his or her own voice giving the relaxation suggestions, following a transcript developed by the therapist. There are resources available that patients can download that include directed imagery alone or directed imagery with music. See resource section after the References.

Guidelines for Improvisational Music Therapy

Meditative Drumming

Overview. Meditative drumming is a subtle and soothing manner of drumming. It allows the drummer to enter into a relaxed and meditative state through playing repetitive rhythms on a hand drum. Patients who need an active method in order to be adequately distracted or achieve a relaxed state may find this type of intervention helpful. The goals for this method are to provide the patient an active method of engagement as a means of distraction to manage stress, anxiety, discomfort, or pain and/or to foster relaxation. The drumming should be calm and calming, as it should not disturb or interfere with the procedure or require much movement or energy from the patient. This method is contraindicated if the patient is not interested in drumming or if the procedure would preclude the patient from engaging in drumming.

Preparation. The environment will be the procedure space provided, which will be predetermined and over which the patient or music therapist will not have control. Since this method allows the patient to self-administer the music, there will be no need for the music therapist to prepare the space. It is vital to inform and educate the procedure team about the music listening protocol. This helps to ensure that the team is supportive and that there are no barriers to the implementation of the protocol for the patient.

What to observe. It is important during the course of the procedure to observe how the patient is managing while playing and notice if tempo, dynamics, or volume need to shift to best meet his or her needs. It may be feasible to observe vital signs via the monitors to which the patient is hooked up, depending on your placement in the room during the procedure. Be sure you are aware of the space needs of the staff conducting the procedure and to keep their work area open.

Procedures. Meet with the patient prior to the procedure or while he or she is being prepped. It is helpful to begin the drumming and help the patient relax prior to the start of the procedure. It is helpful to remind the patient to take slow, deep breaths; this can be accompanied musically as well, to give continuity and provide a rhythm for the patient to focus on. When the procedure is completed, continue to accompany the patient for as long as he or she would like help to maintain a calm and relaxed state.

Adaptations. If the patient is unable to play a hand drum using their hand or finger during the procedure, there may be other instruments that can be used that will not interfere with the procedure. Toning, chanting, humming, or singing could be incorporated into the drumming as well. For procedures that do not allow the patient to move or where movement is restricted, the voice can be utilized as the instrument of choice.

Guidelines for Re-creative Music Therapy

Singing

Overview. Singing can be a great way to ensure that a patient is taking good, solid breaths. In addition, it often provides an effective means of distraction. Singing may be indicated as an intervention if the patient is comfortable using their voice and if it will not in any way interfere with the procedure. The goals of singing during a procedure may be to manage anxiety and provide a means of distraction from discomfort and pain, as well as to ensure that the breathing rate can remain consistent.

Preparation. Prior to the procedure, it is helpful to meet with the patient and determine what song or songs they would like to sing. This ensures that the patient does not have to make decisions while in the midst of the procedure, when it may be difficult for the patient to do so. Songs that are calming, soothing, comforting, or reassuring may be most helpful. For some patients the song(s) may be connected to their faith or simply a song that is familiar. It may be helpful to determine with the patient what message they would like to hear during the course of the procedure. This can help to determine the song(s) to use. It is important that the songs not require too much of the patient, as he or she often needs to be rather still during the procedure.

Discuss with the procedure team where you can stand to accompany the patient, so as to not be in the way of the procedure. It is important to ensure that it is feasible for the patient to sing during the procedure, so this needs to be cleared with the procedure team. This can also serve as an opportunity to inform and educate the procedure team about the intervention and how it benefits the patients. This helps to ensure that the team is supportive and that there are no barriers to the implementation of the intervention for the patient. You will need to ensure that you have also followed the necessary precautions for the procedure. These procedures should be worked out with infection control ahead of time.

What to observe. It is important to observe how the patient is managing the singing experience, and to notice if tempo, dynamics, or volume need to shift to best meet her needs. It may be possible to observe vital signs via the patient's monitor, depending on your placement in the room. Be sure you are aware of the space needs of the staff conducting the procedure and to keep their work area open.

Procedures. Meet with the patient prior to the procedure or while being prepped. Help the patient relax prior to the start of the procedure. Once the procedure begins, start with the song the patient has requested and accompany and sing with the patient. In between songs, it is helpful to remind the patient to take slow, deep breaths. These breaths can be accompanied musically by the therapist in order to give continuity and to help the patient focus on a comfortable rhythm for breathing. When the procedure is completed, continue to sing and accompany the patient for as long as he or she would like help to maintain a calm and relaxed state. Patients may choose to chant a word or phrase that is supportive or comforting.

Adaptations. It may be easier at times for the patient to hum the song(s) rather than sing. Humming can easily be implemented during the procedure, or a patient may alternate between singing and humming during the course of the procedure. Toning or chanting can also be utilized. Toning, chanting, humming, or singing can be utilized to foster a meditative state.

GUIDELINES FOR COMPOSITIONAL MUSIC THERAPY

Songwriting

Overview. Songwriting can be helpful for patients if they have specific words or messages they want or need to hear during the course of the procedure. The goals for this method include managing stress, anxiety, and discomfort; providing a means of self-expression; and empowerment. Songwriting may be contraindicated if the patient does not have time prior to the procedure to work with the music therapist to create the song, or if they feel overwhelmed by the song-writing process while they are thinking and preparing for the procedure. It may also be contraindicated if singing is not feasible during the procedure.

Preparation. As with other methods, it is important to discuss the music therapy intervention with the procedure staff, not only to gain their support and understanding, but also to gain an understanding of the procedure, what to expect, what the space needs of the procedure team are, and where you can be positioned throughout the course of the procedure.

The songwriting process will need to be completed prior to the procedure, and then the song can be sung during the course of the procedure. The song should be simple and should include words and phrases that the patient can easily remember, as he or she will need to sing it from memory.

What to observe. Observe the patient's singing efforts and comfort, as suggested above under "Singing." Adjust tempo, dynamics, or volume to best meet his or her needs. If possible, observe vital signs via the monitors. Be sure to respect the space needs of the staff conducting the procedure and to keep their work area open.

Procedures. Follow the same procedures as presented above under "Singing."

Adaptations. The patient may choose to write a poem that he or she sets to music or makes into a chant. The patient may have key words or phrases that will be helpful and supportive to hear during the procedure and can create a mantra out of them, which can be chanted or sung.

Research Evidence

Music therapists, physicians, and nurses have conducted research surrounding the use of music in surgical and procedural support. Medications administered for sedation during surgical or procedural support can be associated with negative or serious side effects (Chlan, 2009; Vanderboom et al., 2011). These side effects include nausea; compromised respiration (Cheng, 1995; Lin et al., 2012); delirium (Chlan, 2009; Justic, 2000); impacting hemodynamic stability, which is the flow and movement of blood in the body (Vanderboom et al., 2011); and prolonged sedation and recovery (Lang et al., 2000; Martin et al., 2003; Schupp et al., 2005; Vanderboom et al., 2011).

Music has been explored as a nonpharmacological intervention for symptom management, as the medications often utilized for sedation during procedures can have serious side effects (Lang et al., 2000; Martin & Lennox, 2003; Schupp et al., 2005). The use of music in these procedures is designed to help manage the symptoms that patients encounter as a result of the procedures. These symptoms include anxiety (Bampton & Draper, 1997; Bolwerk, 1990; Chlan, 2009; Heiderscheit, Chlan, & Donley, 2011; Miluk-Kolasa et al., 1996; Palakanis, 1994; Vanderboom et al., 2011), stress response (Schneider et al., 2001), mood (Barnason et al., 1995; Chlan, 1995; Clark et al., 2006), vital signs (Chlan, 1995, 1998; Koch, 1998; Smolen et al., 2002; Triller et al., 2006; White, 1992, 1999), and pain or discomfort (Chlan et al., 2000; Dunn, 2004; Ebneshahidi & Mohseni, 2008; Good, 1995; Schupp et al., 2005).

The research surrounding music in surgical and procedural support has focused on how music impacts various symptoms that patients experience in many different surgical and medical procedures. Implementing a nonpharmacological approach in a highly technical environment serves as a tool to improve and enhance patient care (Vanderboom et al., 2011). Music serves a vital role in helping to relax and distract patients in a chaotic and stressful medical environment (Heiderscheit, Chlan, & Donley, 2011).

Receptive Methods

The use of music and music therapy research surrounding surgical and procedural support has utilized primarily receptive methods. Music listening is an ideal intervention as it allows patients to choose what they want to listen to, when they want to listen, and how long they want to listen (Heiderscheit, Chlan, & Donley, 2011). This type of patient-directed approach also does not cause strain or require a great deal of energy. Music can be a comforting and calming stimulus for patients when they have low energy; are experiencing stress, discomfort, and pain; or have limited ability to focus (Heiderscheit, Chlan, & Donley, 2011).

Researchers have utilized music listening to assist patients in managing preoperative anxiety. Updike (1987) found that patients awaiting plastic surgery after listening to Bonny's Music Rx programs for 30 minutes demonstrated significant decrease in blood pressure, heart rate, and mean arterial pressure. Patients also reported an emotional effect, indicating that they recognized that after listening to music, they experienced a more relaxed, calm state. Augustin and Hains (1996) found that patients listening to their preferred music as they awaited surgery helped to significantly reduce heart rate and demonstrated a positive impact on other vital signs as well. They concluded that a music listening intervention is more beneficial than preoperative instruction alone and encourage pre-op staff to offer music listening as an option for surgical patients.

Wang et al. (2002) found in a randomized controlled trial that patients who listened to 30 minutes of music via headphones experienced a 16% decrease in anxiety, when compared to the control group that had headphones and no music or white noise. Lee et al. (2004) discovered that patients who listened to music for 20 to 40 minutes reported significantly lower levels of anxiety than the control group that rested quietly, watched television, or read prior to their surgery. Cooke et al. (2005) explored the use of music listening for surgical patients and found that patients who listened to 30 minutes of music reported significantly lower anxiety levels than the control group that utilized headphones with no music. While music has frequently been explored as a means of managing the preoperative anxiety that patients encounter, research has also explored the use of music intra- and postoperatively as well.

Lin et al. (2012) utilized music listening with older adults undergoing hemodialysis treatments three times a week. Patients in the music group listened to music from playlists they each created on their own, while patients in the control group received the usual care. After one week of music listening during each of the three hemodialysis treatments, patients demonstrated significant decreases in the frequency and severity of adverse reactions to dialysis. Patients also demonstrated decreased respiratory rates, increased finger temperature, and improved oxygen saturation.

Koch et al. (1998) implemented a music listening protocol for patients undergoing urologic surgery to identify what impact it may have on sedative and analgesic requirements. Patients in the experimental group were instructed to bring their preferred music for the surgical procedure, while patients in the control group received usual care. Researchers found that patients in the experimental group utilized significantly less propofol and opiod medication than the control group. Koelsh et al. (2011) also found that patients undergoing elective total hip replacement who listened to instrument music throughout the surgery demonstrated lower propofol consumption and lower cortisol levels than the control group. Steelman (1990) explored the effect of music listening on the anxiety and blood pressure of patients undergoing orthopedic surgery. Patients selected music from nine different prepared audio recordings. They began listening before skin preparation and continued to listen through surgery until the dressings were applied. The control group received routine care and staff utilized verbal distraction during skin preparation. The results indicated that music was comparable to verbal distraction in reducing anxiety, but demonstrated a significant decrease in blood pressure when distraction did not.

Dunn (2004), in a literature review of the use of music to reduce postoperative pain, found that after analyzing 10 studies, while the research methodology in the majority of the studies was poor and could not conclusively prove music effective, patients consistently reported listening to music as a positive experience. Dileo, Bradt, and Murphy (2008) completed a Cochrane Review of music for preoperative anxiety and reported that while many studies have utilized music listening as an intervention to manage anxiety and reduce sedation, there have been several factors that have contributed to the varied results. Studies have utilized small sample sizes, which contribute to difficulties in achieving statistical significance. Additionally, there are variances in study design, length of music listening, intervention method, and intensity of procedures, which contribute to varying results. While many studies have not achieved significance through a music listening intervention, there is still research that indicates a positive and significant impact of music in reducing anxiety and sedation for surgical patients.

Mechanical ventilation (MV) is a lifesaving measure utilized to treat respiratory failure stemming from a variety of causes. While MV is a common procedure in intensive care units (ICU), patients receiving MV experience a great deal of distress and anxiety as a result of the procedure. The distress and anxiety that patients experience can also pose greater risk for complications. Many researchers have explored the use of a music listening intervention to provide patients with a nonpharmacological means of managing their pain, discomfort, and anxiety.

Researchers have found that MV patients who listened to 30 minutes of preferred music experienced a significant decrease in state anxiety (Chlan, 1995, 1998; Wong et al., 2001). Some research has demonstrated that listening to music has significantly decreased heart rate, systolic and diastolic blood pressure, and respiratory rates (Almerud et al., 2003; Wong et al., 2001). Heiderscheit, Chlan, and Donley (2011) describe two cases from a randomized controlled trial utilizing a patient-directed music listening intervention. These two case illustrations provide greater detail regarding the process of assessing an MV patient's preferred music, the successful implementation of a music listening intervention, and how the intervention can be individualized based on patient needs. Chlan and Heiderscheit (2009) developed a music assessment tool (MAT) to utilize in assessing music preferences for patients. Hunter et al. (2010) reported that music therapy was successful in helping patients to manage their anxiety while weaning from MV. They also report high satisfaction rates among patients who received music therapy, as well as their nurses.

Bradt, Dileo, and Grocke (2010) completed a Cochrane Review on the use of music interventions with MV patients. Their review of the research included eight randomized and quasi-randomized controlled trials, which included a total of 213 patients. They reported that the findings of these studies suggest that a music listening intervention is a viable intervention for managing stress and anxiety and may positively impact heart rate, respiratory rate, and anxiety in MV patients. While the research does support the use of music as an effective method, the investigators do recommend that additional research is needed to further explore the effects of music listening with MV patients and that these interventions be provided by a trained or board-certified music therapist.

There are many other surgical and medical procedures with which researchers have explored the use of music and music interventions as a nonpharmacological method of symptom management. These include open heart surgery (Nilsson, 2009); abdominal surgery and hysterectomy (Good et al., 2001; Kain et al., 2000; Taylor et al., 1998); cataract surgery (Cruise et al., 1997); cerebral angiography (Schneider et al., 2001; Vanderboom et al., 2011); caesarean section (Laopaiboon et al., 2009); labor, birth, and delivery (Clark et al., 1981; Geden et al., 1989; Hanser et al., 1983; Kimber et al., 2008); colposcopy (Galaal et al., 2011); colonoscopy (Andrada et al., 2004; Smolen et al., 2002;); sigmoidoscopy (Chlan et al., 2000; Palakanis et al., 1994); and bronchoscopy (Colt et al., 1999; Dubois et al., 1995; Triller et al., 2006).

The research literature continues to grow regarding the effective use of music and music therapy during surgical and medical procedures. As a result, there are meta-analyses (Dileo & Bradt, 2005; Pelletier, 2004; Standley, 1986), reviews of evidence (Chlan, 2009), systematic reviews (Evans, 2002), and various Cochrane Reviews further exploring the effectiveness of music in these areas of medicine. Researchers and clinicians continue to explore how music can be implemented to improve patient care and the patient experience.

Although the current body of research literature utilizes receptive methods, this does not preclude other methods from being applicable in various areas of surgical and procedural support. It is important to note that many of the research studies were conducted by non–music therapists, and many did not employ a music therapist as a member of the research team. These two factors will limit the scope to which music can be utilized in surgery or during a procedure. Additionally, during procedures it may require the patient to be still or sedated, and this will also limit a patient's level of engagement in music or music therapy.

Improvisational, Compositional, and Re-creative Methods

While the research literature does not include studies that utilize improvisational, compositional, and re-creative methods, this does not mean that these methods are contraindicated for surgical and procedural support. It does require careful consideration regarding the patient's needs and what is feasible during the procedure. The music therapy method should in no way interfere with the procedure. The procedure should be able to be conducted and completed as it typically would be. The music therapy method employed is designed to enhance the patient experience and patient care. Be sure, when selecting the method, to review the important considerations for surgical and procedural support denoted earlier in this chapter.

It is important to inform the staff of how music therapy is being utilized and how this is intended to assist the patient to give them a clear understanding of the intervention (Heiderscheit, Chlan, &

Donley, 2011). This can allow the staff to feel prepared in understanding the role of each team member involved in the procedure, and it helps to ensure support for the patient throughout the process. The process of the procedure should be clear, so that questions and clarifications do not need to take place in the midst of the procedure, as this can cause anxiety for the patient and impact patient care.

Summary and Conclusions

The Department of Health and Human Services reports in the National Survey of Ambulatory Surgery (NSAS) Survey, that in 2006 an estimated 53.3 million nonsurgical and surgical procedures were performed (Cullen et al., 2009). With so many procedures being completed each year, there are many opportunities for music therapists to provide support and nonpharmacological means of anxiety and pain management for patients. There is a wide variety of surgeries and procedures conducted, and the level of invasiveness of procedures differs greatly. In order to best meet with needs of patients during procedures, understanding the level of invasiveness is required, as well as having an understanding of the procedure itself and the patient's needs throughout this process.

The current body of research surrounding surgical and medical procedures does demonstrate a positive trend toward the use of receptive methods. Currently, there is no evidence in the research literature utilizing creative, re-creative, and improvisational methods in surgical and medical procedures with adults. While this is absent in the literature surrounding adults, it is evident in procedures for pediatric patients (Loewy, 1997; Standley, 2005). Additionally, these methods may currently be utilized in clinical settings and currently have not been reported in the literature. While various methods of music therapy may be suitable for surgical and procedural support, it is important to determine what method is best suited for the patient and for the given procedure. This requires the music therapist to understand the procedure the patient will be undergoing and then to complete an assessment of the patient's needs before, during, and after this procedure, as well as music preferences.

References

Aldridge, D. (1996). *Music therapy research and practice in medicine: From out of the silence.* Philadelphia, PA: Jessica Kingsley Publishers.

Almerud, S., & Peterson, K. (2003). Music therapy—a complementary treatment for mechanically ventilated intensive care patients. *International Critical Care Nursing, 19*(1), 21–30.

Andrada, J., Vidal, A.. & Aguilar-Tablada, T. (2004). Anxiety during the performance of colonoscopies: Modification using music therapy. *European Journal of Gastroenterology Hepatology, 16,* 1381–1386.

Argstatter, H., Haberbosch, W., & Bolay, H. (2006). Study of the effectiveness of music stimulation during intracardiac catheterization. *Clinical Research in Cardiology, 95*(10), 14–22.

Bampton, P., & Draper, B. (1997). Effect of relaxation music on patient tolerance of gastrointestinal endoscopic procedures. *Journal of Clinical Gastroenterology, 25,* 343–345.

Barnason, S., Zimmerman, L., & Nieveen, J. (1995). The effects of music interventions on anxiety in the patient after coronary artery bypass grafting. *Heart and Lung, 24,* 124–132.

Bolwerk, C. (1990). Effects of relaxing music on state anxiety in myocardial infarction patients. *Critical Care Nursing Quarterly, 13,* 63–72.

Bradt, J., Dileo, C., & Grocke, D. (2010). *Music interventions for mechanically ventilated patients.* (Review). The Cochrane Collaboration. Wiley Publishers; www.cochrane.org

Cheng, E. (1995). The cost of sedating and paralyzing the critically ill patient. *Critical Care Clinics, 11*(4), 1005–1019.

Chlan, L. (1995). Psychophysiologic responses of mechanically ventilated patients to music: A pilot study. *American Journal of Critical Care, 4,* 233–238.

Chlan, L. (1998). Effectiveness of a music therapy intervention on relaxation and anxiety for patients receiving ventilator assistance. *Heart and Lung, 27,* 169–176.

Chlan, L. (2009). A review of the evidence for music intervention to manage anxiety in critically ill patients receiving mechanical ventilatory support. *Archives of Psychiatric Nursing, 23*(2), 177–179.

Chlan, L., Evans, D., Greenleaf, M., & Walker, J. (2000). Effects of single music therapy intervention on anxiety, discomfort, satisfaction, and compliance with screening guidelines in outpatients undergoing flexible sigmoidoscopy. *Gastroenterology Nursing, 23,* 148–156.

Chlan, L., & Heiderscheit, A. (2009). A tool for music preference assessment in critically ill patients receiving mechanical ventilatory support. *Music Therapy Perspectives, 27*(1), 42–47.

Clark, M., Isaacks-Donton, G., Wells, N., Redlin-Frazier, S., Eck, C., Hepworth, J. T., & Chakravarthy, B. (2006). Use of preferred music to reduce emotional distress and symptom activity during radiation therapy. *Journal of Music Therapy, XLIII*(3), 247–265.

Clark, M., McCorkle, R., & Williams, S. (1981). Music therapy assisted labor and delivery. *Journal of Music Therapy, 18,* 88–109.

Colt, H. G., Powers, A., & Shanks, T., (1999). Effect of music on state anxiety scores in patients undergoing fiberoptic bronchoscopy. *Chest, 116*(3), 819–824.

Cooke, M., Chaboyer, W., Schluter, P., & Hiratos, M. (2005). The effect of music on preoperative anxiety in day surgery. *Journal of Advanced Nursing, 52*(1), 47–55.

Cruise, C. J., Chung, F., Yogendran, S., & Little, D. (1997). Music increases satisfaction in elderly outpatients undergoing cataract surgery. *Canadian Journal of Anaesthesia, 44*(1), 43–48.

Cullen, K., Hall, M., & Golosinskiy, A. (2009). Ambulatory surgery in the United States, 2006. National health statistics reports; no 11. Revised. Hyattsville, MD: National Center for Health Statistics. Revised 2009.

Dileo, C. (1999). *Music therapy & medicine: Theoretical and clinical applications.* Silver Spring, MD: American Music Therapy Association.

Dileo, C., & Bradt, J. (2005). *Medical music therapy: A meta-analysis and agenda for future research.* New Jersey: Jeffrey Books,

Dileo C., Bradt J., & Murphy K. (2008). Music for preoperative anxiety (Protocol). Cochrane Database of Systematic Reviews 2008, Issue 1.

Dubois J., Bartter, T., & Pratter, M. (1995). Music improves patient comfort level during outpatient bronchoscopy. *Chest, 108,* 129–130.

Dunn, K. (2004). Music and the reduction of post-operative pain. *Nursing Standard, 18*(36), 33–39.

Ebneshahidi, A., & Mohseni, M. (2008). The effect of patient-selected music on early postoperative pain, anxiety, and hemodynamic profile in cesarean section surgery. *The Journal of Alternative and Complementary Medicine, 14*(7), 827–831.

Evan, D. (2002). The effectiveness of music as an intervention for hospital patients: A systemic review. *Journal of Advanced Nursing, 37*(1), 8–18.

Galaal, K., Bryant, A., Deane, K., Al-Khaduri, M., & Lopes, A. (2011) Interventions for reducing anxiety in women undergoing colonoscopy. Cochrane Database of Systematic Reviews 2011, *12.*

Gardstrom, S., & Hiller, J. (2010). Song discussion as music psychotherapy. *Music Therapy Perspectives, 28*(2), 147–156.

Geden, E. A., Lower, M., Beattie, S., & Beck, N. (1989). Effects of music and imagery on physiologic and self-report of analogued labor pain. *Nursing Research, 38*(1), 7–41.

Ghetti, C. (2012). Music therapy as procedural support for invasive medical procedures: Toward the development of a music therapy theory. *Nordic Journal of Music Therapy, 21*(1), 3–35.

Good, M., Stanton-Hicks, M., Grass, J. A., Anderson, G. C., Lai, H-L., Roykulcharoen, V., & Adler, P. A. (2001). Relaxation and music to reduce postsurgical pain. *Journal of Advanced Nursing, 33*(2), 208–215.

Hanser, S., Larson, S., & O'Connell, A. (1983). The effect of music on relaxation of expectant mothers during labor. *Journal of Music Therapy, 20,* 50–58.

Heiderscheit, A., Chlan, L., & Donley, K. (2011). Instituting a music listening intervention for critically ill patients receiving mechanical ventilation: Exemplars from two patient cases. *Music and Medicine, 3*(4), 239–245.

Justic, M. (2000). Does "ICU psychosis" really exist? *Critical Care Nurse, 20*(3), 28–37.

Kain, Z., Sevarino, F., Alexander, G., Pincus, S., & Mayes, L. (2000). Preoperative anxiety and postoperative pain in women undergoing hysterectomy. A repeated-measures design. *Journal of Psychosomatic Research, 49,* 417–422.

Kimber, L., McNabb, M., McCourt, C., Haines, A., & Brocklehurst, P. (2008). Massage or music for pain relief in labour: A pilot randomized placebo controlled trial. *European Journal of Pain, 12,* 961–969.

Koelsch, S., Fuermetz, J., Sack, U., Bauer, K., Hohenadel, M., Wiegel, M., & Heinke, W. (2011). Effects of music listening on cortisol levels and propofol consumption during spinal anesthesia. *Frontiers in Psychology, 2,* article 58.

Lang, E., Benotsch, E., & Fick, L. (2000). Adjunctive non-pharmacological analgesia for invasive medical procedures: A randomized trial. *Lancet, 355,* 1486–1490.

Lee, D., Henderson, A., & Shum, D. (2004). The effect of music on pre-procedure anxiety in Hong Kong Chinese day patients. *Journal of Clinical Nursing, 13,* 297–303.

Lin, Y., Ly, K., Chen, C., & Chang, C. (2012). The effects of music as therapy on overall well-being of elderly patients on maintenance hemodialysis. *Biological Research for Nursing, 14*(3), 277–285.

Martin, M., & Lennox, P. (2003). Sedation and analgesia in the interventional radiology department. *Journal of Vascular Intervention Radiology, 14,* 1119–1128.

Miluk-Kolasa, B., Matejek, M., & Stupnicki, R. (1996). The effects of music listening on changes in selected physiological parameters in adult pre-surgical patients. *Journal of Music Therapy, 33,* 208–218.

National Institutes of Health. (2012). Definition of invasive procedure. www.cancer.gov/dictionary. Downloaded May 20, 2012.

Nilsson, U. (2009). The effect of music intervention in stress response to cardiac surgery in a randomized controlled trial. *Heart and Lung, 38*(3), 201–207.

Palakanis, K., DeNobile, J., Sweeney, W., & Blankenship, C. (1994). Effect of music therapy on state anxiety in patients undergoing flexible sigmoidoscopy. *Diseases of the Colon and Rectum, 37,* 478–481.

Pelletier, C. (2004). The effect of music on decreasing arousal due to stress: A meta-analysis. *Journal of Music Therapy, 41,* 192–214.

Schneider, N., Schedlowski, M., & Schumeyer, T. (2001). Stress reduction through music in patients undergoing cerebral angiography. *Neuroradiology, 43,* 472–476.

Schupp, C., Berbaum, K., & Berbaum, M. (2005). Pain and anxiety during interventional radiologic procedures: Effect of patients' state anxiety at baseline and modulation by non-pharmocological analgesia adjuncts. *Journal of Vascular Intervention Radiology, 16,* 1585–1592.

Scott, A. (2004). Managing anxiety in ICU patients: The role of pre-operative information provision. *Nursing in Critical Care,* 9(2), 72–79.

Shiel, W., & Conrad-Stoppler, M. (2008). *Webster's New World Medical Dictionary*. Hoboken, NJ: Wiley Publishing, Inc.

Smolen, D., Topp, R., & Singer, L. (2002). The effect of self-selected music during colonoscopy on anxiety, heart rate, and blood pressure. *Applied Nursing Research, 15,* 126–136.

Standley, J. (1986). Music research in medical/dental treatment: Meta-analysis and clinical applications. *Journal of Music Therapy, XXII*(2), 56–122.

Steelman, V. (1990). Intraoperative music therapy: Effects on anxiety, blood pressure. *AORN Journal, 52*(5), 1026–1034.

Taylor, L. K., Kuttler, K. L., Parks, T. A., & Milton, D. (1998). The effect of music in the post-anesthesia care unit on pain levels in women who have had abdominal hysterectomies. *Journal of PeriAnesthesia Nursing, 13*(2), 88–94.

Triller, N., Erzen, D., & Duh, S. (2006). Music during bronchoscopic examination: The physiological effects a randomized trial. *Respiration, 73,* 95–99.

Updike, P., & Charles, D. (1987). Music Rx: Physiological and emotional responses to taped music programs of preoperative patients awaiting plastic surgery. *Annals of Plastic Surgery, 19*(1), 29–33.

Vanderboom, T., Arcari, P., Duffy, M., Somarouthu, B., Rabinov, J., Yoo, A., & Hirsch, J. (2001). Effects of music intervention on patients undergoing cerebralangiography: A pilot study. *Journal of NeuroIntervention Surgery, 10,* 1136–1141.

Wang, S., Kulkarni, L., Dolev, J., & Kain, Z. (2002). Music and preoperative anxiety: A randomized controlled study. *Anesthesia & Analgesia, 94,* 1489–1494.

Winter, M., Paskin, S., & Baker, T. (1994). Music reduces stress and anxiety of patients in surgical holding area. *Journal of Post Anesthetic Nursing,* 340–343.

Wong, H., Lopez-Nahas, V., & Molassiotis, A. (2001). Effects of music therapy on anxiety in ventilator dependent patients. *Heart and Lung, 30*(5), 376–387.

Yung, P., Kam, S., Lau, B., & Chan, T. (2003). The effects of music in managing preoperative stress for Chinese surgical patients in the operating holding area: A controlled trial. *International Journal of Stress Management, 10*(1), 64–74.

Resources

Health Journeys. Dr. Belleruth Naparstek has created and produced a wide array of directed imagery recordings. They can be purchased and downloaded at www.HealthJourneys.com

Wellscapes. This is an iApp that includes five different five-minute videos with guiding and music. Videography is by renowned nature photographer Craig Blacklock, with guiding script and music accompaniment by Annie Heiderscheit. These can be purchased and downloaded at www.csph.umn.edu. Twenty-minute versions are also available as well.

Appendix A

Music Assessment Tool (MAT)*
Chlan and Heiderscheit, 2009
*used with permission

Background Information:

Patient Name: ______________________________
Date: ______________________________
Diagnosis: ______________________________
Age: ________ Education: ______________________________
Vocation: ______________________________
Ethnic background: ______________________________
Religion/Faith practice: ______________________________

Date of ICU admission:

____

Reason for admission:

____
____
____
____

Significant events prior to admission:

____
____
____
____
____
____

Current mood state

____
____
____
____

Any hearing impairment? Specify.

____
____
____
____

PART I: Patient Music Assessment

1. Do you like to listen to music? Yes No

2. Do you play an instrument(s)? Yes No
   If yes, what do you play?

____
____
____
____

3. Are you a professional musician? Yes No

4. Are you a hobbyist musician? Yes No

5. When do you like to listen to music? (Check all that apply)

____	relaxation	____	stress reduction	____	during meals
____	pure enjoyment	____	to pass time	____	w/ family/friends
____	with exercise	____	for prayer	____	during work

Other:

____
____
____
____
____

6. What types of music do you enjoy? (Check all that apply)

____	Classical	____	Religious/Sacred	____	Rock
____	Rhythm & Blues	____	Country	____	Hip-Hop
____	Reggae	____	Jazz	____	Rap
____	New Age	____	World Music	____	Alternative
____	Heavy Metal	____	Oldies (1950–1970)	____	Pop music
____	Other				

____
____
____
____
____

7. Any particular group(s) or artist(s) you prefer?

____
____
____

8. What instruments or instrumental sounds do you like? (Check all that apply)

____	Orchestral	____	Harp	____	Classical guitar
____	Vocal	____	Flute	____	Folk guitar
____	Piano	____	Saxophone	____	Percussion/drumming
____	Brass or horns	____	Clarinet	____	World instruments
____	Oboe	____	Ocean waves	____	Environmental sounds

Other:

____
____
____
____
____

9. Are there any types of music that you DO NOT like?

____
____
____
____
____
____

10. Are there any groups or artists you DO NOT like?

11. Are there any instruments or instrumental sounds that you DO NOT like?

12. Are there any cultural considerations or is culture an important aspect of your music selection?

13. Any other information you would like to share or that I should know?

General Information & Comments:

Chapter 3

Pain Management with Adults

Joy L. Allen

Like music, pain is a universal phenomenon that touches everyone at one time or another. Whether the result of touching a hot stove, falling and scraping a knee, a physical illness, or a tension headache after a stressful day, everyone experiences it. Regardless of the cause, pain serves as a warning. In its most benign form, it warns that something is not quite right. At its worst, it interferes with productivity and well-being, affecting every aspect of an individual's life.

Diagnostic Information

Pain is an unpleasant sensory and emotional experience associated with actual or potential tissue damage or described in terms of such damage (International Association for the Study of Pain, 1979). McCaffery and Beebe (1989) further define pain as "whatever the experiencing person says it is and exists whenever he says it does." It is important for treatment professionals to recognize that the experience of pain is subjective in nature. The definition provided by the International Association for the Study of Pain (IASP) (Merskey & Bogduk, 1994) emphasizes that pain is not a directly observable or measurable phenomenon, but rather a subjective experience. In other words, if two people are subjected to the same painful input, it does not necessarily mean they feel the same degree of pain; each person's perception of pain can be quite distinct. Despite the subjective nature of the pain, it is possible to categorize and describe different types of pain experiences.

Types of Pain

Procedural Pain. Procedural pain refers to pain experienced during a medical procedure and is associated with tissue, muscle, and/or nerve damage. It is caused by the release of chemicals from damaged cells, the inflammatory response, and/or damaged neurons. Procedures might be as simple as a needle stick or stitches or as complex as a chest tube insertion and/or removal, paracentesis, pleuredesis, dressing changes, or minor surgeries. While the patient's perception of pain does not necessarily correlate with the amount of damage, an increase in damage will likely increase the pain experience. Procedural pain may be influenced by a host of interrelated experiences, including the patient's emotional and psychological state, level of anxiety, previous pain experience, and understanding of the procedure (Marsac & Funk, 2008). Patients often report the pain associated with a procedure to be worse than the condition necessitating the procedure (Finley & Schecter, 2003).

Procedural pain is predictive in nature. Medical personnel, and often patients, know what procedures are likely to cause pain and/or discomfort. Because of this, patients can be warned and given medication to reduce the intensity of the pain medication, as well as given or engaged in activities to reduce the severity of the pain experience. Common physical symptoms of procedural pain include temporary increases in blood pressure, respiratory rate, and pulse, as well as perspiration and muscle tension. Emotional symptoms of pain are related to the flight-or-fight response and include the possibility of increased anxiety and fear. Music therapists interested in learning more about interventions for procedural pain are referred to Chapter 2, *Surgical and Procedural Support.*

Acute Pain. Acute pain is defined as "pain of recent onset and probable limited duration. It usually has an identifiable temporal and causal relationship to injury or disease" (Ready & Edwards, 1992). Acute pain begins suddenly and is usually described as sharp, stinging, and/or intense in quality. It serves as a warning of a threat to the body and is associated with soft tissue damage. Surgery, infections, ligament strains, broken bones, burns, and labor and delivery are common events or circumstances associated with acute pain. Acute pain may be mild and short-lived, or it might be severe and last for weeks. However, when the underlying cause of the pain has been treated or healed, acute pain subsides and individuals return to premorbid functioning levels. Acute pain often responds to treatment with analgesic medications and lasts no longer than six months.

Acute pain is the most common reason individuals seek medical care (Fox et al., 2000). It is a common occurrence in medical settings, with an estimated 25 million Americans experiencing acute pain due to injury or surgery per year (American Pain Foundation, 2012). Despite advances in pain management protocols, 11%–20% of postoperative patients report experiencing severe pain (Apfelbaum, Chen, Mehta, & Gan, 2003), a percentage that has remained stable in the last decade (Hutchinson, 2007). Poorly managed acute pain can cause serious medical complications, impair recovery from injury or procedures, result in extended hospital stays, and progress to chronic pain (Carr et al., 1992). Patient satisfaction with care is strongly tied to their experiences with pain during hospitalization. Evidence suggests that higher levels of pain and depression are linked to poor satisfaction with care in ambulatory settings (Bair, 2007).

Chronic Pain. The International Association for the Study of Pain (1986) defines chronic pain as pain that "persists beyond the normal tissue healing time, which is assumed to be three months." Chronic pain can be caused by any number of diseases or injuries, from sprains and strains to cancer. Some cases of chronic pain can be traced back to a specific injury; others have no apparent cause. Common conditions associated with chronic pain include migraines, cancer (from tumor pressing on nerves or organs, inflammation, or treatment side effects), degenerative conditions (osteoporosis and osteoarthritis), fibromyalgia, multiple sclerosis, and neuropathic pain (Fine, 2011; Leadley, Armstrong, Lee, Allen & Kleijnen, 2012). Chronic pain can be mild or excruciating, episodic or continuous, inconvenient or completely debilitating. Words often used to describe chronic pain include constant, nagging, dull, aching, throbbing, or burning. The unpredictable nature of chronic pain can lead to severe emotional distress.

The American Pain Society (2011) classifies chronic pain into four separate categories.

- *Pathophysiology:* secondary to the functional changes associated with or resulting from disease or injury. Examples can be pain secondary to multiple sclerosis, kidney disease, degenerative conditions such as osteoporosis and osteoarthritis, and certain types of cancer-related pain.
- *Nociceptive:* due to ongoing tissue injury. Examples of nociceptive pain include tension headaches, arthritis, back pain not associated with nerve damage, pelvic pain from joint instability, endometriosis, prostate pain, irritable bowel syndrome, and general muscle pain.
- *Neuropathic:* resulting from damage to the brain, spinal cord, or peripheral nerves; pain relievers may be less effective. Examples of neuropathic pain include phantom limb pain, peripheral neuropathy, sciatica, central pain syndrome, and certain types of advanced cancer pain.
- *Mixed:* undetermined causes. Can also be referred to as idiopathic pain. Examples include fibromyalgia and TMJ disorders.

Untreated pain can become more complex in its pathophysiology than the pain caused by the original injury or disease (Fine, 2011). Structural and functional alterations in the nervous system take place, making the pain an entirely separate condition (Baliki, Geha, Apkarian, & Chialvo, 2008). The extent and severity of chronic pain may be more important than the underlying etiology (Gureje, Von Korff, Simon, & Gater, 1998). The IASP (2011) reports that one in five people suffers from moderate to severe chronic pain and that one in three has lifestyle limitations due to their pain. Chronic pain affects Americans more than diabetes, heart disease, and cancer combined (American Academy of Pain Medicine, 2006) and costs billions of dollars in health care and lost work productivity each year (Committee on Advancing Pain Research, Care, and Education, 2011).

Worrisome epidemiological trends are leading to a pain crisis in our society. With increased age come more pain-related problems. The number of people who will need treatment for pain from back disorders, degenerative joint diseases, rheumatological conditions, visceral diseases, and cancer is expected to rise (Brokcoff, 2001). Unavoidable nerve damage secondary to surgical procedures will cause chronic pain in 15%–50% of patients (Kehlet, Jensen, & Woolf, 2006). Nerve damage or neuropathic pain in cancer patients, often side effects of treatment, represent about 20% of all cancer-related pains. The elderly are affected more than the young, and for the most chronic pain conditions, women are affected more than men (Committee on Advancing Pain Research, Care, and Education, 2011).

Needs and Resources

Inadequately managed pain can lead to adverse physical and psychological outcomes for patients and their families. The potential physical, emotional, behavioral, social, and spiritual impacts of pain are outlined below.

Physical. Acute and chronic pain is associated with several physical complications. Physiological responses to acute pain include increased blood pressure, increased respiratory rate, increased pulse, dilated pupils, muscle tension, and perspiration. Long-term elevation of these physiological measures can lead to further health complications, as chronic pain is a statistically significant predictor of hypertension (Bruehl, Chung, Jirjis, & Biridepalli, 2005). Pain can also lead to disruptions in sleep, with the degree of sleep disturbance directly related to the severity of pain (Marin, Cyhan, & Miklos, 2006). Approximately 50%–98% of individuals with chronic pain suffer from sleep disturbances (McCracken & Iverson, 2002; Morin, Gibson, & Wade, 1998). Pain can also lead to guarding of the painful area. Overprotection of a body part for extended periods of time can result in physical abnormalities from disuse. This includes muscle atrophy, muscle tightness or spasms, loss of elasticity of ligaments and tendons, brittle bones, and further pain (Galer & Dworkin, 2000). Pain can lead to sexual dysfunction, including difficulty with arousal, confidence, performance, positions, and fear of worsening pain (Ambler, Williams, Hill, Gunary, & Cratchley, 2001).

Emotional. Acute pain can lead to increases in anxiety, fear, and distress. Chronic pain can result in similar emotional experiences, as well as more complicated emotional issues. Research indicates that individuals with chronic pain are more likely to develop psychological disorders (Gureje, Von Korff, Simon, & Gater, 1998). Increased rates of major depressive disorder (Ohayon & Schatzberg, 2003), as well as increased rates of suicide ideation and suicide attempts (Ratcliffe, Enns, Belik, & Sareen, 2008), have been associated with chronic pain. Furthermore, 50% of individuals with chronic pain consider suicide as a viable cure (MacDonald, 2000; Thomas & Johnson, 2000). Additionally, individuals with neuropathic pain are likely to suffer from panic/anxiety disorders (Bouhassira, Lanteri-Minet, Attal, Laurent, & Touboul, 2008). Changes in identity and losses within self-esteem and self-image have also been associated with chronic pain (Fenwick, Chaboyer, & St. John, 2012).

Cognitive/Behavioral. Behavioral responses to acute pain are often present. These include restlessness, poor concentration, apprehension, and distress. Physical changes in the brain related to chronic pain have been shown to have specific effects on cognitive processes or brain structure/function. Dick and Rashiq (2007) found that up to two-thirds of patients with chronic pain have impairments in memory and attention. Other changes have been associated with various sensory and affective measures of pain, including perception of chronic pain (Grachev, Fredrickson, & Apkarian, 2000).

Social. Individuals with acute and chronic pain suffer from reduced quality of life, based on measures of functionality (McCarberg, Nicholson, Todd, Palmer, & Penles, 2008). This includes interruptions in social activities, personal relationships, employment status, and daily activities (Breivik, Collett, Ventafridda, Cohen, & Gallacher, 2006; McCarberg, Nicholson, Todd, Palmer, & Penles, 2008; Smith et al., 2001). Patients with chronic pain are more likely to report work disability and lowered work productivity (Gureje, Von Korff, Simon, & Gater, 1998; Stewart, Ricci, Chee, Morganstein, & Lipton, 2003). Family coping and functioning are impacted, including increases in marital conflict and feelings of anger, anxiety, resentment, and despondency among family members (Snelling, 1994). One in four individuals with chronic pain report that relationships with family and friends are strained or broken (IASP, 2011).

Spiritual. Unmanaged pain can lead to spiritual suffering. Individuals with chronic pain report feelings of hopelessness and helplessness, and begin to question whether or not they can survive the ordeal (Fenwick, Chaboyer, & St. John, 2012).

Resources

The pain cycle has been developed to illustrate the connection between physical and psychological components of pain. When a person experiences pain, it can lead to activity avoidance, which leads to progressive deconditioning and muscle tension, which leads to decreasing activity and further deconditioning, which leads to more pain, which leads to anger/anxiety/fear/distress, which leads to impoverished mood, which leads to depression, which leads to increased perception of pain. As this cycle continues, hopelessness sets in and spiritual suffering begins. The goal of pain management is to break this cycle of pain.

Therapists can help the individual experiencing pain to identify and control the cycle of pain. Strategies that have been most helpful include monitoring daily activity and mood, using problem-solving techniques, challenging some of the recurrent worried thoughts, engaging in a gradual exercise program, watching body cues, maintaining a daily routine and schedule, learning to pace activities, watching diet and caloric intake, getting involved in distracting activities with others, sharing emotions associated with the pain, and contacting others for help when needed. Therapists can also be helpful in reviewing steps to prevent a relapse. With time, the person with pain can become more "smart" about the pain in working toward better control, anticipating good and bad days, and not dwelling on those things that are out of the person's control (American Pain Society, 2013).

Music Therapy

The goal of music therapy services for pain management is to address the immediate needs of the patient by providing a nonpharmacological technique to decrease the patient's pain perception (Bailey, 1986; Magill, 2001). Music therapy is applied not only to soothe and relax, but also to promote expression of thoughts, fears, grief, and anger (Bailey, 1986; Dileo & Bradt, 1999; Magill, 2001; O'Callaghan, 1996). Music therapists in medical settings are trained to address the psychosocial as well as the clinical issues faced by patients and their families.

Music therapy works by interfering with the brain's perception of pain, reducing anxiety, reducing muscle tension, and stimulating endorphins (Bailey, 1986; Dileo & Bradt, 1999; Magill-Levreault, 1993;

Saperston, 1999). Additionally, Dileo & Bradt (1999) state that music therapy may function to reduce or eliminate pain by serving as a means for mood enhancement, as a mechanism for providing choice and control, as an outlet for self-expression, as a method for cognitive reframing, and/or as a vehicle for social support.

Referral and Assessment

Acute Pain

Unrelieved pain is a major yet preventable public health problem. In response to the growing need for pain management standards, The Joint Commission (formerly known as the Joint Commission on Accreditation of Healthcare Organizations, JCAHO) developed national pain assessment and management standards in the United States (Dahl & Gordon, 2002). These standards require accredited health care facilities to be committed to assessing, treating, and responding to changes in a patient's pain. This includes recognition of the following: efforts to address pain must be interdisciplinary; assessment must be ongoing and incorporate physical, emotional, cultural, and spiritual domains; therapy should be evidence-based and employ pharmacological and nonpharmacological techniques; pain strategies should address the entire continuum of care; patient and family should be educated on strategies to improve pain management; and evaluation of outcomes should be ongoing (Paice, 2010).

The treatment setting and related policies and procedures determine the referral process for music therapy services. In some medical settings, any member of the treatment team, including the patient and family members, may make a referral for music therapy services. In other medical settings, referrals may be automatically generated based on established criteria. For example, a setting may have computer-generated referrals for anyone who has self-reported pain at a "4" or greater or anyone exhibiting nonverbal indicators of pain. Acute pain management clinical practice guidelines recommend psychological-based interventions, such as music therapy, for those patients who manifest anxiety or fear, have inadequate pain relief after appropriate pharmacological interventions, or experience chronic or recurrent pain (Jacox et al., 1992). It is important for the music therapists to establish consistent criteria for referral and educate treatment team members on such criteria. This includes educating treatment team members on the effectiveness of music therapy for addressing acute pain.

Chronic Pain

The research literature (Flor, Fyrich, & Turk, 1992; Turk & Okifuji, 1998) and various organizations (American Society of Anesthesiologists, 1997; Commission on the Accreditation of Rehabilitation Facilities, 1999) support the use of an interdisciplinary rehabilitative approach to the management of chronic pain. This includes a process in which health care professionals from diverse treatment approaches collaborate to diagnose and treat patients suffering from debilitating pain. The Rehabilitation Accreditation Commission defines a chronic pain management program as a program that "provides coordinated, interdisciplinary team services to reduce pain, improve functioning, and decrease the dependence on the health care system of persons with chronic pain syndrome" (Commission of the Accreditation of Rehabilitation Facilities, 1998; 1999). Team members may include physicians (neurologists, psychiatrists, rheumatologists, anesthesiologists), nurses, pharmacists, case managers, social workers, physical therapists, vocational counselors, psychologists, and related professions (International Association for the Study of Pain, 2009; Stanos, 2012; Stanos & Houle, 2006).

In many developed countries, a variety of pain treatment facilities exist for the management of chronic pain. The International Association for the Study of Pain (2009) has outlined and defined the characteristics of these facilities as follows: multidisciplinary pain center (largest and most complex of the pain treatment facilities, usually attached to medical school or teaching hospital, has a wide range of health care specialists and researchers); multidisciplinary pain clinic (similar to multidisciplinary pain center; however, does not include research and teaching activities); and pain clinic (distinguished from above centers by the absence of interdisciplinary assessment and management of chronic pain). Information is not currently available on the percentage of pain centers or clinics that employ music therapists or refer chronic pain patients to music therapy to address the physical, emotional, or spiritual needs of those living with chronic pain.

Assessment

The American Pain Society (2006) recommends a six-step assessment of pain. The first step is the initial pain evaluation. This step focuses on the physical aspects of pain, including the location, quality, and severity of the pain, as well as the triggers and fluctuations in the pain experience. The second step focuses on assessing the physical and psychosocial impact of pain. Specific areas include general activity level, sleeping patterns, mood, and relationship patterns. The third step gathers pain-related history. This includes any comorbidities, as well as pain treatment history. The fourth step focuses on a physical examination. The fifth step focuses on treatment goals. This includes having the patient state what level of pain relief is acceptable to them. This is particularly important if complete resolution of pain is not achievable. The sixth step focuses on treatment follow-up. This step determines the effectiveness of the pain management plan, including patient adherence to the plan as well as perceived problems with the plan.

Several tools are available to assess and evaluate pain intensity. Self-report measures are the most reliable way to assess pain intensity in cognitively intact adults (Wells, Pasero, & McCaffery, 2008). In the clinical setting, this is most often done by using the zero to 10 numerical rating scale or the zero to 5 Wong-Baker FACES scale (McCaffery & Pasero, 1999). The numerical rating scale consists of a straight horizontal line numbered at equal intervals from zero to 10, with anchor words of "no pain" for zero, "moderate pain" for 5, and "worst pain" for 10. The FACES scale consists of six faces showing progressive pain intensities, beginning with a smiling face and ending with a crying face.

Although not as widely used, multidimensional self-report assessment tools can provide information on pain characteristics and effects on a patient's daily life (Chapman & Syrjala, 2001). The Brief Pain Inventory consists of a series of questions addressing the pain experience over a 24-hour period. It has been found useful in quantifying pain intensity and associated disability in a wide range of populations (Breitbart et al., 1997; Chapman & Syrjala, 2001; Cleeland, 1985). The McGill Pain Questionnaire assesses sensory, affective, and evaluative components of the pain experience. The self-report questionnaire was designed to provide quantitative measures of clinical pain that can be treated statistically (Melzack, 1975).

In addition to self-report measures, physiological and behavioral responses to perceived pain should be assessed (Carr et al., 1992). Physiological responses include increases in respiratory rate, heart rate, and blood pressure. Behavioral responses include splinting, grimacing, moaning or grunting, distorted posture, and reluctance to move. A lack of physiological responses or an absence of pain-related behavior(s) should not be used as an indicator of the absence of pain (Wells, Pasero, & McCaffery, 2008).

When the patient is unable to self-report pain, other less reliable measures must be used to identify the existence and probable intensity of pain. These include the following: conditions or procedures that are likely to cause pain, including surgery and wound care; nonverbal indicators of pain, including affect, muscle tension, and motor agitation/excessive motor movement; and consultation with family members to determine any pre-existing conditions associated with pain or behaviors indicative of pain (McCaffery & Pasero, 1999; Pasero & McCaffery, 2005).

Behavioral assessment tools are helpful in identifying the existence of pain and evaluating interventions. One example of such a scale is the Behavioral Pain Scale, developed for use with critically ill ICU patients (Payen et al., 2001). The Behavioral Pain Scale evaluates and scores the categories of behavior: facial expressions, with scores ranging from 1 for relaxed to 4 for grimacing; upper-limb movement, with scores ranging from 1 for no movement to 4 for permanently retracted; and ventilator compliance, with scores ranging from 1 for tolerating ventilator to 4 for unable to control ventilation. It is important to note that this scale is not a pain intensity score, but it is useful in determining the effectiveness of interventions to address the probable presence of pain.

Clinicians, including music therapists, need to remember that all pain assessment tools should be appropriate to the given patient. Special consideration should be given to the cultural, educational, and developmental age of the patient. Research indicates underreporting of pain secondary to fear, cultural beliefs, cognitive impairments, stoicism, and fear of addiction or side effects of treatment (Berry & Dahl, 1998; McCaffery & Pasero, 1999).

Music Therapy Assessment

While a formal music therapy assessment for the treatment of pain is not available, several music therapy research studies have reported on assessment strategies in the treatment of pain. Magill-Levreault (1993) suggested that music therapists assess the patient's medical condition, including functional ability, coping ability, and prior musical experiences. Music therapists may consider the description, source, level, and meaning of pain as well as whether the patient believes that the pain can be controlled (Bailey, 1986; Loewy, 1999; Magill, 2001). The assessment process is centered on the patients' needs, wishes, and goals, with an effort to work in the physical, psychosocial, emotional, and spiritual components of the total pain experience in a supportive environment. In turn, this can modify the suffering components and influence overall pain perception (Magill, 2001).

Overview of Methods and Procedures

The following methods and procedures are most commonly implemented to address the physical, emotional, social, and/or spiritual needs of patients experiencing acute or chronic pain. These have not been sequenced to reflect relative significance, effectiveness, or complexity.

Receptive Music Therapy

- Music Listening: The individual listens to selected music.
- Song Communication: The client selects songs based on themes, thoughts, and/or wishes they would like to express.
- Music-Assisted Relaxation: The therapist designs and guides the patient through music-centered relaxation routines.
- Music and Imagery: The patient is led through a short relaxation induction and then images freely while listening to live, improvised music.
- Bonny Method of Guided Imagery and Music: Individual form of psychotherapy in which the client images to specifically designed music programs while in an altered state.
- Entrainment: Type of therapist-led improvisation designed to symbolically represent a patient's pain experience, with gradual shifting to healing or pain relief.

Improvisational Music Therapy

- Song Improvisation: The client creates lyrics and or melody in the moment, musically supported by therapist.
- Referential Improvisation: The client explores musical sounds to express an experience, feeling, idea, event, or relationship.

Re-creative Music Therapy

- Therapeutic Singing: The client uses his voice to reproduce preferred music, incorporating deep breathing.

Compositional Music Therapy

- Songwriting: The therapist provides appropriate structure to engage the client in writing of original lyrics and/or accompaniment.

GUIDELINES FOR RECEPTIVE MUSIC THERAPY

Music Listening

Overview. Listening to selected music during treatment and/or during episodes of increased anxiety or discomfort is a common application of music for pain management. The goals of this method are to decrease any treatment-related distress as well as distract the patient from any discomfort or potential discomfort.

Depending on the facility or treatment setting, the music therapist might play an auxiliary or consultant role in the establishment of a listening library. This includes selecting music from various genres that are conducive to a relaxation experience. In other facilities, the music therapist might serve as a consultant whereby she meets with patients considered at high risk for anxiety or treatment noncompliance secondary to increased discomfort or fear. During this time, they work with the patient to develop a music program of familiar, relaxing music to play during treatment sessions. Types of treatment sessions may include physical therapy sessions, wound care, burn care, or ventilator weaning.

Preparation. The music therapist will need to have a large selection of songs and/or instrumental music available from which the patient can choose. This includes music from various genres and time periods. Songs should be chosen for their therapeutic value, focusing on tempi close to those of the natural heartbeat and supportive themes. Appropriate selections can be found in jazz, rhythm and blues, classical, New Age, country, slow rock, Big Band, and/or pop music. Music playback equipment will need to be provided. Some hospitals and facilities have a selection of portable devices for patient use; others may encourage patients to bring in personal equipment. Proper staff will need to be notified if personal equipment is being used to ensure and electronic devices meets safety and infection control requirements.

What to observe. The therapist and/or staff should watch for any visible signs of decreased distress and/or increased relaxation.

Procedures. Approach the patient and assess music preferences. Helpful questions may include the following: What types of music do you listen to for pleasure? Is there a particular style of music that you find relaxing? Particular artist(s) or song(s) that you enjoy listening to? Are there any songs that you listen to when you need comfort or reassurance? If the patient has time and resources, it is beneficial to encourage them to bring in personal selections. During the music listening experience, the patient should be encouraged to listen to the music, breathing in time to the beat, if appropriate. After the music listening experience, the music therapists should follow up with the patient to determine the success of this experience, noting any changes that might be helpful in future situations. This is particularly true if music listening is being used during medical treatment such as wound care or physical therapy.

If creating a music program to use during physical activity and/or physical therapy, the music therapist should ensure that the program has music for the various phases of the exercise program. This includes selections for a warm-up and for the cooldown. Specific exercises can be coordinated to musical selections to encourage patient compliance.

Song Communication

Overview. Song communication focuses on the patient selecting songs for the therapist to play and sing with them. Depending on implementation procedures, this method can be useful to promote a sense of control, enhance decision-making opportunities, provide an outlet for self-expression, enhance spirituality, or to facilitate attention towards a more positive experience. At a more advanced level, this technique can be used as a way to communicate feelings, wishes, emotions, or messages to others. Lastly, song communication can be used for assessment purposes, as choices can be directed toward emotional, social, and spiritual coping mechanisms.

This technique is contraindicated for patients experiencing high levels of pain, in the moment. If the therapist is intending to use this technique for insight-oriented experiences, he/she must be comfortable with verbal processing techniques.

Preparation. The therapist should have a wide repertoire of songs, from a variety of genres. It is helpful to provide the patients with a list of potential songs, categorized by genres, as a starting point. Additionally, when possible, it is helpful to provide patients with lyric sheets, allowing them to hear and see the lyrics simultaneously. Several resources provide the therapist with song titles matched to specific themes. While this might be helpful for a beginning therapist or a starting point for creating a songbook, the risk is the development of preconceived notions of a song and subsequent patient meanings to a song. It is important to remember that songs hold different meanings for every individual based on the situation. Engaging the patient in a discussion regarding their choice opens the therapeutic space for accessing, exploring, and connecting.

What to observe. The therapist also needs to watch for signs of fatigue or increased discomfort. Additionally, the therapist should watch the patient's body language and facial expressions for any visible reactions to the lyrics, message, mood, or emotions portrayed in the song. The therapist should be mindful of any emerging themes or messages.

Procedures. The first step is inviting the patient to choose a song. This can be done in a number of different ways, depending on the overall goal of the experience. On a more supportive level, the therapist might ask the client to choose something they would like to hear or enjoy hearing. On a deeper level, they might be asked to choose a song that captures how they feel in the moment, what they need in the moment, or what has meaning to them in the moment. Next, the therapist plays the song chosen. It is okay to invite the patient to participate in any way they feel comfortable. Some patients may choose to sing with the therapist, while others might enjoy a more passive role. After the song has concluded, the therapist can engage the patient in a discussion, being mindful to balance supportive questions/reflection with more probing questions. Grocke and Wigram (2007) suggest the following order of questions:

- First-level questions: Ask about the music to gain information about the patient's preferences as well as if the patient is open to exploring specific lyrics or overall themes.

Examples include: "What did you like about the song?" "What do you like about the composer?"

- Second-level questions: Probe the meaning of the song to the patient to uncover parallels with the client's current life situation. Examples include: "Do any lyrics stand out to you?" "Does the song remind you of anything significant to you?"
- Third-level questions: Connect the meaning of the song with what is happening in the patient's life at the moment. Examples include: "How did that song make you feel?" "Is there something in your current situation that is described in that song?"

It is important to remember that some patients might immediately open up to the song choice and its connection to their current life situation, while others might feel vulnerable. At the end of the discussion, the therapist can choose, depending on the client's presenting state and available time, to continue the experience with another song or end the session by thanking the patient for sharing with them.

Adaptations. Song communication can be modified to incorporate remembrance of positive events. For patients experiencing pain, focusing on more pleasant memories or specific events of pleasure can help focus and reframe the current difficulties they are experiencing. While this technique may not have lasting effects, it may decrease the pain perception to a level that is more acceptable and bearable as well as counteract increases in anxiety, fear, and distress often exacerbated by the experience of pain.

Music-Assisted Relaxation

Overview. In music-assisted relaxation, the therapist designs and guides the patient through a music-centered relaxation routine. The purpose might be to address pain perception, pain related insomnia, or emotional needs such as anxiety, fear, and/or distress. A psychoeducational approach should be applied, with emphases on working with the patient to create a routine they will be able to independently implement in time of need. While advanced training is not needed to implement this technique, it is essential that the therapist have supervision during the learning process.

Preparation. The therapist should be familiar with a variety of recorded music suitable for relaxation experiences. The most effective music for relaxation experiences is characterized by a steady pulse; supportive base line; predictability in melodic, harmonic, and rhythmic elements; few dynamic changes; and repetition. Individual preferences can be taken into account. The therapist should also take the length of the music experience into consideration. In acute care settings, it is very difficult to have uninterrupted sessions for more than 15–20 minutes. Given the procedural steps that need to be implemented within this time, it is suggested that selections average from four to six minutes in length. The length of the music can be gradually increased as the patient becomes more comfortable with this technique. Based on the experience level and training level of the therapist as well as the potential association with voices, it is recommended that the therapist choose instrumental versus vocal pieces. This eliminates any concerns over a patient projecting a human persona onto the music. Several suitable pieces can be found within classical, New Age, and jazz music.

In addition to appropriate music selections, the therapist should be prepared to implement a variety of relaxation experiences, including, but not limited to, progressive muscle stretching, breathing exercises, autogenics, and imagery. Each of these will be briefly described below.

Progressive muscle stretching focuses on physically stretching large muscle groups throughout the body. It is recommend for patients who need to experience a physically active form of relaxation, those who have pent-up energy, and those who respond best to concrete instructions. This technique is similar to progressive muscle relaxation; however, it is more suitable for medical patients for whom tensing muscles is contraindicated. In this technique, the therapist leads the patient through body stretches, beginning with the feet/ankles and finishing with the neck and/or jaw muscles.

Breathing exercises focus on encouraging deep breathing, set to a tempo close to that of the natural heart rate. Breathing exercises are particularly helpful for those patients who are anxious and taking shallow breaths, those who have no prior experience with relaxation methods, or those with short attention spans. During implementation, it is helpful for the therapist to model breathing patterns by exaggerating their own breath for the patient to hear.

Autogenics is a method that emphasizes awareness of one's autonomic nervous system. The goal is to teach the patient to become more aware of their physiological responses and to direct those responses to change into a relaxed state. This is accomplished through a series of "I" or "my" statements. This technique is great for establishing a sense of control. It is contraindicated for those with an underlying cardiac condition.

Imagery uses the patient's imagination to "escape" the current situation and transport them to a place, time, or experience that is more pleasant. In acute-care settings, it is best that the therapist solicit information from the client about where they go to relax, a favorite place to visit, or a time in their life when they remember feeling peaceful. From this information, the therapist can direct an imagery experience to re-create the experience for the patient. It is important to keep the images simple and uncomplicated, as well as incorporate the various senses. Common experiences include oceans, open field with sun shining, and meadows. Imagery is contraindicated for those patients who experience periods of confusion.

What to observe. Physiological responses need to be monitored at all times. For those patients with medical monitoring equipment, this would include heart rate, respiratory rate, and pulse. Additional physiological responses include muscle tension, facial grimaces, and vocalizations.

Procedures. The therapist begins with assessing the patient's needs, resources, preferences, and preferred outcome. This includes having the patient rate their pain and/or anxiety of level on a scale from 1 to 10. Next, the therapist determines what type of music and relaxation experience to implement. For those patients with advanced knowledge of relaxation techniques, it may be helpful to include them in the decision-making process. This information will direct the therapist to the type of relaxation experiences and corresponding music selections to use. With medical patients, it is helpful to inform them of the experience that will be implemented. For example, "I will lead you through a progressive muscle stretching experience, followed by listening to a selection of music. The entire time, I will be monitoring you for relaxation responses and I will process with you afterward as to what worked for you." Next, an environment conducive to a relaxation experience should be established, using the following guidelines:

- Uninterrupted space: The therapist should inform nursing staff and, if possible, place a sign on the door stating a session is in progress. If the patient is in a semiprivate room, the roommate should be informed of the session and asked to minimize interruptions. If appropriate, they may be invited to join the experience. Phones should be disconnected or silenced, as well as all electronic equipment.
- Comfortable position for the patient: The therapist should help the patient get in as comfortable a position as possible. To foster this, it may be necessary to lower the bed, adjust pillows and blankets, reposition the patient's body and reposition any tubes pulling on the patient.
- Darkening room: It is helpful to turn off overhead lights, particularly if they are fluorescent lights. If natural light is too bright, closing curtains might be beneficial.
- Setting up music: When using recorded music, it is imperative to check the reproductive quality and volume prior to starting the music-assisted relaxation experience. This includes making sure a specific track is cued and ready to be played when needed.

Once the environment is established, the therapist is ready to start the music-assisted relaxation experience. Start by verbally reassuring the client that they are in a safe place and that this time is just for them. Next, begin the relaxation experience. While directing the relaxation experience, the therapist should be mindful of the following: voice is midrange at a volume the patient can hear and pace is consistent and at a tempo close to that of the natural heartbeat. It is important that the therapist sound natural, and not as though they are reading off a script. At the end of the relaxation induction, the therapist should direct the client to listen to the music and allow it to bring to them what it is that they need.

After the music listening experience, the therapist will need to bring the patient back to the here-and-now, slowly reacclimating them back into the environment. This may include bringing their awareness back to the sounds in the environment and physical sensations such as the support of the bed against their back. Once they are acclimated, the therapist should process the music-assisted relaxation experience with the patient.

In processing the experience, the therapist should ask the patient to once again rate their pain and/or anxiety level. They should inquire as to any feelings, sensations, and/or images the patient experienced as well as their reactions to such. Reactions to the various steps of the experience can be explored. Did they find the relaxation experience helpful? Was the music helpful? All of this can help the therapist and patient determine any changes that might need to be made. The therapist should determine if a relaxation routine can be established for self or family implementation.

Adaptations. Several variances can be made to the music-assisted relaxation routine based on the therapist's level of experience. These include choreographing music to the relaxation experience, separate selections of music for the relaxation experience and music listening experience, and more advanced imagery techniques. It is possible to use this technique with family members present as well as train them in how to implement aspects of this technique for their loved ones. Additionally, recordings of beneficial relaxation routines can be made and provided to the patient and/or family to use during episodes of increased discomfort or during episodes of pain related insomnia.

Music and Imagery

Overview. In this approach, the patient is led through a short relaxation induction and then images freely while listening to live, improvised music. The aim is to stimulate imagery while relaxing the mind and the body for healing purposes. This technique can address the physical as well as the emotional and/or spiritual components of the pain experience. In this approach, the music takes a more central role, with the patient's imagery evoked by the improvised music, as compared to other approaches that have music as the background to a human voice guiding the patient into a state of relaxation. This technique is valuable in addressing emotional and spiritual elements of the pain experience, self-expression, and reducing distress. Therapists wishing to use this approach need advanced training in music psychotherapy and/or training in the Bonny Method of Guided Imagery and Music.

This approach is contraindicated for those patients who are cognitively unable to process the experience, those clients with severe hearing deficits, and those in situations where the therapist is unable to control possible interruptions.

Preparation. When preparing to engage a client in a music and imagery experience, it is important for the therapist to control interruptions. Treatment team members can be verbally informed, or a sign can be placed outside the patient's door. Electronic devices, including phones, should be silenced, and lights should be dimmed. The therapist should be in a position from which they are able to see a patient's body from head to toe.

What to observe. During this experience, the therapist will need to watch for any signs of increased discomfort or distress. Physiologically, these may include increased muscle tension, heart rate, or respiratory rate. Additional signs may include facial grimacing or vocal grunting.

Procedures. Procedural steps can be divided into five sections: opening conversation, short relaxation induction, music experience, post-listening discussion, and patient follow-up. Given the need for advanced training to successfully implement this technique, procedural steps will be described on a general level.

At the beginning of each session, the therapist engages clients in a conversation, focusing on the history, past experiences, and coping strategies related to presenting pain and/or anxiety. If appropriate, clients are asked to describe their experience in sensory terms as well as to describe any physical and/or emotional reactions and any associated images or metaphors. The therapist should have the client rate their pain and/or anxiety using the standard numeric rating scale of 1–10.

Following the opening conversation, clients should be led through a short relaxation induction, intended to address physical comfort, reduce stress, and focus awareness on the music. This induction should be based on client responses during the opening conversation. It may include a breathing exercise, progressive body stretches, autogenics (repeating verbal phrases focused on a particular effect to facilitate a deeper state of relaxation), and/or directed imagery (e.g., ball of energy massaging each part of your body). The induction should conclude with the therapist directing the participant to "allow the music to bring you whatever you need."

During the music experience portion of the session, music is improvised by the therapist on an acoustic guitar and/or keyboard, based on the presenting needs of the client. The use of live, improvised music facilitates the imagery process, as the music is generally created with mood, tempo, and timbre that meet the patient's needs. While chordal patterns, style, and picking patterns may vary, repetitive and predictable chord structures with tempi close to those of the natural heartbeat should be maintained. Additionally, the music should be controlled in dynamics and tempo so that it is not intense or arousing. Specific elements within the music should be used to re-create and resolve specific sensory experiences the patient described in the opening conversation. For example, tension and resolution can be re-created musically. Without being so directed, if a client chooses to report on their images during the music listening, the therapist should direct the participant to notice specific aspects of the actual image. At the end of the music listening experience, the therapist should ask the client to bring their awareness back into the room so that a transition could be made from music listening to post-listening discussion.

During the post-listening discussion, the therapist should ask the client to fully describe any images they may have experienced during the music listening and their reactions to those images, as well as to relate those images to their overall pain and/or anxiety experience. Images may be auditory, visual, sensory or related to memories. Prior to concluding the session, clients should again be asked to rate their pain and/or anxiety level using the standardized rating scale.

During the follow-up visit, patients should be asked if they had reflected on the music and imagery experience, and, if so, to describe that reflection and any associated connection to their overall experience. They should be asked if the music and imagery experience had any lasting effects on their pain and/or anxiety levels. If appropriate, the therapist should give additional suggestions on how they could use aspects of this technique during future exacerbations.

Adaptations. When appropriate, this technique can incorporate friends and/or family members. When doing so, the therapist should remain focused on the patient, ensuring that the experience matches the patient's needs in the moment. During the postlistening discussion, family and/or friends can be asked to share their personal experience, and any connections with the patient can be explored.

Bonny Method of Guided Imagery and Music

Overview. This is an individual form of psychotherapy in which the client images to specifically designed music programs while in an altered state. The Bonny Method of Guided Imagery and Music (BMGIM), refers to the specific method developed by Helen Bonny (Bruscia, 2000). It is a form of therapy that allows one to imagine, explore, and more fully experience possible life choices in a safe and supportive environment. This technique is not intended for inpatient or acute pain experiences, but rather for individuals living with chronic pain. Short (2002) suggests that guided imagery and music with medical patients typically includes ventilation of emotions, insight into problem relations or negative patterns of behaviors, symbolic transformation of body parts, and increased feelings of physical and mental health in addition to emotional reactions related to self-concept. BMGIM is an advanced practice technique that requires specialized training. Additional information, including information on training programs, can be found through the Association for Music and Imagery.

BMGIM is used to address the emotional and spiritual needs of chronic pain sufferers and is contraindicated for those who are not medically stable. This includes those in acute care settings. Additionally, BMGIM is contraindicated for patients with challenges related to reality orientation, those who lack appropriate interpersonal boundaries, and those with intellectual impairments.

Procedures. Sessions involve a preliminary conversation, a relaxation induction, guided music-imaging, return to an alert state, and a postlude discussion. Given the advanced nature of this technique, an overview of each of these steps will be provided; however, specific instructions on how to implement will not be.

The preliminary conversation serves to identify the goal, concern, theme, and/or conflict that are relevant to the individual for that session. Once the overall theme is decided upon, the type of listening experience, the induction and focus, and the music program are selected.

The purpose of the relaxation induction is to prepare the individual physically and emotionally for the imagery experience. The type of induction for each session is based on the nature of the presenting problem, theme, and music selection. Inductions may include breathing exercises, progressive body stretches, autogenics (repeating verbal phrases focused on a particular effect to facilitate a deeper state of relaxation), and/or directed imagery (e.g., ball of energy massaging each part of your body). The induction concludes with the therapist providing a starting image based on the theme and chosen music.

During the music imaging experience, an individual images while listening to music in a relaxed state, assisted by verbal interventions by the therapist, all aimed at helping each individual explore and work through the selected theme. As the music imaging experience comes to a close, the therapist helps the individual return to the here-and-now and the session transitions into the postlude discussion.

The purpose of the postlude is to process, work through, and/or consolidate the music-imaging experience. The therapist works with the individual to process and reflect on the experience in an effort to find connections and meaning. Alternatively, the therapist explores the experience even further or consolidates the experience to closure. The specific approach taken during the postlude is based on the overall direction of the session as decided on in the prelude.

Entrainment

Overview. Entrainment is a type of improvisation designed to symbolically represent a patient's pain experience with gradual shifting to healing or pain relief. While the therapist improvises music, the technique is receptive, as the patient is receiving the music during the actual entrainment session. Dileo (1999) states that this method is most appropriate for those patients with high levels of perceived pain; with pain that does not respond well to medication; with medical conditions for which adequate pain medication is not an option; motivated to actively participate in the music therapy process; whose belief system supports alternative methods of pain treatment; and who may be experiencing pain-related suffering. It is best to implement this technique in outpatient settings.

This technique is contraindicated for those who are medically fragile, those with boundary issues, and those who do not have the cognitive ability to participate in the process (Dileo, 1999). Entrainment is a technique, which requires advanced training and supervision.

Preparation. The therapist will need to have a variety of melodic and percussive instruments available. The session room should be soundproof, if possible, and have enough space to foster patient and therapist comfort.

What to observe. Throughout the experience, the therapist will need to be aware of changes in physiological parameters as well as changes in affect. The therapist should also be aware of the specific elements of the pain and healing improvisation, ensuring that there is a gradual shift and musical resolution is possible.

Procedures. The experience begins with the therapist asking the patient to describe their pain in an effort to identify musical sounds that match the pain as closely as possible. Specific questions the therapist may ask involve the intensity, rhythm, and brightness of the pain. The McGill Pain Questionnaire may be helpful in the process, as it captures sensory aspects of the pain experience. As the patient is describing their pain, the therapist explores with musical sounds to capture the experience, relying on patient feedback to find the sounds that most closely resemble the patient's experience of pain. This process will take time, as it is important for the patient to have their pain experience fully captured in the auditory image being created by the therapist. After the auditory image of pain is created, the therapist works with the patient to create musical sounds of healing. The same process is used during this process.

Once the musical sounds are created, the patient is led through a short relaxation induction and directed to give their attention to the improvisation led by the therapist. The improvisation is a gradual process, beginning with sounds that signify the onset of pain and progressing to the full pain experience. Once the patient signifies, or the therapist determines via patient body language that the patient has fully embraced the pain sounds, the therapist begins to gradually shift the improvisation to incorporate the sounds of healing. The improvisation ends with the improvisation of healing sounds designed by the patient.

At the end of the experience, the therapist processes with the patient on the experience. Recordings of the experience may be used independently; however, the therapist and patient need to continually reassess the suitability of the musical sounds for the patient, as it is not uncommon for there to be shifts in the pain experience. In addition to possible physiological benefits, entrainment has several possible psychological benefits. The process of creating sounds to represent pain and healing experiences may provide the client with an increased sense of control, outlet for self-expression, validation of feelings, emotions, and experiences, and the ability to communicate with family and loved ones on a multidimensional level.

Guidelines for Improvisational Music Therapy

Song Improvisation

Overview. Song Improvisation is when the therapist musically supports the client creating lyrics or melody lines, in the moment. This technique usually occurs spontaneously and is not preplanned by the therapist. It is particularly useful for clients who need to access, explore, or fully experience an emotion and/or reaction. It is an inherently creative process, allowing the client to connect to their emotional, creative self vs. their cognitive self. It shares comparisons with free association. However, unlike free association, the therapist provides musical direction to keep the client within the experience. This technique requires advanced clinical skills, particularly in clinical improvisation. With individuals experiencing acute or chronic pain, song improvisations can provide an outlet for self-expression and an opportunity to communicate with family/friends or a higher power. Additionally, song improvisation can allow client's the opportunity to explore identity and self-esteem issues related to the pain experience.

Song improvisation is contraindicated for clients not comfortable with using their voice, as this is a particularly intimate part of their being. Furthermore, it is contraindicated for patients who have difficulty using their voice or supporting their breath or voice secondary to medical procedures or precautions. Precautions should also be taken with clients exhibiting disorientation or confusion. This technique is most effective when used in individual versus group or family sessions. It is also contraindicated for those patients that are not medically stable to explore emotions, feelings, or reactions.

Preparations. The therapist will need a guitar or keyboard to facilitate musical support. In some situations, a client with a musical background may choose to play an accompaniment. The therapist should be in close physical proximity to the client, for observational purposes.

What to observe. The therapist should be aware of emotional and physiological reactions during the experience. This will help direct musical responses of the therapist. Additionally, the therapist needs to watch for signs of fatigue, increased discomfort, or exhaustion, particularly if using this technique with hospitalized patients.

Procedures. Song improvisation generally begins one of two ways. The first is when the therapists enters a patient's space and, during the assessment process, determines the patient is "stuck" on a particular experience, feeling, or emotion. This may present as the patient perseverating on few words, a few key words, or a particular issue/experience. This is an opportunity for the therapist to musically support the client, either vocally reflecting those words and/or musically reflecting the portrayed emotions or feelings. This process of musical support and/or reflection continues, with the therapist offering musical empathy, structuring, redirection, and/or elicitation in direct response to the patient's musical offerings. The song improvisation ends when it appears as though the patient has expressed or explored what they needed to and is ready to end.

The second way song improvisations can begin is when, through the assessment process, the therapist determines that the client is open to using musical creativity to freely explore what needs to be said or heard. This type of song improvisation may start with the client choosing a musical accompaniment that matches their current emotions and/or feelings. The therapist can explore several patterns and styles of chordal accompaniments with the client, with the goal of finding one that resonates with them. The therapist would then improvise with this pattern. If needed, the therapist might start with just having the client freely explore vocal sounds. This can help the client get into the experience before adding words. During this process, the therapist should musically support the client, offering musical reflection, empathy, structuring, elicitation, or redirection, as appropriate. If the client chooses to add words, the therapist would continue musical support. The song improvisation ends when the client has explored and expressed what they needed to, or when fatigue prevents continuation.

Gardstrom (2007) provided several examples of music facilitation skills to use during improvisation experiences. A selection of these is listed below:

- Empathy Techniques
  - Imitate a client's response
  - Synchronize with a client's playing
  - Incorporate a musical motif of the client into one's improvising
  - Pace one's improvising with the client's energy level
  - Reflect the moods, attitudes, and feelings exhibited by the client
- Structuring Techniques
  - Establish and maintain a rhythmic ground
  - Establish and maintain a tonal center
- Elicitation Techniques
  - Use repetition as an invitation for the client to respond
  - Model desired musical responses
  - Make spaces in one's improvising for the client's improvising

- Interject music into the spaces made by the client
- Redirection Techniques
    - Introduce musical change to redirect the client's playing
    - Intensify elements within the improvisation

After the song improvisation ends, the therapist will need to decide whether verbally processing the experience is necessary. In many cases, the experience speaks for itself and additional processing is not necessary.

Referential Improvisation

Overview. In referential improvisation, the client explores musical sounds to express an experience, feeling, idea, event, or relationship. This type of music experience can foster self-expression and identity exploration and validate personal experiences as well as exploration of self in relation to others. The therapist can suggest referents based on emotions, feelings, and/or experiences related to the pain experience. Creating and hearing these experiences provides a different sensory experience for the patient, which can open the door for healing to occur. The music therapist should have advanced training in improvisational techniques, including improvisation assessment and evaluation.

Instrumental improvisation is not recommended for patients admitted to the hospital. The energy level required to play as well as the potential volume of the experience are of great concern for inpatient medical settings. Additionally, most facilities prefer a bare number of musical instruments be transported to patient rooms, as infection control procedures are usually in place.

Preparation. The therapist should have a selection of quality rhythm and melodic percussive instruments from which the patient can select. Recording equipment is also helpful, for playback of the improvisation to the client.

What to observe. The therapist should be aware of emotional and physiological reactions during the experience, including changes in affect, energy level, and body positioning. This will help direct musical responses of the therapist. Additionally, the therapist needs to watch for signs of fatigue, increased discomfort, or exhaustion, particularly if using this technique with patients receiving medical treatment.

Musically, the therapist should be aware of instrument choices and playing of the instruments, and the relationship of various musical elements in the improvisational experience.

Procedures. The improvisational experience should begin with the therapist selecting instruments to present to the client. The client should be given ample time to explore each instrument, encouraging characteristic and noncharacteristic playing of the instruments. This allows the patient to experience the variety of sound potentials for each instrument. Once this is done, the therapist and client will have to decide the individual roles within the improvisation. Considerations include solo, duo, or group play. The therapist and/or client deciding on a specific theme for the improvisation follow this. Possibilities include specific emotions, events, feelings, relationships, or ideas related to the pain experience. When the improvisation experience is ready to begin the therapist should record the experience for later playback. During the improvisation, the therapist should engage in musical facilitation skills, as appropriate.

After the improvisation ends, the therapist should process with the client. This should begin with a focus on the musical sounds created and corresponding reaction to them. Next, the therapist should work with the client to make any connections between the client's interpretation of the musical sounds and the referent provided at the beginning of the improvisation. During this time, if appropriate, the therapist can replay the improvisation for the client. The therapist should support the client in making any connections to the musical sounds, referent given, and client's current life situation.

GUIDELINES FOR RE-CREATIVE MUSIC THERAPY

Therapeutic Singing

Overview. Singing involves the client using their voice to reproduce preferred music. It is not unusual for individuals experiencing pain to display shallow breathing patterns. Singing can encourage patients to take deep breaths, while regulating their respiratory rate. The goal of this technique is the self-monitoring of physiological signs of pain, as well as increased self-expression. Live music is beneficial to teach patients self-regulation techniques. Once established, the therapist can assist the client in selecting appropriate recorded music. This technique is particularly beneficial for those patients needing an active method for pain management and/or those who enjoy singing.

Preparation. The therapist should have a wide repertoire of songs, from a variety of genres. It is helpful to provide the patients with a list of potential songs, categorized by genres, as a starting point. Additionally, the therapist should provide patients with lyric sheets, allowing them to hear and see the lyrics simultaneously. The therapist will need to instruct the patient on diaphragmatic breathing. Diaphragmatic breathing can slow the breathing rate and decrease oxygen demand, and requires less effort and energy for the patient to breathe. If lying in bed, the patient can be instructed as follows: Lie on a flat surface or in bed, with knees bent and head supported; use a pillow under the knees to support the legs; place one hand on the upper chest and the other just below the rib cage—this will allow the patient to feel their diaphragm move as they breathe; breathe in slowly through the nose so that the stomach moves out against the hand; tighten your stomach muscles, letting them fall inward as you exhale through pursed lips. If the patient is in a chair, the following instructions should be used: Sit comfortably, with your knees bent and your shoulders, head, and neck relaxed; breathe in slowly through the nose so that your stomach moves out against the hand—the hand on your chest should remain as still as possible; place one hand on the upper chest and the other just below the rib cage—this will allow you to feel your diaphragm move as you breathe; tighten the stomach muscles, letting them fall inward as you exhale through pursed lips.

What to observe. The therapist should be aware of baseline physiological parameters, including heart rate and respiratory rate. Throughout the experience, the therapist should be aware of changes in physiological signs as well as changes in affect.

Procedures. The therapist should begin by assessing patient preferences and establish baseline physiological parameters. The therapist, in conjunction with the patient, may do modeling of diaphragmatic breathing. Once diaphragmatic breathing is established, the therapist should encourage the patient to use vocal sounds while exhaling. Next, the therapist can encourage partner song singing, wherein the therapist starts the musical phrase and the client completes it. This will alternate therapist/patient breathing patterns and allow for singing of a continuous musical phrase. When using previously composed songs, it is often necessary for the music therapist to alter the tempo to achieve desired benefits. An example of partner song singing can be provided using the song "Swing Low, Sweet Chariot." The therapist will take a deep breath and sing "Swing." While the therapist is singing "Swing," the client is taking a deep breath, preparing to vocalize "Low." While the patient is vocalizing "Low," the therapist is taking a deep breath and preparing to vocalize the "Sweet." The focus is on the regulation of breath via a consistent and predictable melodic phrasing and rhythm. Once this is accomplished, the therapist can focus on having the patient establish the melodic phrase and rhythm and sing independently.

Guidelines for Compositional Music Therapy

Songwriting

Overview. With this method, the therapist provides an appropriate structure to engage the patient in the writing of original lyrics and/or accompaniment. Songwriting is a great way to foster the decision-making process while providing a valuable tool for the exploration of feelings, beliefs, wishes, and emotion as well as a tool to encourage communication. In acute pain situations, it may be used as a way to focus the patient on a more pleasant stimulus while enhancing a sense of control. In chronic pain clients, it may be used to address the emotional, social, and spiritual components of the pain experience.

In order to engage a patient in songwriting, the therapist should be a solid musician with the ability to play a variety of musical styles. Furthermore, they should be comfortable with changing leadership roles with the client, with a flexible give-and-take to ensure that it is the client's experience, not the therapist's interpretation of the experience or the therapist's need for a finalized "product." The therapist should be comfortable with verbal processing techniques, particularly those needed to enhance or deepen the patient's experience. Open-ended questions, timely reflection of statements, and probing are useful within this experience.

Songwriting is contraindicated for those patients exhibiting or experiencing high levels of physical or emotional distress or who are disoriented or confused.

Preparation. In addition to the therapist having a guitar and/or keyboard available, it is also necessary to have something with which to write down the lyrics and chords. If desired, a recording device is helpful for those opportunities when a patient may want to record the final product.

What to observe. The therapist should be mindful of the choices the patient makes during the experience, focusing on any insights and/or incongruities present.

Procedures. Wigram (2005) developed the Flexible Approach to Songwriting in Therapy (FAST). This working model outlines the possibilities within each stage of songwriting. Aspects of the FAST model are outlined below:

- Introduction to Songwriting
    - Improvising incorporating story creation or client's life story
    - The therapist proposes idea in discussion
- Formulation of Lyrics
    - Brainstorming themes (client and therapist)
    - Words are spontaneously suggested (client or therapist)
    - Words related to client issues are suggested (client or therapist)
    - Client brings precomposed lyrics
- Development of Music
    - Improvised (client and therapist)
    - Improvised melody over structured harmonic frame (client and/or therapist)
    - Clients create melody and harmony
    - Therapist offers ideas in short fragments or chords of melody and harmony, accepted or rejected by client
- Writing Down a Song
    - Lyrics only
    - Lyrics and melody
    - Lyrics, melody, and basic guitar/piano chordal harmonic structure
- Performing a Song
    - The song is performed by client and therapist together
    - The song is performed to staff and other clients

    - The song is performed to family and friends
- Recording of Song
    - The song is recorded by client and therapist

Throughout the experience, the therapist needs to be mindful of the client's word choices, including where they place themselves within the song. Additionally, the therapist may need to shape the client's words into a verse. While doing so, they need to make sure they capture what the client communicates, not what they think the client is communicating. This can be done verbally with such statements as: "What I hear you saying is this ...?" "Do the words capture what you were communicating, or does something need to be changed?" "Would you like this to go like this or should we change the order of this?"

Adaptations. Story songs are a specific type of songwriting. A story song is an imaginative story created by a client with the support of the music therapist, through music that depicts the client's situation or understanding of his or her situation. This may be done vocally, instrumentally, or as a combination of vocals and instruments. The musical structure of a story song is similar to that of a story and includes the following elements: recitative, theme, conflict, variations, and resolutions (Rubin-Bosco, 2007). The creation of story songs can take several sessions, so it is best to use this technique with chronic pain patients being seen in an outpatient setting. Story songs are a great way to support clients in their process of accessing, exploring, and expressing their experience of pain and can easily be adapted for group situations.

Research Evidence

Research on music therapy and pain indicates that music therapy techniques are effective for a variety of procedural, acute, and chronic conditions. Furthermore, music therapy is more effective than music medicine interventions and, when used in combination with analgesics, has been found to reduce the dependency on pain medication (Dileo & Bradt, 2005). The following is a review of literature on music therapy in the management of adult pain, separated by music therapy methods employed.

Receptive Music Therapy

The earliest studies on the effectiveness of music therapy for pain management involve receptive music therapy methods. Bright (1972) suggested using music for relaxation purposes before attempting physical therapy in older adults. Masler (1986), in a review of the literature on music therapy and pain, reported that music could be used to teach pain management techniques to promote awareness of the body and in turn reduce pain. Cook (1986) researched the benefits of music therapy with inpatient cancer patients. She found that listening to classical music was effective in decreasing analgesic intake with cancer patients as well as addressing insomnia. Beck (1991), in a study investigating the therapeutic effects of music therapy, found that cancer patients who listened to music twice per day reported a significant decrease in their need for pain medication. Robb, Nichols, Rutan, Bishop, and Parker (1995), in an investigation on music assisted relaxation, found the following characteristics of music were most desirable for relaxation purposes: slow to moderate tempo at or below the resting heart rate (60–72 bpm); rhythm should be smooth, flowing, and without sudden changes; melodies should be slow, sustained, and progress by step; pitch should be low, as high pitches tend to elicit tension; dynamics should be soft to moderately loud. Lastly, Magill (2001) stated that music therapy techniques for pain management provide resources that can soothe and relax, promote comfort and inner peace, enhance communication and enhance the development of improved coping skills.

More recent studies have investigated the effects of listening to live music on pain perception.

Madson and Silverman (2010) investigated the effects of live, patient preferred music on relaxation, anxiety, pain perception, and nausea in adult solid organ transplant patients. Results indicated significant improvement in self-reported measures of relaxation, anxiety, pain and nausea. Furthermore, the researchers reported increased positive verbalization and increased positive affect. In a similar study, Chaput-McGovern and Silverman (2012) investigated the effects of live, patient preferred music on measures of relaxation, anxiety, and pain in post-operative oncology patients. Results indicated live music listening significantly decreased pain perception and anxiety levels while increases measures of relaxation.

A few studies have investigated the use of song communication in the management of pain. Colwell (1997) reported on the use of song choice with a chronic pain patient. She concluded that song choice aided in distracting the patient, increased relaxation, and decreased use of narcotics for pain management. Krout (2001) investigated the effects of single session music therapy sessions to address the needs of hospice patients. Results indicated that song choice was a type of music intervention useful to decrease pain perception and increase physical comfort in hospice patients. Lastly, Ghetti (2011) investigated the effects of music therapy with transplant patients. She reported that active engagement through song choice significantly decreased pain perception and negative affect of liver and kidney transplant patients.

Several studies have investigated the effectiveness of music and imagery techniques for pain management. Bonny (1986) stated that music enhances the flow of images and that kinesthetic, visual, or emotional images can be used in treating various diseases. Imagery nurtures creativity and is a means through which feelings, ideas, associations, and perceptions of pain can be realized, identified, and processed (Magill-Levreault, 1993). The use of live, improvised music facilitates the imagery process as the music is generally created with the mood, tempo, and timbre that meet the patient's needs. Imagery used in conjunction with carefully selected music can reduce pain and effect muscle relaxation; it can also be used to explore inner feelings, memories, and life issues (Bonny, 1986; Rider, 1985). Jacobi (1995) investigated the effects of BMGIM with rheumatoid arthritis sufferers. Individuals received ten BMGIM sessions which resulted in significantly decreased pain perception and psychological distress. Allen (2001) found that music-assisted relaxation significantly decreased pain and anxiety in postoperative older adults in a rehabilitation setting. Allen (2008) explored the use of music and imagery for addressing advanced cancer pain in hospitalized cancer survivors. She found that music-evoked imagery decreased pain perception as well as addressed the emotional and spiritual components of the pain experience.

There is limited literature addressing entrainment for pain management. Rider (1985) found that entrainment was more effective than preferred music in producing desired physiological changes. Dileo & Bradt (1999), in an overview of entrainment and pain related suffering, reported that entrainment allows for patient confrontation with the pain along with increased awareness that there are sounds that heal. Furthermore, they reported that the patient's externalization of the pain and the therapist's resonance with the patient's pain experience provide necessary healing components. Lastly, Dimaio (2010) explored entrainment and the creation of healing music with hospice patients. She reported that entrainment can address a client's pain, include the client in the process, offer dignity by emphasizing the client's experience of pain, and offer hope in decreasing that perception of pain.

Improvisational Music Therapy

A very limited number of studies were found in relation to improvisational methods for pain management in the adult medical patient. Krout (2001), in an examination of single-session music therapy with hospice patients, reported improvisation as one method used in decreased pain perception. Accordingly, improvisation may be effective for enhancing physical comfort and relaxation in hospice patients. Magill (2011) investigated bereaved caregivers reflections on the role of music therapy. Results indicated vocal and instrumental improvisational techniques were beneficial in exploring feelings and issues that frequently compounded the pain experience.

Re-creative Music Therapy

A few studies have examined the benefits of therapeutic singing on the pain experience. Krout (2001), in an investigation of the effectiveness of single music therapy sessions, found singing beneficial in decreasing pain and increasing physical comfort in hospice patients. Kenny and Faunce (2004) investigated the effects of group singing on mood, coping, and perceived pain in chronic pain patients. Results indicated that group singing increased active coping skills and decreased pain perception. Lichtensztejn (2009) investigated the clinical use of piano with patients experiencing pain related breathing distress. She reported that actively engaging in singing decreases pain, as it encourages patients to regulate their breathing while letting go of their pain. Lastly, Skingley and Vella-Burrows (2010) investigated the therapeutic effects of singing for older adults. Results indicated that singing was an effective tool for decreasing pain perception of osteoarthritis patients in a nursing home setting.

Compositional Music Therapy

Songwriting may be an effective tool in addressing a patient's pain experience, however there is limited research investigating its effectiveness. Krout (2001), while investigating the effects of single music therapy sessions, found songwriting effective in decreasing pain and increasing the comfort of hospice patients. Magill (2001), in research on the benefits of music therapy with advanced cancer pain, mentioned songwriting as a valuable technique to explore to address the total pain experience. Lastly, Curtis (2011), in an investigation on the effects of university community project, reported that songwriting was one method used to decrease pain, facilitate relaxation, and increase quality of life in palliative care patients.

Summary and Conclusions

Pain can be an overwhelming experience that impacts physical, psychological, interpersonal, and spiritual well-being. Pain and music share several characteristics. Both are multifaceted phenomena that manifest and affect people in different ways. Furthermore, pain and elements within music can be described with similar adjectives: tightening, tension and release, resonating, evocative, etc. Music therapy can offer patients a nonthreatening, physically noninvasive treatment with the potential for accessing inner resources while generating desired outcomes. It can be an effective therapy, giving patients an active role in their treatment and a form of symbolic expression. This allows patients to safely explore and experience a unique way of healing.

Research on music therapy and pain overwhelmingly favors music listening interventions as well as interventions to address acute pain conditions. As we are facing a health care crisis in regard to chronic pain, music therapy research needs to investigate the effectiveness of various music therapy methods in addressing the physical, social, emotional, and spiritual needs of chronic pain patients. This includes various methods of music therapy in addressing the chronic pain experience.

References

Allen, J. (2001). The effects of music therapy, preferred music listening, and standard treatment on perceived pain and anxiety of post-operative older adults in a rehabilitation setting. Unpublished manuscript.

Allen, J. (2008). Music-evoked imagery in the treatment of oncological pain. Unpublished manuscript.

Ambler, N., Williams, A., Hill, P., Gunary, R., & Cratchely, G. (2001). Sexual difficulties of chronic pain patients. *Clinical Journal of Pain, 17*(2), 138–142.

American Academy of Pain Medicine (n.d.). *Facts and figures on pain.* Glenview, IL: American Academy of Pain Medicine. Retrieved from: http://www.painmed.org/patientcenter/facts_on_pain.aspx

American Pain Foundation (2012). *Pain facts & figures.* Retrieved from: http://www.painfoundation.org/media/resources/pain-facts-figures.html. Accessed August, 2012.

American Pain Society. (2006). *Pain Control in the Primary Care Setting.* Glenview, IL: American Pain Society

American Society of Anesthesiologists, Task Force on Pain Management, Chronic Pain Section. (1997). Practice guidelines for chronic pain management. *Anesthesiology, 86*(4), 995–1004.

American Society of Anesthesiologist. (1997). Practice guidelines for chronic pain management. *Anesthesiology, 86*(4), 995-1004.

Apfelbaum, J., Chen, C., Mehta, S., & Gan, T. (2003). Postoperative pain experience: Results from a national survey suggesting postoperative pain continues to be undermanaged. *Anesthesia & Analgesia, 97,* 534–540.

Bailey, L. (1986). Music therapy in pain management. *Journal of Pain and Symptom Management, 1*(1), 25–28.

Bair, M., Kroenke, K., Sutherland, J., McCoy, K., Harris, G., & McHorney, C. (2007). Effects of depression and pain severity on satisfaction in medical outpatients: analysis of the Medical Outcomes Study. *Journal of Rehabilitative Research Development, 44*(2), 143–152.

Baliki, M., Geha, P., Apkarian, A., & Chialvo, D. (2008). Beyond feeling: Chronic pain hurts the brain, disrupting the default-mode network dynamics. *Journal of Neuroscience, 28*(6), 1398–1403.

Beck, S. (1991). The therapeutic use of music for cancer-related pain. *Oncology Nurse Forum, 18,* 1327–1337.

Berry, P., & Dahl, J. (1998). *Barriers to adequate pain management: An Ishikawa (Fishbone) diagram.* University of Wisconsin–Madison: Institutionalizing Pain Management Project

Bonny, H. (1986). Music and healing. *Music Therapy, 6,* 3–12.

Bouhassira, D., Lanteri-Minet, M., Attal, N., Laurent, B., & Touboul, C. (2008). Prevalence of chronic pain with neuropathic characteristics in the general population. *Pain, 136*(3), 380–387.

Breivik, H., Collett, B., Ventafridda, V., Cohen, R., & Gallacher, D. (2006). Survey of chronic pain in Europe: Prevalence, impact on daily life, and treatment. *European Journal of Pain, 10*(4), 287–333.

Bright, R. (1972). *Music in geriatric care.* Sydney: Agnus & Robertson.

Brokoff, D. (2001). Chronic pain: A new disease. *Hospital Practice , 35*(7), 45.

Bruehl, S., Chung, O., Jirjis, J., & Biridepalli, S. (2005). Prevalence of clinical hypertension in patients with chronic pain compared to nonpain general medical patients. *Clinical Journal of Pain, 21*(2), 147–153

Bruscia, K. (2000). A manual for level one training in guided imagery and music. Unpublished.

Carr, D.B., Jacox, A.K., Chapman, C.R., Ferrell, B., Fields, H.L., Heidrich, G (III)., Hester, N.K., Hills, C.S. Jr., Lipman, A.G., McGarvey, C.L., Miaskowski, C.A., Mulder, D.S., Payne, R., Schechter, N., Shapiro, B.S., Smith, R.S., Tsou, C.V. & Vecchiarelli, L. (1992) Acute pain management: Operative or medical procedures and trauma. Clinical practice guideline. Rockville, MD: Agency for Health Care Policy and Research, Public Health Service, US Department of Health and Human Services, AHCPR Pub. No. 92-0032

Chapman, C. & Syrjala, K. (2001). Measurement of pain. In J. Loese, S. Butler, C. Chapman, & D. Turk (eds), *Bonica's management of pain*, 3rd edition. (pp. 310-328). Baltimore, MD: Williams & Wilkins.

Chaput-McGovern, J., & Silverman, M. (2012). Effects of music therapy with patients on post-surgical unit: A pilot study determining maintenance of immediate gains. *The Arts in Psychotherapy, 39*(5), 417–422.

Colwell, C. (1997). Music as distraction and relaxation to reduce chronic pain and narcotic ingestion: A case study. *Music Therapy Perspectives, 15*(1), 24–31.

Commission on Accreditation of Rehabilitation Facilities. (1998). *Standards manual for and interpretive guidelines for medical rehabilitation.* Tucson, AZ: Commission on Accreditation of Rehabilitation Facilities.

Commission on Accreditation of Rehabilitation Facilities. (1999). *Standards manual for and interpretive guidelines for medical rehabilitation.* Tucson, AZ: Commission on Accreditation of Rehabilitation Facilities.

Committee on Advancing Pain Research, Care, and Education. (2011). *Relieving pain in America: A blueprint for transforming prevention, care, education, and research.* Washington, DC: Institute of Medicine of the National Academies.

Cook, J. (1986). Music as an intervention in the oncology setting. *Cancer Nursing, 9,* 23–28.

Curtis, S. (2011). Music therapy and the symphony: A university community project in palliative care. *Music & Medicine, 3*(1), 20–26.

Dahl J.& Gordon D. (2002). The Joint Commission standards: A progress report. *American Pain Society Bulletin, 12*(1), 11–12.

Dick, B., & Rashiq, S. (2007). Disruption of attention and working memory traces in individuals with chronic pain. *Anesthesia and Analgesia, 104*(5), 1223–1229.

Dileo, C., & Bradt, J. (1999). Entrainment, resonance, and pain-related suffering. In C. Dileo (Ed.), *Music therapy and medicine: Theoretical and clinical applications* (pp. 181–188). Silver Spring, MD: American Music Therapy Association.

Dileo, C., & Bradt, J. (2005). *Medical music therapy: A meta-analysis and agenda for future research.* Cherry Hill, NJ: Jeffery Books.

DiMaio, L. (2010). Music therapy entrainment: A humanistic music therapist's perspective of using music therapy entrainment with hospice patients experiencing pain. *Music Therapy Perspectives, 28*(2), 106-115.

Finley, G., & Schechter, N. (2003). Sedation. In N. Schechter, C. Berde, & M. Yaster (Eds.), *Pain in infants, children, and adolescents,* (2nd ed.) (pp. 563–577) Philadelphia, PA: Lippincott Williams & Wilkins.

Fenwick, C., Chaboyer, W., & St. John, W. (2012). Decision-making processes for the self-management of persistent pain: A grounded theory study. *Contemporary Nurse, 42*(1), 53–66.

Fine, P. (2011). Long-term consequences of chronic pain: Mounting evidence for pain as a neurological disease and parallels with other chronic disease states. *Pain Medicine, 12,* 996–1004.

Flor, H., Fyrich, T., & Turk, D. (1992). Efficacy of multidimensional pain treatment centers: A meta-analytic review. *Pain, 49,* 221–230.

Fox, C., Berger, D., Fine, P., Gebhart, G., Grabois, M., Kulich, R., Lande, S., McCarberg, B., & Portenay, R. (2000). Pain assessment and treatment in the managed care environment. A position statement from the American Pain Society. Glenview, IL: American Pain Society. Retrieved from: http://www.painanddisability.com/pain/pain_assessment.html

Galer, B., & Dworkin, R. (2000) *A clinical guide to neuropathic pain.* Minneapolis, MN: The McGraw-Hill Companies, Inc.

Gardstrom, S. (2007). *Music therapy improvisation for groups: Essential leadership competencies.* Gilsum, NH: Barcelona Publishers.

Ghetti, C. (2011). Active music engagement with emotional-approach coping to improve well-being in liver and kidney transplant patients. *Journal of Music Therapy, 48*(4), 463–485.

Grachev, I., Fredrickson, B., & Apkarian, A. (2000). Abnormal brain chemistry in chronic back pain: An in vivo proton magnetic resonance spectroscopy study. *Pain, 89*(1), 7–18.

Grocke, D. & Wigram, T. (2007). *Receptive methods in music therapy: Techniques and clinical applications for music therapy clinicians, educators, and students.* Philadelphia, PA: Jessica Kingsley.

Gureje, O., Von Korff, M., Simon, G., & Gater, R. (1998). Persistent pain and well being: A World Health Organization study in primary care. *Journal of the American Medical Association, 280*(2), 147–151.

Hutchinson, R. (2007). Challenges in acute postoperative pain management. *American Journal of Health System Pharmacy, 64*(6 Suppl), S2–S5.

International Association for the Study of Pain, Task Force on Guidelines for Desirable Characteristics for Pain Treatment Facilities. (2009). *Desirable characteristics for pain treatment facilities.* Glenview, IL. International Association for the Study of Pain. Retrieved from: http://www.iasp-pain.org/AM/Template.cfm?Section=General_Resource_Links&Template=/CM/HTMLDisplay.cfm&ContentID=3011

International Association for the Study of Pain Subcommittee on Taxonomy. (1986). Classification of chronic pain. Descriptions of chronic pain syndromes and definitions of pain terms. Prepared by the International Association of Pain, Subcommittee on Taxonomy. *Pain Supplement, 3,* S1–S226.

International Association for the Study of Pain. (1979). The need for a taxonomy. *Pain* 6(3), 246-248.

Jacobi, E. (1995). The efficacy of The Bonny Method of Guided Imagery and Music as experiential treatment in the primary care of persons with rheumatoid arthritis. *Dissertation Abstracts International: Section B: The Sciences & Engineering, 56*(2–B), 1110.

Jacox, A., Ferrell, B., Heidrich, G., Hester, N., and Miaskowski, C (1992). A guideline for the Nation: Managing acute pain. *American Journal of Nursing* 92(5), 49-55.

Kehlet, H., Jensen, T. S., & Woolf, C. J. (2006). Persistent postsurgical pain: Risk factors and prevention. *Lancet, 367*(9522), 1618–1625.

Kenny, D., & Faunce, G. (2004). The impact of group singing on mood, coping, and perceived pain in chronic pain patients attending a multidisciplinary pain clinic. *Journal of Music Therapy, 41*(3), 241–258.

Krout, R. (2001). The effects of single-session music therapy interventions on the observed and self-reported levels of pain control, physical comfort, and relaxation of hospice patients. *American Journal of Hospice & Palliative Medicine, 18*(6), 270–283.

Leadley, R., Armstrong, N., Lee, Y., Allen, A., & Kleijnen, J. (2012). Chronic diseases in the European Union: The prevalence and health cost implications of chronic pain. *Journal of Pain & Palliative Care Pharmacotherapy, 26*(4), 310–325.

Lichtensztejn, M. (2009). The clinical use of piano with patients suffering from breathing distress related to pain. In R. Azoulay & J. Loewy (Eds.), *Music, the breath and health: Advances in integrative music therapy* (pp. 213–222). New York: Satchnote Press.

Logan, H. (1998). Applied music-evoked imagery for the oncology patient: Results and case studies of a three month music therapy pilot program. Unpublished manuscript.

Loewy, J. (1999). The use of music psychotherapy in the treatment of pediatric pain. In C. Dileo (Ed.), *Music therapy and medicine: Theoretical and clinical applications,* (pp. 189-206). Silver Spring, MD: American Music Therapy Association.

McCaffery, M. & Beebe, A. (1989). *Pain: Clinical manual for nursing practice.* St. Louis, MO: C.V. Mosby.

McCaffery, M., & Pasero, C. (1999). Assessment: Underlying complexities, misconceptions, and practical tools. In M. McCaffery & C. Pasero (Eds.), *Pain: Clinical Manual 2* (pp. 35–102). St. Louis, MO: Mosby.

McCarberg, B., Nicholson, B., Todd, K., Palmer, T., & Penles, L. (2008). The impact of pain on quality of life and the unmet needs of pain management: Results from pain suffers and physicians participating in an internet survey. *American Journal of Therapeutics, 15*(4), 312–320.

McCracken, L., & Iverson, G. (2002). Disrupted sleep patterns and daily functioning in patients with chronic pain. *Pain, Research, & Management, 7*(2), 75–79.

McDonald, J. (2000). A deconstructive turn in chronic pain treatment: A redefined role for social work. *Health and Social Work, 25*(1), 51–58.

Madson, A., & Silverman, M. (2010). Effect of music therapy on relaxation, anxiety, pain perception, and nausea in adult solid organ transplant patients. *Journal of Music Therapy, 47*(3), 220–232.

Magill, L. (2011). Bereaved family caregivers' reflections on the role of music therapy. *Music and Medicine, 3*(1), 56-63.

Magill, L. (2001). The use of music therapy to address the suffering in advanced cancer pain. *Journal of Palliative Care, 17*(3), 167–172.

Magill-Levreault, L. (1993). Music therapy in pain and symptom management. *Journal of Palliative Care, 9*(4), 42–48.

Magill, L., Coyle, N., Handzo., G., & Loscalzo, M. (1997). Cancer and pain: A creative, multidimensional approach in working with patients and families. In J. Loewy (Ed), *Music therapy in pediatric pain*, (pp. 107 – 114). Cherry Hill, NJ: Jeffrey Books.

Marin, R., Cyhan, T., & Miklos, W. (2006). Sleep disturbance in patients with chronic low back pain. *American Journal of Physical Medicine & Rehabilitation, 85*(5), 430–435.

Marsac, M., & Funk, J. (2008). Relationships among psychological functioning, dental anxiety, pain perception, and coping in children and adolescents. *Journal of Dentistry for Children, 75*(3), 243–251.

Masler, P. (1986). The effect of music on the reduction of pain: A review of the literature. *The Arts in Psychotherapy, 13*, 215-219.

Melzack, R. (1975). The McGill Pain Questionnaire: Major properties and scoring methods. *Pain, 1*(3), 277–299.

Mersky, H., & Bodguk, N. (eds). (1994). *Classification of chronic pain, 2nd edition, IASP task force on taxonomy.* Seattle, WA: International Association of the Study of Pain Press

Michel, D. (1995). A survey of music therapists using music for pain relief. *The Arts in Psychotherapy, 22*, 49–51.

Morin, C., Gibson, D., & Wade, J. (1998). Self-reported sleep and mood disturbances in chronic pain patients. *Clinical Journal of Pain, 14*(3), 311–314.

O'Callaghan, C. (1996). Pain, music creativity, and music therapy in palliative care. *American Journal of Hospice and Palliative Medicine, 13*(2), 43–49.

Ohayon, M., & Schatzberg, A. (2003). Using chronic pain to predict depressive morbidity in the general population. *Archives of General Psychiatry, 60*(1), 39-47.

Paice, J. (2010). Pain at the end of life. In B. Ferrell, & N. Coyle (Eds.), *Oxford textbook of palliative care*, (3rd ed.) (pp. 161–185). New York: Oxford University Press.

Pasero, C., & McCaffery, M. (2005). No self-report means no pain-intensity rating. *American Journal of Nursing, 105*(10), 50–53.

Payen J, Bru O, Bosson J, Lagrasta A, Novel E, Deschaux I., Lavagne, P., & Jacquot, C. (2001). Assessing pain in critically ill sedated patients by using a behavioural pain scale. *Critical Care Medicine, 29*(12), 2258—2263.

Ratcliffe, G., Enns, M., Belik, S., & Sareen, J. (2008). Chronic pain conditions and suicidal ideation and suicide attempts: An epidemiological perspective. *Clinical Journal of Pain, 24*(3), 204–210.

Ready, R., & Edwards, W. (Eds). (1992). *Management of acute pain: A practical guide.* Seattle, WA: International Association for the Study of Pain.

Rider, M. (1999). Homeodynamic mechanisms of improvisational music therapy. In C. Dileo (Ed.), *Music therapy and medicine: Theoretical and clinical applications* (pp. 107–114). Silver Spring, MD: American Music Therapy Association.

Rider, M. (1985). Entrainment mechanisms are involved in pain reduction, muscle relaxation, and muscle mediated imagery. *Journal of Music Therapy, 12*(4), 183–192.

Robb, S., Nichols, R., Rutan, R., Bishop, B., & Parker, J. (1995). The effects of music-assisted relaxation on preoperative anxiety. *Journal of Music Therapy, 32*(1), 2–21.

Rubin-Bosco, J. (2007). Resolution vs. re-enactment: A story song approach to working with trauma. In J. V. Loewy & A. Frisch Hara (Eds.), *Caring for the caregiver: The use of music and music therapy in grief and trauma* (pp. 118-127). Silver Spring, MD: American Music Therapy Association

Saperston, B. (1999). Music-based individualized relaxation training in medical settings. In C. Dileo (Ed.), *Music therapy and medicine: Theoretical and clinical applications* (pp. 41–51). Silver Spring, MD: American Music Therapy Association.

Short, A. (2002). Guided imagery and music (GIM) in medical care. In K. Bruscia & D. Grocke (Eds.), *Guided imagery and music: The Bonny Method and beyond (pp. 151-170).* Gilsum, NH: Barcelona Publishers.

Skingley, A., & Vella-Burrows, T. (2010). Therapeutic effects of music and singing for older people. *Nursing Standards, 24(*19), 35–41.

Smith, B., Elliott, A., Chamber, W., Cairns Smith, W., Hannaford, P., & Penny, K. (2001). The impact of chronic pain in the community. *Family Practice, 18*(3), 292–299.

Snelling, J. (1994). The effect of chronic pain on the family unit. *Journal of Advanced Nursing, 19,* 543–551.

Standley, J. (2000). Music research in medical treatment. In Standley, J. (Ed.), *Effectiveness of music therapy procedures: Documentation of research and clinical practice, 3rd Ed.* (pp. 1–64). Silver Spring, MD: American Music Therapy Association.

Stanos, S. (2012). Focused review of interdisciplinary pain rehabilitation programs for chronic pain management. *Current Pain & Headache Reports, 16*(2), 147–152.

Stanos, S., & Houle, T. (2006). Multidisciplinary & interdisciplinary management of chronic pain. *Physical Medicine Rehabilitation Clinics of North America, 17*(2), 435–450.

Stewart, W., Ricci, J., Chee, E., Morganstein, D., & Lipton, R. (2003). Lost productivity time and cost due to common pain conditions in the US workforce. *Journal of the American Medical Association, 290*(18), 2443–2454.

Thomas, S., & Johnson, M. (2000). A phenomenological study of chronic pain. *Western Journal of Nursing Research, 22*(6), 683–705.

Turk, D., & Okifuji, A. (1998). Efficacy of multidisciplinary pain centres: An antidote to anecdotes. *Baillière's Clinical Anaesthesiology, 12*, 103–119.

Wells, N., Pasero, C., & McCaffery M. (2008). Improving the Quality of Care Through Pain Assessment and Management. In R. Hughes (Ed.), *Patient safety and quality: An evidence-based handbook for nurses*. Rockville, MD: Agency for Healthcare Research and Quality (US); available from: http://www.ncbi.nlm.nih.gov/books/NBK2658/

Wigram, T. (2005). Songwriting methods – Similarities and differences: Developing a working model. In F. Baker and T. Wigram (Eds.), *Songwriting: Methods, techniques, and clinical applications for music therapy clinicians, educators, and students* (pp. 246–264. Philadelphia, PA: Jessica Kingsley.

Chapter 4

Adults in Critical Care

Jeanette Tamplin

Diagnostic Information

In this chapter, the term "critical care" is taken to mean any type of hospital environment that manages immediate life-threatening conditions following medical trauma. Such medical trauma may include, but is not limited to, brain injury, spinal cord injury, stroke, and multi-organ failure. The critical care environment may include trauma patients in coma, low awareness states (LAS), early post-traumatic amnesia (PTA), and mechanically ventilated patients. As paediatrics, burns, and cardiac care are dealt with in other chapters in this series, they will not be covered in this chapter.

The settings for work with critical care patients can include intensive care units (ICU) in acute hospitals, high-dependency units (HDU) in rehabilitation hospitals, and other wards in acute hospitals, such as neurology or acute spinal wards. These settings are very medically focused, as their primary purpose is to maintain and support life. The critical care environment is also typically very noisy due to high levels of nursing intervention, machine noises, ventilators, staff talking, and visiting families. There is a growing body of evidence on the detrimental effect of noise on recovery and sleep in the ICU (BaHammam, 2006; Hardin, 2009; Lawson et al., 2010; Parthasarathy & Tobin, 2006). Physiological effects secondary to noise and sleep deprivation include cardiovascular stimulation, increased gastric secretion, pituitary and adrenal stimulation, suppression of the immune system and wound healing, and possible contribution to delirium and decreased cognitive function (BaHammam, 2006). Environmental and social isolation negatively impact recovery for patients in critical care, and this provides a strong case for music therapy intervention in this setting.

There is an expanding body of literature surrounding environmental enrichment for people in low awareness states. Research suggests that stimulation provided from the surrounding environment causes increased synapse activity, which may ameliorate cognitive impairments and aid the treatment of brain injury (Fan, Liu, Weinstein, Fike, & Liu, 2007). Music therapy provides an ideal medium for appropriate environmental enrichment. Patients are enticed to respond to a wide variety of musical cues and stimuli, and these responses are maximised and reinforced musically when they occur.

The aim of this chapter is to provide detailed information on music therapy interventions for patients with impaired levels of consciousness and mechanically ventilated patients, while distinguishing these from music medicine interventions. There is currently very little information or research on the use of music therapy interventions with trauma patients in critical care. However, there are numerous publications in the nursing literature that examine the effects of nurse-initiated use of recorded music with mechanically ventilated and other ICU patients (often inaccurately described as "music therapy"). The therapeutic needs for patients in critical care differ according to diagnoses, clinical presentation, and therapeutic need. This chapter will divide the critical care population into three subgroups in order to provide greater clarity: (1) coma and LAS, (2) early PTA, and (3) mechanical ventilation.

Coma and Low Awareness States

Damage to the brain, and particularly the brain stem, usually results in a period of unconsciousness, or coma. Levels of consciousness vary along a continuum from total loss of consciousness (coma), to various stages of impaired consciousness (LAS, PTA), to full consciousness (Bates, 1993). Consciousness involves being alert, awake, and aware of surroundings and self, and is characterised by two fundamental elements: arousal and awareness. Arousal is a brain stem function and consists of more primitive reflex responses to stimuli (Davis & White, 1995). Awareness involves thought or cognitive processing of environmental stimulation and is demonstrated through purposeful behaviour. At the extreme end of the continuum of consciousness (after death) is coma: the absence of both arousal and awareness of self and environment even when externally stimulated (Plum & Posner, 1980). The comatose patient does not open the eyes, follow commands, or speak (Ponsford, Sloan, & Snow, 1995). Low awareness states (LAS) are composed of two broad categories: vegetative state (VS) and minimally conscious state (MCS). Vegetative state has been described as wakefulness without awareness (Giacino & Kalmar, 1997), that is, despite evidence of wakefulness, there are no discernible indications of consciousness. In contrast, MCS is characterised by minimal but definite behavioural evidence of self or environmental awareness (Giacino et al., 2002). The clinical presentation of people in LAS can include periods of wakefulness, fluctuating arousal levels, lack of verbal comprehension, reflex movements, and severe physical impairments (making nonverbal forms of communication difficult). Behavioural presentation can be difficult to interpret, and this is the main cause for the high level of misdiagnosis between MCS and VS.

Early rehabilitation has been associated with better outcomes following severe brain injury (Mackay, Bernstein, & Chapman, 1992; Oh & Seo, 2003), and consequently it has been suggested that where possible and appropriate, early rehabilitation should be conducted within the ICU (Elliott & Walker, 2005). Patients in LAS are often denied early rehabilitation. This can be because of a belief that a patient must reach a certain level of responsiveness to benefit or because rehabilitation interventions are left until the patient is admitted to a specialist rehabilitation unit (Shiel et al., 2001). Music has an inherent temporal organization, which can be used to influence the neural organization required for arousal, awareness, and orientation for people in altered states of consciousness (Thaut, 2005). This organizing quality of rhythm in music can be used to facilitate neural reorganization and subsequently increase patient engagement, both with musical stimuli and in social interaction. In addition, music has a strong influence on emotion: attention, perception, memory, executive function, and learning are all enhanced by appropriate affective states.

It should be noted here that medically induced coma presents similarly to trauma-induced coma; however, the needs of this population are different. A medically induced coma is used to protect the brain from swelling by reducing the metabolic rate of brain tissue, as well as the cerebral blood flow. By putting the patient in a medically induced coma, or deep state of unconsciousness, the brain is able to rest, swelling is more likely to decrease, and pressure on the brain is thus reduced. Therefore, music therapy interventions aimed at increasing arousal from such patients are contraindicated. There is, however, a potential role for music therapy in keeping the medically induced coma patient calm and reducing the distress caused by an unfamiliar environment and physical sensations.

Post-Traumatic Amnesia

Following brain injury, when the patient emerges from coma, they typically pass through a phase of generalised cognitive disturbance called post-traumatic amnesia (PTA). During this phase, the patient becomes more responsive but remains confused (Forrester, Encel, & Geffen, 1994; Geffen, Encel, &

Forrester, 1991; Ponsford et al., 1995). PTA is classified and measured according to two primary symptoms: inability to orientate to the environment and inability to recall new experiences or learn new information. The length of PTA (which includes the period of coma) can vary from minutes to months. As the brain swelling subsides and complications resolve, the patient begins to emerge from PTA and is then ready to begin intensive rehabilitation (Artiola I Fortuny, Briggs, Newcombe, Ratcliffe, & Thomas, 1980). By this stage, the PTA patient usually no longer requires life-supporting medical intervention and will have been transferred out of the intensive care or high-dependency unit. However, during the early stages of PTA, the patient may still be in a critical condition and may also be appropriate for music therapy intervention.

Patients in PTA are often distressed as a result of poor orientation to time, place, and person. Their awareness is limited and perception of the environment and other incoming stimuli is often distorted. This confusion can cause anxiety and may lead to aggressive verbal and physical behaviour. Additionally, fatigue, both physical and cognitive, is a significant characteristic of PTA. As a result, poor attention and concentration and a low threshold for stimulation are common (Ponsford et al., 1995). When these thresholds are exceeded, patients may become overaroused. A patient who is overaroused may exhibit challenging behaviours such as pulling at intravenous tubes or bandages, dismantling objects, irritability, excessive movement, self-stimulatory behaviour, aggression, agitation, and restlessness (Baker & Tamplin, 2006).

Mechanical Ventilation

Mechanical ventilation is a method to mechanically assist or replace spontaneous breathing in the case of respiratory failure (Torpy, Campbell, & Glass, 2010). Respiratory failure is classified as hypoxemic (insufficient oxygen in the blood) or hypercapnic (too much carbon dioxide in the blood). The most common reason for mechanical ventilation withair critically ill is hypoxemic respiratory failure (Yende & Wunderink, 2002), which is associated with almost all acute lung diseases. This type of respiratory failure can be caused by pneumothorax or atelectasis (collapsed lung), pulmonary edema (buildup of fluid in the lungs causing shortness of breath), pneumonia, pulmonary fibrosis (scarring or thickening of lung tissue), early acute respiratory distress syndrome, and smoke inhalation. Hypercapnic respiratory failure can result from head trauma, spinal cord injury, and acute chronic obstructive pulmonary disease (COPD) exacerbation. Respiratory failure can also result from acute lung injury, respiratory muscle fatigue, neuromuscular disease, and coma (Tobin, 2006).

Insertion of a tube into the throat is required for mechanical ventilation. This may be inserted through nose or mouth (endotracheal) or directly into the throat (tracheostomy). This tube has two main purposes: It provides an unobstructed airway, and its small balloon cuff seals off the trachea, protecting the patient from aspiration and allowing accurate air flow measurement by the ventilator.

Needs and Resources

Coma and Low Awareness States

The depth and duration of coma and PTA are indicators of expected degree of recovery (Brooks, Aughton, Bond, Jones, & Rizvi, 1980; Shores, 1989). It is thus important to accelerate recovery from coma to improve a patient's long-term prospects for rehabilitation. By commencing rehabilitation as soon as possible postinjury, the potential for spontaneous recovery is enhanced, and the functional loss of physical range of movement is minimized.

Patients in coma and LAS need an appropriate level of sensory stimulation, as they are simultaneously at risk for both over- and understimulation from their environment. The capacity for selective attention is diminished during coma, causing difficulty with filtering irrelevant stimuli. Thus overstimulation, such as the constant noise of nearby machines and medical interventions, may cause confusion, anxiety, and further retreat in an already disoriented person. On the other hand, there is a risk for sensory deprivation through limited physical movement and minimal human contact. Sensory deprivation can decrease the structure, function, and chemistry of the brain (Neville & Bavelier, 2002), causing further cognitive deficits and thus hindering recovery. The human brain is extremely responsive to external stimuli and is able to develop and adapt through utilization (Bach-Y-Rita, 2003). Thus sensory stimulation is often employed with severely brain-injured patients to increase arousal and awareness through stimulating the reticular activating system (Canedo, Grix, & Nicoletti, 2002). Sensory stimulation programs have been used both to promote arousal and to measure responsiveness and coma scale scores. Most of these programs involve the five senses, and include pain-inducing stimuli and presentation of lights, sounds, smells, and tastes. A recent Cochrane Review found no strong evidence to support or rule out the effectiveness of multisensory stimulation programs for patients in coma or vegetative state (Lombardi, Taricco, De Tanti, Telaro, & Liberati, 2009). This was primarily due to poor methodological quality, and variation in outcome measures, study design, and conduct of the included studies.

In a critique of sensory stimulation programs, Wood (1991) promoted the concept of sensory regulation, highlighting the potential for sensory overload to activate the habituation response. According to Wood, the use of stimuli that are meaningful to the patient, presented in a regulated sensory environment, may be more likely to promote increased awareness and orientation to the environment than systematic stimulation of the five senses. Music may be considered a meaningful stimulus for two reasons: It may be familiar, and it is able to match and respond to physical cues. Advances in neuroscience have led to greater understanding of how the brain responds to music. Attention and perceptual activity are influenced by physiological factors that can in turn be influenced by the rhythmic and melodic qualities of music. Music may increase bilateral cerebral arousal levels by activating music processing areas in the brain (Morton, Kershner, & Siegel, 1990). Thus music therapy may increase awareness for patients in LAS and promote the regaining of consciousness in comatose patients. Music therapy may directly affect the injured brain by activating the centres for emotion processing and stimulating the reticular activating system in the brain stem that regulates arousal and attention. As part of the arousal response pattern, the reticular activating system also affects muscle tone and movement. Thus music can stimulate muscle contraction and create cortical arousal effects in the cerebrum.

Boyle and Greer (1983) conducted the first study on music therapy with LAS. Employing a single case design, they used operant conditioning with recorded music as a reward for learned behaviours (pressing a switch) that demonstrated patient-initiated movement. The advantage of using such a behavioural approach is that variables can be controlled (e.g., recorded music) and results may be more objective (e.g., pillow-pressing). The advantage of using live, improvised music in a humanist approach is that the music can be altered in the moment to match patient responses and encourage active participation and communication. Humanistic music therapy interventions described in the literature employ melodic vocal improvisation based on the patient's physiological rhythms (respiration rate). Subjective reported outcomes have included changes in heart and respiration rate, voluntary movement, EEG measures, and regaining of consciousness (Aldridge, Gustorff, & Hannich, 1990; Gustorff, 1995; Tamplin, 2000). There is little empirical research evaluating this type of intervention. In particular, measures to reduce risk of bias and chance influencing results are needed, such as the use of control subjects and random allocation.

Clinical guidelines for music therapy intervention in LAS have been proposed based on current understandings from neuroscience and music psychology (Baker & Tamplin, 2006; Magee, 2005). Music therapists working in the critical care setting need to be aware of appropriate levels of stimulation, how to assess patients in LAS, indicators for when to cease intervention, and the distinction between assessment and treatment in this population. In particular, consistent, replicable responses from LAS patients to meaningful stimulation needs to be distinguished from reflexive, or non–cognitively mediated, responses. Given that most patients in LAS have a very limited capacity for active participation in music therapy, predominantly receptive methods are employed with this population. There is potential for improvisational music therapy approaches with therapist-improvised music taking cues from and responding to the physiological responses of the patient. For example, music therapy for patients in a MCS (as distinguished from VS) focuses on stimulating consistent, replicable responses from the patient and maximising these responses when they occur.

Post-Traumatic Amnesia

Patients in PTA need to feel safe and reassured. Due to diminished cognitive ability to make sense of their environment, everything can appear unfamiliar and frightening. This combination of confusion and fear can lead to, or exacerbate, an already heightened level of agitation. Therefore, the needs of PTA patients are to increase orientation to their environment and decrease agitation levels. Maximum rate of recovery occurs when PTA patients are relaxed and have plenty of rest (Ponsford et al., 1995).

It is important to note that patients in PTA are hyperaroused and are at risk of overstimulation due to an "oversensitive" filter, which rejects both relevant and irrelevant information (Baker 2001). Therefore, only small amounts of stimulation can be tolerated, and activities that require the use of cognitive skills are contraindicated. A patient in PTA may be able to follow only parts of a conversation and may quickly become distressed when confused. Therefore, questions that require complex thinking or lengthy conversations should be avoided.

PTA is generally seen as a time for rest, and minimal stimulation or therapeutic intervention is recommended. Music therapy may thus seem contraindicated due to the potentially stimulating nature of music. However, research has shown that a regulated and informed music therapy intervention can increase orientation and decrease agitation for patients in PTA (Baker, 2001a, 2001b). This has positive implications for decreasing length of time in PTA, thus improving prognosis for recovery. Music therapy for PTA patients in the critical care setting tends to focus on behavioural symptoms such as agitation, impulsivity, and disorientation that place PTA patients at greatest risk in terms of medical management. The cognitive and memory issues tend to be addressed later in the rehabilitation stage.

To date, only one study has examined the effects of music therapy with PTA patients (Baker, 2001a, 2001b). Participants listened to preferred music (live and recorded) or no music and were tested for agitation and orientation before and after each condition using the Agitation Behaviour Scale and the Westmead PTA Scale. Participants were exposed to all three conditions twice in randomised order over six days. Results showed significant increases in orientation and significant decreases in agitation following both music conditions and no change following the control (no music) condition. No difference was found between the effect of live and recorded music. This lack of difference may reflect unique benefits for live and recorded music. Recorded music may be more familiar than a live rendition, however, participants were more able to recall the live music, which may imply greater engagement and therefore greater potency in evoking changes in orientation and agitation.

Orientation to the environment is a significant goal for these patients. As mentioned previously, it has been demonstrated that listening to familiar music can improve orientation for patients in PTA. It assists patients to recognize a familiar element of their environment, and in doing so, they are more likely to engage appropriately with their surroundings. At the same time, the familiarity of the music often assists in alleviating anxiety, which in turn assists in managing agitation. By listening to and focusing on the music, patients can be distracted from their confusion.

Patients often automatically move in time with music, which may help to organize agitated movement patterns. The organizational effects of temporally regulated auditory stimuli on subsequent motor behavior occur, at least initially, precognitively, and do not require the patient to make overt conscious efforts to synchronize (Baker & Tamplin, 2006). Given the need to minimize stimulation with this population, receptive music therapy methods are most commonly used. Most methods that require active music-making or cognitive contributions from the patients are contraindicated.

Mechanical Ventilation

There is a high prevalence of anxiety in the ICU caused by mechanical ventilation (Chlan, 2003; Pochard et al., 1995). Significant distress and anxiety has been reported by mechanically ventilated patients due to discomfort, the sensation of breathlessness, frequent suctioning, inability to talk, and fear and uncertainty about prognosis (Wong, Lopez-Nahas, & Molassiotis, 2001). The process of weaning from ventilation may cause additional fear and anxiety (Boles et al., 2007). Sedation is frequently used to manage anxiety in critical care, but can cause further complications such as venous thrombosis (blood clots in the veins), weakening the immune system, and causing pressure damage to the nerves and skin through lack of movement (Hunter et al., 2010). Nonpharmacologic approaches to anxiety management may be effective, but as yet, little research has been conducted on the use of music therapy in mechanical ventilation.

There is a growing body of literature and research on the use of music-based interventions that involve playing recorded music to the patient (White, 2000), but this differs significantly from music therapy methods that are inherently interactive in nature. Music therapists are trained to assess patient needs and develop therapeutic, and often "live" music-based interventions to address these needs. In addition to the music, the development of a therapeutic relationship with the patient is central to providing emotional support, enhancing a sense of control, and being able to respond in the moment to the patient's physical and emotional responses (Bradt, Dileo, & Grocke, 2010). A recent Cochrane Review found that music listening may have a beneficial effect on heart and respiratory rates and state anxiety for mechanically ventilated patients (Bradt et al., 2010). However, of the eight studies included in the review, only one study used live music with a trained music therapist. Thus it is not possible at this time to establish whether music therapy interventions are more effective than listening to prerecorded music. The consistency of method in the remaining seven studies included in the review (a single session of listening to prerecorded music) adds to the strength of the review findings. However, questions relating to optimal dosage recommendations remain unanswered. Other studies have shown that listening to prerecorded music can reduce levels of pain perception and blood pressure in critical care and mechanically ventilated populations (Chlan, 1995; White, 2000; Wong et al., 2001).

Music medicine research provides a solid foundation on which to build music therapy research with mechanically ventilated patients. It has established that music listening does no harm with this population. However, the use of patient-preferred music may play an important role in influencing positive outcomes, and, consequently, if music is used that the patient dislikes, negative outcomes may result. A recent meta-analysis of music medicine and medical music therapy research indicated that music therapy interventions with medical populations are significantly more effective than music medicine interventions on a range of outcome measures (Dileo & Bradt, 2005). Possible reasons cited by the authors for this difference include individualization of music therapy interventions to specific needs, more active engagement of the patient in music-making, and a more systematic process of assessment, treatment, and evaluation.

As mechanically ventilated patients in critical care have a limited capacity for active participation in music therapy, receptive methods are predominantly employed with this population. The endotracheal or tracheostomy tube, inserted into the throat to provide ventilation, prohibits verbal communication, so singing and/or verbal processing of the music are not possible. However, depending on physical ability, there may also be potential for patients to participate in creative/improvisational music therapy using small, handheld instruments.

Assessment and Referral

The three subgroups of critical care patients described in this chapter each present with differing etiology and clinical presentation. As such, assessment will focus on different areas of need for each subgroup. However, a common music therapy referral form for patients in critical care may be used. The referral form should include standard information such as patient name, medical record number, admission date, referral date, and a section for diagnostic information. A section called "reason for referral," or something similar, can provide a checklist of possible reasons for referral to music therapy. These would include, but are not limited to, assessment of awareness, sensory stimulation, decreasing agitation, promoting sleep, increasing orientation, decreasing anxiety, pain management, encouraging purposeful behavior, and providing opportunities for creative expression.

Coma and LAS

Music therapists may have a unique role to play in the assessment of patients in LAS. Accurate distinction between VS and MCS is difficult, evidenced by a 37%-43% misdiagnosis rate (Andrews, Murphy, Munday, & Littlewood, 1996; Beaumont & Kenealy, 2005; Childs, Mercer, & Childs, 1993), but has significant implications for funding, treatment, prognosis, and medico-legal judgments (Giacino et al., 2002). Distinguishing between purposeful and reflexive responses is particularly difficult using purely behavioral observation due to the small and inconsistent nature of responses typical of this population (Gill-Thwaites & Munday, 2004). The use of specialized assessment tools and procedures designed to quantitatively measure levels of consciousness may be helpful (Giacino et al., 2002). Some commonly used generic instruments include:

- Glasgow Coma Scale (GCS) (Teasdale & Jennett, 1974)
- Glasgow Outcome Scale (GOS) (Jennett & Bond, 1975)
- Coma Recovery Scale-Revised (CRS) (Giacino & Kalmar, 2006)
- Disability Rating Scale (DRS) (Rappaport, Hall, Hopkins, & Belleza, 1982)
- Wessex Head Injury Matrix (WHIM) (Shiel et al., 2000)
- Rappaport Coma/Near Coma Scale (Rappaport, Dougherty, & Kelting, 1992)
- Ranchos Los Amigos Scale (Hagen, Malkmus, & Axen, 1989),
- Sensory Modality Assessment and Rehabilitation Technique (SMART) (Gill-Thwaites & Munday, 2004)

Previous music therapy research using generic assessment tools (CRS and DRS) to assess the effect of music therapy interventions with LAS patients found these lacking in sensitivity (Formisano et al., 2001). Magee and colleagues have recently developed a specific music therapy assessment tool for low awareness states: MATLAS (Daveson, 2010; Daveson, Magee, Crewe, Beaumont, & Kenealy, 2007; Magee, 2007). This standardized instrument has been designed to be sensitive enough to measure the subtle responses of patients in LAS to music therapy intervention and has been successfully used to differentiate between MCS and VS diagnoses (Magee, 2005). Specialized assessor training is required prior to use of the tool and training courses are provided by the Royal Hospital for Neuro-disability in London (www.rhn.org.uk/events/courses-and-training). The MATLAS assesses 14 behavioral response categories covering the five commonly assessed behavioral domains; motor, communication, arousal, auditory, and visual responses. "Each item is categorized into levels of observed behavioral responses with a numerical grading," where zero indicates "no response" (Magee, 2007, p. 321). Definitions of observable behaviors for each level are provided in the MATLAS Assessment Manual. These categories are combined to provide three summed categories. Category 1, "essential diagnostic criteria," combines five behavioral response categories relating directly to diagnostic features of VS and MCS and synthesizes these into a single diagnostic descriptive statement. Category 2 describes patient musical parameter preference and behavioral response type, and category 3 provides clinical information that can be used for goal-setting and treatment planning. A MATLAS assessment is usually conducted over four sessions within 8 to 10 days and involves the controlled presentation of live music, both familiar and novel, using a range of musical stimuli and instruments (Daveson et al., 2007). For example, "the item 'Responses to auditory stimuli' records localizing and tracking behaviours. ... The auditory stimuli presented vary from simple single musical sounds to more complex musical stimuli that can be subtly manipulated in parameters such as pitch and volume" (Magee, 2007 , p. 322). Music's independence from language renders it an ideal medium to use in both assessment and therapeutic intervention with patients who are not capable of verbal communication. It has been suggested that key elements of music, such as pulse, tempo, and rhythm, are able to influence physiological outcomes through entrainment of the respiratory and cardiovascular systems (Magee, 2005). In addition, the nonverbal capacity and emotional power of music are the crucial aspects used therapeutically to engage patients and stimulate behavioral and communicative responses.

Post-Traumatic Amnesia

As discussed in the previous section, PTA patients in the critical care setting are usually referred for music therapy to address behavioral symptoms such as agitation, impulsivity, and disorientation, as these place PTA patients at greatest risk in terms of medical management.

In Australia, orientation is usually assessed using the Westmead PTA Scale (Shores, Marosszeky, Sandanam, & Bachelor, 1986). This scale consists of seven orientation questions and five memory questions to produce a score out of 12. When a person achieves a score of 12 for three consecutive days, they are considered to have emerged from PTA. Another widely used orientation scale used in PTA is the Galveston Orientation and Amnesia Test (GOAT; Levin, O'Donnell, & Grossman, 1979). Agitation can be measured through observation or by completing a behavioural checklist such as the Agitated Behaviour Scale (Corrigan, 1989), which has high validity and inter-rater reliability (Corrigan & Bogner, 1994). The Agitated Behaviour Scale contains 14 items describing agitated behaviours. The rater is required to assign each item a score of between 1 and 4 and add the scores together to obtain an overall score. A total score of 14 indicates an absence of agitation, and 56 is the highest possible agitation score. Any score greater than 36 is indicative of severe agitation. This scale can be used to track agitation from pre- to postsession and/or over time.

Mechanical Ventilation

The primary reason for referring mechanically ventilated patients to music therapy is anxiety management. State anxiety can be assessed using standardized tools such as the State-Trait Anxiety Measure (STAI; Spielberger, Gorsuch, Lushene, Vagg, & Jacobs, 1983), the Beck Anxiety Inventory (BAI; Beck & Steer, 1990), and the Hospital Anxiety and Depression Scale-Anxiety (HADS-A; Zigmond & Snaith, 1983). Other outcome measures may include sedative drug intake and physiological outcomes such as heart rate, respiratory rate, blood pressure, airway pressure, and oxygen saturation.

Overview of Music Therapy Methods

Music therapists in critical care units commonly use the following methods and procedures. These have not been sequenced to reflect relative significance, effectiveness, or complexity.

Receptive Music Therapy

- Presentation of Familiar Music: Music therapist provides live or recorded music for client to listen to.

Improvisational Music Therapy

- Therapist-Improvised Music: Music therapist improvises music based on the changing physiological rhythms and responses of the patient in an attempt at creating mutuality.
- Client/Therapist Vocal/Instrumental Improvisation: Active musical participation from both client and therapist.

Re-creative Music Therapy

- Lyric completion: The use of live, familiar music to prompt song line completion.

Guidelines for Receptive Music Therapy

Receptive music therapy traditionally encompasses techniques in which the patient is a recipient of the music experience, as distinct from active music-making (Grocke & Wigram, 2007). According to Bruscia (1998), in receptive music therapy experiences, the patient listens to music and responds silently or in another modality. However, for some of the interventions included the following section on receptive music therapy, the therapeutic goal is to actively engage the patient and stimulate purposeful (sometimes musical) responses. This may seem to be the antithesis of receptive music therapy, but these interventions are positioned in the following section due to the presentation of familiar music to the patient, as opposed to music improvised or re-created with the patient.

Assessment of music preferences can be challenging in the critically-ill population due to communication difficulties or inability. If the patient has CDs or an MP3 player in their room, this may be used to form an initial picture of the patient's musical tastes. Consultation with the patient's family and friends may be able to further complete this picture. If none of the above are possible, determine the patient's age and begin by using popular songs from their young adult life that are therapeutically appropriate.

Presentation of Familiar Music: Coma Patients

Overview. Receptive music therapy with coma patients uses live (or recorded) presentation of familiar music with the goal of increasing awareness and orientation. Contraindications with coma patients may include any physiological changes that might indicate a negative reaction, such as significant increases in respiration or heart rate. In addition, dislike or lack of affiliation with the music offered may discourage engagement and promote further retreat for patients in reduced states of consciousness. It is also possible that some familiar music may bring up memories or emotions that the unconscious patient is unable to cognitively or verbally process.

Preparation. In order to minimize the risk for overstimulation, the music needs to be deconstructed and then gradually reconstructed. This may include altering the tempo, simplifying the melody and/or rhythm, reducing or even eliminating harmony and accompaniment, and minimizing use of attack or dynamic change. These alterations should be practiced extensively (outside of the session) prior to implementation to ensure the ability to adapt musical parameters as needed during the session based on patient responses.

What to observe. Observation of the heart rate or breathing rate and the physical presentation of the patient should be conducted both prior to commencement and during the session, as well as any behavioural changes that may indicate awareness of the musical stimuli, such as eye opening, orientation toward the sound source, and increases or changes in movement.

Procedures. Appropriate receptive music therapy methods may include singing/playing familiar songs (and adaptations of these, involving word substitution and song parody) and/or listening to carefully selected recorded music. Live music presentation is preferable in most cases, due to the potential for altering musical elements to increase therapeutic applicability. Using the principles of entrainment, start the music (selected from the patient's preferences) at a tempo that matches the patient's breathing rate. Always start with the most uncomplicated, deconstructed musical stimuli, for example, a simple unaccompanied melody with no complex rhythms and minimal dynamic variation. This can be reconstructed and built on gradually as the patient begins to demonstrate increasing awareness and no signs of overstimulation.

Adaptations. Live adaptations of patient-preferred songs can increase therapeutic applicability. For example, heavy rock or metal songs can be played live with minimal or no accompaniment, with a slower tempo and quieter but engaging dynamics. This aims to decrease the stimulating aspects of the music, without removing its familiar but engaging properties.

Presentation of Familiar Music: LAS Patients

Overview. Receptive music therapy with LAS patients uses live (or recorded) presentation of familiar music to engage the patient and stimulate expressive, behavioural, and physiological responses. Goals with the LAS population include assessing level of awareness and responses to verbal material and developing a consistent yes/no response. If patients in LAS are presenting with agitated behaviours, the receptive music therapy methods described for PTA patients in the following section may also be implemented with LAS patients in critical care. There is also the potential for familiar music to trigger memories and emotional responses in the nonverbal LAS patient that are not able to be processed and resolved.

Preparation. Patient-selected, familiar music should be used where possible and contrasted with novel, unfamiliar music. If the patient is able to communicate a reliable yes/no response, this can be used to ascertain musical preferences. If not, use the procedure described above to determine musical preferences.

What to observe. For patients in LAS, observe for any indication of awareness of the musical stimuli, such as changes in breathing rate, movement or facial gestures, eye opening, eye contact, visual tracking, localising, orientation toward the sound source, attempts to vocalise, and any other possible communication attempts. Responses to meaningful stimulation need to be consistent and replicable as opposed to reflexive, non–cognitively mediated, responses. For the patient aiming to develop a consistent yes/no response, initially monitor ability to accurately follow movement instructions (to generate a nonverbal yes/no response). Next, monitor the number of correct vs. incorrect responses on concrete choice-making tasks.

Procedures. During the session, provide a range of musical experiences to stimulate and assess responses from the patient in LAS. Magee (2005) offers suggestions for manipulating the music in terms of pitch (high or low), volume (loud or soft), attack (sudden or gradual), and form (repetition, novel or familiar material) in order to assist the development of appropriate communication strategies. For patients in LAS with receptive communication disorders, specific pitch range, intensity level, or melodic contour may significantly aid comprehension. Use familiar instruments, pictures of the patient's favourite artists, and musical repertoire with which the patient will be familiar. Also, determine any particular musical dislikes. These are useful to contrast with preferred songs in choice-making activities and can assist in determining receptive communication abilities. Visual discrimination tasks may require the patient to look at a particular picture or instrument in answer to a question. Other communication responses, such as eye pointing, eye blinking (e.g., two blinks for yes, one blink for no), thumbs up/down, and use of alternative communication devices may be trialed and practiced in music therapy sessions. Playing the patient's chosen song/instrument can positively reinforce choices and communication attempts.

Adaptations. Compare the patient's response to live versus recorded versions of preferred songs. Develop guidelines for music listening activities that can be used by family and friends to enhance interactions. This will also provide significant others with opportunities to practice and reinforce the patient's communication strategies.

Presentation of Familiar Music: PTA Patients

Overview. Receptive music therapy with PTA patients uses familiar music (preferably live) to target the following therapeutic goals: decrease agitated physical movements (e.g., repetitive limb movement, pulling at tubes/restraints); distract the patient from their distress or confusion; encourage relaxation and/or sleep; and/or orient the patient to time and place. During the critical care phase, the primary goal for most patients is to decrease agitation and encourage rest and sleep. Orientation is a secondary goal, as most PTA patients in critical care are not alert enough or cognitively ready to focus on orientation goals.

Overstimulation may lead to fatigue and increases in agitation. PTA patients should not be encouraged to actively participate in music (by singing, playing, or moving to the music), as, again, this may cause overstimulation. However, spontaneous participation is not contraindicated as long as agitation and fatigue are closely monitored. If it appears that the music is agitating the patient significantly, the session should be terminated.

Preparation. If the patient is unable to communicate musical preferences, use the procedure described above to determine the music to be used in sessions. A period of observation and assessment of the patient's agitation level should be conducted prior to commencing any music therapy intervention with PTA patients in critical care. Formal assessment tools such as the previously discussed Agitated Behavior Scale (Corrigan, 1989) may be used, or an informal observational assessment of agitation level. This assessment will inform the music therapist's decisions about the presentation of the music, e.g., whether musical accompaniment is indicated or not. As a general guideline, the music should be played in a calming and relaxing manner, with minimal or no accompaniment, to avoid overstimulating the patient. The environment should be prepared so that minimal competing stimuli are present and any unnecessary noises in the room are eliminated. Family members who wish to be present for the session should be instructed to observe quietly and not encourage active participation from the patient. The number of additional people in the room should be kept to a minimum: ideally, only one or two observers. The session should also not be disrupted unnecessarily. This may mean consulting with medical and nursing staff prior to the session to ensure that the team understands the therapeutic goals of the session and the need to ensure minimal disruption and stimulation.

What to observe. Presession observations of agitation should be recorded. Symptoms of agitated behavior in the critical care environment may include restlessness, excessive and/or repetitive movement, moaning, and/or pulling at tubes/restraints. During the presentation of music, these same observations should be monitored and any changes in behavior or presentation noted. Behaviors such as making eye contact, smiling, vocalizing, and moving to the music indicate an increase in engagement and meaningful interaction with others. A period of observation should also be recorded postsession to reveal any lasting effects of the intervention.

Procedures. Live and recorded music can be effective for work with PTA patients. The advantage of using live music is that the music can be modified therapeutically, according to behavioral presentation. Sessions should last no longer than 15 minutes (approximately three songs), and music should be presented at a low volume so as to avoid overstimulation. Familiar music should be used where possible; however, often the patient will not be able to disclose this information due to memory and/or communication impairments. Family members and friends may be able to indicate the patient's music preferences, and it may also be possible to examine the patient's music collection if they have CDs or an MP3 player in their room. Familiar music can improve orientation through capturing the patient's attention and the recognition of something well-known. Familiar music is also reassuring and helps to decrease distress and anxiety, which in turn helps to manage agitation. Familiar music is thought to lead to optimal arousal rather than maximal levels of arousal (Baker, 2002, 2009; Soto et al., 2009) whereas nonpreferred music may overstimulate patients. Finally, using the same songs each session (unless it is obvious that the patient is responding negatively to them) will bring familiarity, consistency, and predictability to the therapy sessions.

Adaptations. In a live performance, a song can be played very differently from its original recorded version. The musical elements of dynamics, tempo, timbre, and accompaniment can all be modified. This means that if a patient's music preferences may be deemed overstimulating in their original recorded format, the music can still be used by adapting the musical elements. Accompaniment can be minimized (or even eliminated) and dynamics and tempo can be reduced, thus ensuring a calming and relaxing presentation of the music. Last, if, during the session, the patient appears to be agitated or increasing in agitation, the music presentation can be modified in the moment by decreasing the volume and/or speed of the music and maybe even humming rather than singing words.

Presentation of Familiar Music: Mechanically Ventilated Patients

Overview. Presentation of familiar music with mechanically ventilated patients is often used to decrease anxiety. It may also be employed as a pain management strategy, to provide emotional support, and to enhance the mechanically ventilated patient's sense of control. Contraindications may include increased heart rate or breathing rate, or any physiological changes that might indicate a negative reaction (Bradt et al., 2010). In addition, dislike of the music offered may agitate the patient and subsequently, rather than alleviating anxiety, may increase the stress response.

Preparation. If the patient is alert and aware, nonverbal communication, such as head nodding, may be used in response to the therapist's verbal suggestions for songs or musical excerpts played by the therapist. If the patient is not conscious, use the procedure described previously to determine music preferences.

Although music should be patient-selected, there are also qualities of the music that should be taken into account when selecting music for this population. Sedative or calming music should be used when aiming to decrease anxiety. This includes music that is characterized by a slow tempo, with no abrupt changes or sharp timbres. Further, music that evokes strong emotional reactions (either positive or negative) that may be caused by memories associated with the music should be avoided when selecting music to reduce stress and anxiety (Dileo & Bradt, 2007).

What to observe. Prior to commencement of the session, monitor the heart rate or breathing rate and the physical presentation of the patient. Look for any observable signs of stress or anxiety such as facial expression, clenched fists, etc. Monitor these same signs during and after the presentation of music.

Procedures. Using the principles of entrainment, start with music (selected from patient preferences) at a tempo that matches the patient's breathing rate. Over the course of the session, begin to decrease the pace of the music and use songs that are more lyrically and musically soothing. Encourage the patient to focus on the positive lyrical messages in the songs where appropriate. Patients may also be instructed to close their eyes and focus intentionally on releasing tension and anxiety.

A simple form of music-assisted relaxation may also be employed with this population. Progressive muscle relaxation, guided verbally by the music therapist, can be accompanied by supportive, relaxing, instrumental accompaniment. This may be effective prior to the presentation of live, familiar music.

Adaptations. As discussed previously, live presentation of familiar songs can be played very differently from the original recorded versions through modification of dynamics, tempo, timbre, and accompaniment. This means that if a patient's music preferences may be deemed overstimulating in their original recorded format, songs can still be used by adapting the musical elements to present the songs in a more therapeutic manner. Accompaniment can be minimized (or even eliminated), dynamics and tempo can be reduced, and the songs can be presented in a calming and relaxing style.

GUIDELINES FOR IMPROVISATIONAL MUSIC THERAPY

Therapist-Improvised Music: Coma Patients

Overview. In improvisational music therapy with coma patients, the music therapist improvises music based on the changing physiological rhythms and responses of the patient with the goal of stimulating awareness, orientation, and responsiveness. Contraindications may include any physiological changes that might indicate a negative reaction, such as significant increases in respiration or heart rate. Increases in agitated movement need to be considered carefully. An increase in movement indicates greater arousal; however, if this increase in movement signifies overstimulation, it may be contraindicated.

Preparation. Sessions for patients in a reduced state of consciousness are best conducted in a sensory-regulated environment. This reduces the possibility for overstimulation from additional, competing stimuli. A sensory-regulated environment involves minimizing any unnecessary stimulation—for example, turning off a television or music player—and ensuring that any necessary nursing interventions are completed prior to or after the session where possible.

As with receptive music therapy interventions with coma patients, it is important to minimize the risk for overstimulation by deconstructing the music initially. Examples of how this may be accomplished include altering the tempo, simplifying the melody and/or rhythm, reducing or even eliminating harmony and accompaniment, and minimizing use of attack or dynamic change. To ensure flexibility in adapting musical parameters based on patient presentation, these alterations should be practiced extensively (outside of the session) prior to implementation.

What to observe. Therapists should observe for any indication of awareness of, or responses to, the musical stimuli, such as changes in breathing rate, movement or facial gestures, eye opening, eye contact, visual tracking, localising, orientation toward the sound source, fine motor movements, head turning, attempts to vocalise, and any other possible communication attempts. Due to the minimal nature of responses in this population, it may increase objectivity to have a second therapist also observe the session and record patient responses.

Procedures. Improvise music based on the patient's physiological rhythms, i.e., breathing pattern or heart rate. Use of the voice (wordless singing) is highly indicated for this population due to its inherently human quality. A preverbal, emotionally focused, tonal language has the capacity to connect with the unconscious patient and stimulate communication at emotional, social, and cognitive levels (Jochims, 1994).

The music should be based on a pulse, but to be perceived as rhythmic, the pulse needs to be uneven in chronological time (in contrast to the fixed pulses of machine noises that surround patients in critical care). The pulse of the improvisations can be timed with the patient's expirations, and repeating melodic phrases provide predictability and familiarity. Music interventions need to be kept very short (five to six minutes) and simple in terms of rhythm, harmony, and dynamic change, so as not to overstimulate the patient. Tonality of improvisations should be culturally appropriate to the individual, for example, use of non-Western scales and harmonies may be indicated. The aim of improvisation in this context is to stimulate the patient to respond to the music. Such responses may include physiological changes, movement, or vocal responses. This aim to stimulate the patient to respond to the music indicates an attempt at creating mutuality in the improvisation and thus distinguishes this technique from a receptive intervention where the therapist improvises music for the patient to listen to with the aim of relaxation or orientation.

Adaptations. It may be helpful to use excerpts from familiar song melodies, or adaptations of these, in musical improvisations with the aim of stimulating memories, emotions, and awareness. There is potential for negative effects, however, if the patient has a distressing memory or emotional response to the familiar material and is unable to process or express this.

Client/Therapist Vocal/Instrumental Improvisation: LAS Patients

Overview. Creative or improvisational music therapy involves active musical participation from both client and therapist. Pragmatic skills such as listening, turn-taking, imitation, repetition, and creative expression can thus be practiced in music therapy with LAS patients without the need for verbal communication. Improvisational music therapy for this population may target the following goals:

- to assess social awareness
- to assess nonverbal communication skills
- to increase vocalizations
- to provide a nonverbal outlet for emotional expression
- to encourage purposeful physical movement

Improvisational music therapy provides an ideal nonverbal setting in which to assess interaction and social awareness through encouraging turn-taking and imitation of rhythmic or melodic phrases and other musical parameters such as tempo and dynamics in music-making. Through musical interaction on a nonverbal level, the patient can also be encouraged to express immediate feeling states and supported to explore these. The music therapist can provide musical support for this expression and, by using reflecting techniques in clinical improvisation, can match the mood or emotional tone of the patient's vocalizations. As with receptive music therapy, improvisational music therapy intervention with LAS patients may generate an increase in agitated behavior if the patient is overstimulated. It is possible that the music may stimulate emotional responses that the patient is subsequently unable to fully process. There is also potential for the patient to become frustrated if unable to participate actively in the music when encouraged by the music therapist.

Preparation. Music therapy sessions are best conducted in a sensory-regulated environment. This reduces the possibility for overstimulation or confusion from competing stimuli. Thus any unnecessary stimulation should be minimized, for example, turning off a television or music player and ensuring that any necessary nursing interventions are completed prior to or after the session where possible.

Infection control is an important consideration, particularly for an at-risk, hospitalized population. All instruments should be decontaminated after each session with a particular patient, using hospital-grade, antibacterial disinfectant to minimize the possibility for transfer of infectious agents between patients. Also, any instruments provided for patient use should be adapted where necessary. This may mean consultation with an occupational therapist about patient positioning, the need for stretching prior to playing, and the best instruments or instrument adaptation to offer based on the patient's current movement capabilities. The weight and size of instruments also needs to be considered. Foam padding or splints may assist patients with poor grasp strength to hold on to some instruments.

What to observe. This will depend on the goal for intervention (listed above). When assessing level of social awareness, first observe for any indication of awareness of the musical stimuli, such as changes in breathing rate, movement or facial gestures, eye opening, eye contact, visual tracking, localising, orientation toward the sound source, attempts to vocalise, and any other possible communication attempts. Look for any patterns in the way the patient responds, for example, vocalising at the pitch of the music being played or vocalising only during the presentation of music. These behaviours demonstrate awareness and intentionality in interaction. As discussed previously, consistent, replicable responses to meaningful stimulation need to be distinguished from reflexive, or non–cognitively mediated, responses. Due to the minimal nature of responses in this population, it may increase objectivity to have a second therapist also observe the session and record patient responses. Observe the physical responses of the patient to music. Look for finger or toe tapping to the pulse of the music. In terms of social awareness, take note of whether the patient is able to participate in turn-taking during improvisations. Also note whether the patient is able to imitate vocal sounds, pitches, melodic fragments, or rhythms, and any indication of purposeful movements during improvisations.

Procedures. The music therapist should provide a safe and inviting musical environment that encourages the patient in LAS to express musically. Musical improvisation activities can be semistructured or completely spontaneous and interactive, and may use vocalization or instrumental play. The therapist should provide musical holding patterns during instrumental improvisation with LAS patients, as it may take some time for the patient to respond. The therapist can offer musical instruments that require different movement patterns to encourage the development of purposeful physical movements. Immediate aural, visual, and kinesthetic feedback is received by the patient if the movement has been performed correctly, which acts as a positive reinforcement for correct movement patterns. Music is also able to motivate and energize a patient to participate in improvisation, even when physically demanding. This encourages longer periods of participation in activities that target purposeful physical movement.

Adaptations. Music technology may be employed to increase accessibility of music-making for patients with very limited range of movement and strength. This may include use of adaptive devices such as electronic switches or banana keyboards to activate MIDI instruments or touch-activated, virtual instrument applications on tablet computers.

Therapist Improvised Music: Mechanically Ventilated Patients

Overview. Music improvisation can be used to provide emotional support and enhance sense of control for mechanically ventilated patients. In musical improvisations, the music therapist is able to respond musically to the patient's physical and emotional musical responses in the moment. Mechanically ventilated patients in critical care often have a limited capacity for active participation in music therapy due to physical limitations. As discussed previously, the tracheal or tracheostomy tube, inserted into the throat to provide ventilation, prohibits verbal communication, so singing and/or verbal processing of the music are not possible. However, depending on physical ability, it may be possible for these patients to participate in musical improvisation using small, handheld instruments, portable keyboards, or other adaptive technology.

If the patient does not feel comfortable participating in musical improvisation or feels unsuccessful in music-making attempts, this may be contraindicative to the goal of increasing the patient's sense of control. The music therapist needs to be aware of this possibility and support the patient to regain a sense of control through whatever means possible, including a decision not to participate. Gentle encouragement and the development of patient-therapist rapport through receptive music therapy interventions may be used to pave the way to more active music therapy interventions such as improvisation.

Preparation. Assess the patient's physical abilities, including strength and range of movement, prior to the session or through discussion with other members of the multidisciplinary team. Bring a range of suitable instruments/music-making devices to the session to increase the choices available to the patient.

What to observe. Look out for changes in the music improvised by the patient over time. Does their music become more confident, adventurous, or expressive as they become more comfortable in the method? If so, how is this change expressed musically?

Procedures. Decide what instruments will be provided. If the patient is using melodic instruments, the therapist should improvise using modes or pentatonic scales to prevent discordant notes. The use of musical holding patterns allows the patient time to respond and provides a sense of security for the patient, which will encourage initiation and exploration of musical ideas.

Adaptations. Adaptive music technology may be employed to increase accessibility of music-making for mechanically ventilated patients, particularly those with a spinal cord injury. Switches or banana keyboards can be set up to activate MIDI instruments, and iPads or other tablet computers with virtual instruments can be used to make music with very limited strength and range of movement.

Guidelines for Re-creative Music Therapy

Lyric Completion: LAS Patients

Overview. Lyric completion is the use of live, familiar music to prompt song line completion. Initially, the goal for developing verbal responses in LAS patients may simply focus on achieving voice consistently at target places in song (usually at the end of song lines). When this goal has been achieved, the patient may be prompted to focus on target sounds, i.e., to achieve correct placement of the articulators for target phoneme production. Finally, the target word may be extended into a target phrase. The patient may become frustrated or upset if unable to complete words to familiar songs.

Preparation. Prepare musical material that the patient is likely to know from memory. Well-known, familiar, cultural songs are ideal, as well as carefully selected patient-preferred songs. The music therapist should be very competent at playing these songs. Considerable modification of timing is required for this method.

What to observe. The therapist should record the following: percentage of appropriately timed vocalizations/verbalizations; percentage of accurately produced words; and/or the maximum number of words per phrase.

Procedures. Using well-known, familiar songs, identify where the target words are located. This may be explained to the patient if it is deemed that they can cognitively process the information. The cues to stimulate target word production should be primarily musical and nonverbal. These cues may include pauses or gaps in the music, musical lead-in or anacrusis, ritardando, use of repetition, changes in facial expression, and/or nonverbal breathing prompts. Additional verbal cues may be added if appropriate. Appropriately placed pauses need to be inserted in songs to create space for the patient to vocalize or attempt word/phrase production. The use of musical holding patterns during extensive pauses will allow time for the patient to respond and provide a sense of continuity in the music.

Adaptations. When the patient is successfully achieving single words at the end of song lines, target words in the middle of phrases or aim for multiple word phrase completion.

WORKING WITH CAREGIVERS

Music therapists may work with family members and caregivers to provide ideas for shared leisure activities involving music. This is particularly significant for family members of nonverbal patients. Interacting in musical activities that are personally meaningful may enhance the time spent with their loved one. By providing guidelines for how to involve their loved one in music choices, active listening, and responses to the music, a shared musical experience may be facilitated. This may be more fulfilling for both patient and caregiver than just putting on a CD in the background.

RESEARCH EVIDENCE

Very little research has been conducted on the efficacy of music therapy interventions with critical care populations. One early music therapy study examined operant conditioning with three LAS patients. Recorded music was used as a reward for switch-pressing and demonstrated patient-initiated movement (Boyle & Greer, 1983). There is little empirical research evaluating live music therapy interventions. Formisano (2001) used standardised tools, in addition to video analysis with blinded assessors, to evaluate the effect of improvisational music therapy in 34 patients in LAS. The assessment tools used included Glasgow Outcome Scale (Jennett & Bond, 1975), Disability Rating Scale (Rappaport et al., 1982), Coma Recovery Scale (Giacino, Keznarsky, & De Luca, 1991), and Post-Coma Scale (Formisano, Vinicola, & Carlesimo, 1996). Although data from the evaluation scales were inconclusive, blinded observations from the video footage suggested improvements in psychomotor initiative (inertia) and decreases in psychomotor agitation. Aldridge and colleagues (1990, 1995) have also reported effects of live, improvised singing on heart rate, respiration, EEG measures, and voluntary movements. However, these publications did not report any measures taken to reduce risk of bias and chance influencing results. Well-designed studies, using control subjects and random group allocation, are greatly needed in this area.

To date, only one study has examined the effects of music therapy with PTA patients (Baker, 2001a, 2001b). Results of this randomized, controlled trial demonstrated significant increases in orientation and decreases in agitation following familiar music listening, but no change following the control condition (no music). A recent Cochrane Review found only one unpublished music therapy study using patient-selected, live music interventions with mechanically ventilated patients (Bradt et al., 2010). Results of this study suggested that the music therapy intervention significantly decreased heart and respiration rates (Phillips, 2007). Several music medicine studies have shown that listening to prerecorded music can reduce state anxiety, levels of pain perception, and blood pressure in critical care and mechanically ventilated populations (Bradt et al., 2010; Chlan, 1995; White, 2000; Wong et al., 2001).

Summary and Conclusions

Although the three subgroups of critical care patients described in this chapter each present with differing etiology and clinical presentation, there are some areas of similarity and shared need. Regulation of the sensory environment is vital due to the growing body of evidence on the detrimental effect of noise on recovery and sleep in critical care settings. Increased heart rate, poorer immune function, and impairments in cognitive function are just a few of the negative effects cited. The application of music therapy to promote rest and sleep in a sensory-regulated environment is therefore strongly indicated. The environmental enrichment literature also supports the application of music therapy for patients in low awareness states. Through a rich and musically stimulating environment, patients are enticed to respond, and these responses are musically reinforced.

A range of possible indications for music therapy intervention with critical care patients has been presented in this chapter. These include, but are not limited to: assessment of awareness, sensory stimulation, decreasing agitation, promoting sleep, increasing orientation, decreasing anxiety, pain management, encouraging purposeful behavior, and providing opportunities for creative expression. Receptive and improvisational techniques are the primary modes of music therapy intervention with this clinical population due to the minimal range of responses possible for most patients.

The music therapy methods described in this chapter have been employed in clinical practice based on the foundations of neuroscience and music psychology research. Our understanding of how music is processed in the brain at a neurological level (in terms of arousal, awareness, and attention) and at a psychological level (in terms of anxiety, pain perception, and sense of control) continues to grow. Efficacy research on music therapy interventions with this population is urgently needed, however. In particular, research utilizing scientifically robust design and methodology is required. It is hoped that the methods described in this chapter will inspire music therapists not only to work with patients in critical care, but also to conduct empirical research that will contribute to the knowledge base informing this work.

Acknowledgment

I would like to acknowledge and thank Janeen Bower for her valuable feedback in the preparation of this chapter.

References

Aldridge, D., Gustorff, D., & Hannich, H. J. (1990). Where am I? Music therapy applied to coma patients. *Journal of the Royal Society of Medicine, 83*(6), 345–346.

Andrews, K., Murphy, L., Munday, R., & Littlewood, C. (1996). Misdiagnosis of the vegetative state: Retrospective study in a rehabilitation unit. *British Medical Journal, 313*(7048), 13–16.

Artiola I Fortuny, L., Briggs, M., Newcombe, F., Ratcliffe, G., & Thomas, C. (1980). Measuring the duration of PTA. *Journal of Neurology, Neurosurgery and Psychiatry, 43*, 377–379.

Bach-Y-Rita, P. (2003). Theoretical basis for brain plasticity after a TBI. *Brain Injury, 17*(8), 643–651.

BaHammam, A. (2006). Sleep in acute care units. *Sleep and Breathing, 10*(1), 6–15.

Baker, F. (2001a). The effects of live, taped and no music on people experiencing posttraumatic amnesia. *Journal of Music Therapy, 38*(3), 170–192.

Baker, F. (2001b). Rationale for the effects of music therapy on agitation and orientation levels of people in posttraumatic amnesia. *Nordic Journal of Music Therapy, 10*(1), 32–41.

Baker, F., & Tamplin, J. (2006). *Music therapy methods in neurorehabilitation: A clinician's manual.* Philadelphia, PA: Jessica Kingsley Publishers.

Bates, D. (1993). The management of medical coma. *Journal of Neurology, Neurosurgery and Psychiatry, 56,* 589–598.

Beaumont, J. G., & Kenealy, P. M. (2005). Incidence and prevalence of the vegetative and minimally conscious states. *Neuropsychological Rehabilitation, 15*(3–4), 184–189.

Beck, A. T., & Steer, R. A. (1990). *Manual for the Beck Anxiety Inventory*. San Antonio, TX: Psychological Corporation.

Boles, J. M., Bion, J., Connors, A., Herridge, M., Marsh, B., Melot, C., et al. (2007). Weaning from mechanical ventilation. *European Respiratory Journal, 29*(5), 1033–1056.

Boyle, M. E., & Greer, R. D. (1983). Operant procedures and the comatose patient. *Journal of Applied Behavior Analysis, 16*(1), 3–12.

Bradt, J., Dileo, C., & Grocke, D. (2010). Music interventions for mechanically ventilated patients. (Review). *Cochrane Database of Systematic Reviews, 12,* CD006902.

Brooks, D. N., Aughton, M. E., Bond, M. R., Jones, P., & Rizvi, S. (1980). Cognitive sequelae in relationship to early indices of severity of brain damage after severe blunt head injury. *Journal of Neurology, Neurosurgery and Psychiatry, 43,* 529–534.

Bruscia, K. (1998). *Defining music therapy* (2nd ed.). Gilsum, NH: Barcelona Publishers.

Canedo, A., Grix, M. C., & Nicoletti, J. (2002). An analysis of assessment instruments for the minimally responsive patient (MRP): clinical observations. *Brain Injury, 16*(5), 453–461.

Childs, N. L., Mercer, W. N., & Childs, H. W. (1993). Accuracy of diagnosis of persistent vegetative state. *Neurology, 43*(8), 1465–1467.

Chlan, L. (1995). Psychological responses of mechanically ventilated patients to music: A pilot study. *American Journal of Critical Care, 4*(3), 233–238.

Chlan, L. (2003). Description of anxiety levels by individual differences and clinical factors in patients receiving mechanical ventilatory support. *Heart & Lung, 32*(4), 275–282.

Corrigan, J. D. (1989). Development of a scale for assessment of agitation following traumatic brain injury. *Journal of Clinical and Experimental Neuropsychology, 11*(2), 261–277.

Corrigan, J. D., & Bogner, J. A. (1994). Factor structure of the agitated behavior scale. *Journal of Clinical and Experimental Neuropsychology, 16*(3), 386–392.

Daveson, B. (2010). An audit about music therapy assessments and recommendations for adult patients suspected to be in a low awareness state. *Journal of Music Therapy, 47*(4), 408–422.

Daveson, B., Magee, W., Crewe, L., Beaumont, G., & Kenealy, P. (2007). The music therapy assessment tool for low awareness states. *International Journal of Therapy and Rehabilitation, 14*(2), 33–45.

Davis, A. E., & White, J. J. (1995). Innovative sensory input for the comatose brain-injured patient. *Psychosocial and Environment Considerations in Critical Care, 7*(2), 351–361.

Dileo, C., & Bradt, J. (2005). *Medical music therapy: A meta-analysis and agenda for future research.* Cherry Hill, NJ: Jeffrey Books.

Dileo, C., & Bradt, J. (2007). Music therapy: Applications to stress management. In P. Lehrer & R. Woolfolk (Eds.), *Principles and practice of stress management*. New York: Guilford Press.

Elliott, L., & Walker, L. (2005). Rehabilitation interventions for vegetative and minimally conscious patients. *Neuropsychological Rehabilitation, 15*(3/4), 480–493.

Fan, Y., Liu, Z., Weinstein, P. R., Fike, J. R., & Liu, J. (2007). Environmental enrichment enhances neurogenesis and improves functional outcome after cranial irradiation. *European Journal of Neurosciences, 25*(1), 38–46.

Formisano, R., Vinicola, V., & Carlesimo, G. A. (1996). Assessment scale for patients with prolonged disturbances of consciousness (post-coma scale). In J. Ponsford, R. Snow, & V. Anderson (Eds.), *Proceedings of the 5th Conference of the International Association for the Study of Brain Injury* (pp. 110–113). Melbourne, Nov. 15–17: Australian Academic Press.

Formisano, R., Vinicola, V., Penta, F., Matteis, M., Brunelli, S., & Weckel, J. W. (2001). Active music therapy in the rehabilitation of severe brain-injured patients during coma recovery. *Annali Dell'Istituto Superiore di Sanita, 37*(4), 627–630.

Forrester, G., Encel, J., & Geffen, G. (1994). Measuring PTA: An historical review. *Brain Injury, 8*(2), 175–184.

Geffen, G., Encel, J., & Forrester, G. (1991). Stages of recovery during post-traumatic amnesia and subsequent everyday memory deficits. *Neuroreport: An International Journal for the Rapid Communication of Research in Neuroscience, 2,* 105–108.

Giacino, J. T., Ashwal, S., Childs, N., Cranford, R., Jennett, B., Katz, D. I., et al. (2002). The minimally conscious state: Definition and diagnostic criteria. *Neurology, 58*(3), 349–353.

Giacino, J. T., & Kalmar, K. (1997). The vegetative and minimally conscious states: A comparison of clinical features and functional outcomes. *Journal of Head Trauma Rehabilitation, 12*(4), 36–51.

Giacino, J. T., & Kalmar, K. (2006). Coma Recovery Scale—Revised. *The Center for Outcome Measurement in Brain Injury.* Retrieved from http://www.tbims.org/combi/crs.

Giacino, J. T., Keznarsky, M. A., & De Luca, J. (1991). Monitoring rate of recovery to predict outcome in minimally conscious patients. *Archives of Physical Medicine and Rehabilitation, 72*(11), 897–901.

Gill-Thwaites, H., & Munday, R. (2004). The sensory modality assessment and rehabilitation technique (SMART): a valid and reliable assessment for vegetative state and minimally conscious state patients. *Brain Injury, 18*(12), 1255–1269.

Grocke, D., & Wigram, T. (2007). *Receptive methods in music therapy: Techniques and clinical applications for music therapy clinicians, educators and students.* Philadelphia, PA: Jessica Kingsley Publishers.

Gustorff, D. (1995). "Herr G." In G. Ansdell (Ed.), *Music for life: Aspects of creative music therapy with adult clients* (pp. 59–64). Philadelphia, PA: Jessica Kingsley Publishers.

Hagen, C., Malkmus, D., & Axen, K. (1989). *Levels of cognitive functioning.* Downey, CA: Ranchos Los Amigos Hospital, Inc.

Hardin, K. A. (2009). Sleep in the ICU: Potential mechanisms and clinical applications. *Chest, 136*(1), 284–294.

Hunter, B. C., Oliva, R., Sahler, O. J. Z., Gaisser, D. A., Salipante, D. M., & Arezina, C. H. (2010). Music therapy as an adjunctive treatment in the management of stress for patients being weaned from mechanical ventilation. *Journal of Music Therapy, 47*(3), 198–219.

Jennett, B., & Bond, M. (1975). Assessment of coma outcome after severe brain damage. *The Lancet, 305*(7905), 480–484.

Jochims, S. (1994). [Establishing contact in the early stage of severe craniocerebral trauma: Sound as the bridge to mute patients]. *Rehabilitation (Stuttg), 33*(1), 8–13.

Lawson, N., Thompson, K., Saunders, G., Richardson, J., Brown, D., Ince, N., et al. (2010). Sound intensity and noise evaluation in a critical care unit. *American Journal of Critical Care, 19*(6), e88–e98.

Levin, H. S., O'Donnell, V. M., & Grossman, R. G. (1979). The Galveston Orientation and Amnesia Test: A practical scale to assess cognition after head injury. *The Journal of Nervous and Mental Disease, 167*(11), 675–684.

Lombardi, F. F. L., Taricco, M., De Tanti, A., Telaro, E., & Liberati, A. (2009). Sensory stimulation for brain-injured individuals in coma or vegetative state. (Review). *Cochrane Database of Systematic Reviews, 2009*(1).

Mackay, L. B., Bernstein, P., & Chapman, E. (1992). Early intervention in severe head injury: Long-term benefits of a formalized program. *Archives of Physical Medicine and Rehabilitation, 73*(7), 635–641.

Magee, W. L. (2005). Music therapy with patients in low awareness states: Approaches to assessment and treatment in multidisciplinary care. *Neuropsychological Rehabilitation, 15*(3–4), 522–536.

Magee, W. L. (2007). Development of a music therapy assessment tool for patients in low awareness states. *Neurorehabilitation, 22*(4), 319–324.

Morton, L. L., Kershner, J. R., & Siegel, L. S. (1990). The potential for therapeutic applications of music on problems related to memory and attention. *Journal of Music Therapy, 27*(4), 195–208.

Neville, H., & Bavelier, D. (2002). Human brain plasticity: Evidence from sensory deprivation and altered language experience. *Progress in Brain Research, 138,* 177–188.

Oh, H., & Seo, W. (2003). Sensory stimulation programme to improve recovery in comatose patients. *Journal of Clinical Nursing, 12*(3), 394–404.

Parthasarathy, S., & Tobin, M. J. (2006). Sleep in the intensive care unit. *Applied Physiology in Intensive Care Medicine, 2*(2.2), 147–156.

Phillips, S. D. (2007). The effect of music entrainent on respiration of patients on mechanical ventilation in the intensive care unit. Unpublished Master's thesis, Florida State University, Florida.

Plum, F., & Posner, J. B. (1980). *The diagnosis of stupor and coma.* Philadelphia, PA: FA Davis Company.

Pochard, F., Lanore, J. J., Bellivier, F., Ferrand, I., Mira, J. P., Belghith, M., et al. (1995). Subjective psychological status of severely ill patients discharged from mechanical ventilation. *Clinical Intensive Care, 6*(2), 57–61.

Ponsford, J., Sloan, S., & Snow, P. (1995). *Traumatic brain injury: Rehabilitation for everyday adaptive living.* London: Lawrence Erlbaum Associates Ltd.

Rappaport, M., Dougherty, A., & Kelting, D. L. (1992). Evaluation of coma and vegetative states. *Archives of Physical Medicine and Rehabilitation, 73*(7), 628–634.

Rappaport, M., Hall, K., Hopkins, K., & Belleza, T. (1982). Disability Rating Scale for severe head trauma: Coma to community. *Archives of Physical Medicine and Rehabilitation, 63*(3), 118–123.

Shiel, A., Burn, J. P. S., Henry, D., Clark, J., Wilson, B. A., Burnett, M. E., et al. (2001). The effects of increased rehabilitation therapy after brain injury: Results of a prospective controlled trial. *Clinical Rehabilitation, 15*(5), 501–514.

Shiel, A., Horn, S., Wilson, B. A., Watson, M., Campbell, M. J., & McLellan, D. L. (2000). The Wessex Head Injury Matrix (WHIM) main scale: A preliminary report on a scale to assess and monitor patient recovery after severe head injury. *Clinical Rehabilitation, 14*(4), 408–416.

Shores, E. A. (1989). Comparison of the Westmead PTA Scale and Glasgow Coma Scale as predictors of neuropsychological outcome following extremely blunt head injury. *Journal of Neurology, Neurosurgery and Psychiatry, 52,* 126–127.

Shores, E. A., Marosszeky, J. E., Sandanam, J., & Bachelor, J. (1986). Preliminary validation of a clinical scale for measuring the duration of post-traumatic amnesia. *The Medical Journal of Australia, 144*(11), 569–572.

Spielberger, C. D., Gorsuch, R. L., Lushene, R., Vagg, P. R., & Jacobs, G. A. (1983). *Manual for the State-Trait Anxiety Inventory (STAI).* Palo Alto, CA: Consulting Psychologists Press.

Tamplin, J. (2000). Improvisational music therapy approaches to coma arousal. *Australian Journal of Music Therapy, 11,* 38–51.

Teasdale, G., & Jennett, B. (1974). Assessment of coma and impaired consciousness. *The Lancet, 304*(7872), 81–84.

Thaut, M. H. (2005). *Rhythm, music and the brain: Scientific foundations and clinical applications.* New York: Taylor & Francis Group.

Tobin, M. J. (2006). *Principles and practice of mechanical ventilation* (2nd ed.). New York: McGraw-Hill.

Torpy, J. M., Campbell, A. D., & Glass, R. M. (2010). Mechanical ventilation. *The Journal of the American Medical Association, 303*(9), 902.

White, J. M. (2000). State of the science of music interventions. Critical care and perioperative practice. *Critical Care Nursing Clinics of North America, 12*(2), 219–225.

Wong, H. L., Lopez-Nahas, V., & Molassiotis, A. (2001). Effects of music therapy on anxiety in ventilator-dependent patients. *Heart & Lung, 30*(5), 376–387.

Wood, R. L. (1991). Critical analysis of the concept of sensory stimulation for patients in vegetative states. *Brain Injury, 5*(4), 401–409.

Yende, S., & Wunderink, R. (2002). Causes of prolonged mechanical ventilation after coronary artery bypass surgery. *Chest, 122*(1), 245–252.

Zigmond, A. S., & Snaith, R. P. (1983). The hospital anxiety and depression scale. *Acta Psychiatrica Scandinavica, 67*(6), 361–370.

Chapter 5

Cardiac Care

Christine Pollard Leist

Diagnostic Information

Cardiovascular disease is characterized by a buildup of plaque in the cardiovascular system of the body. Cardiovascular disease may result in incidence of heart disease and cerebrovascular accident (CVA or stroke). According to the American Heart Association, approximately 82 million adults have one or more types of cardiovascular disease. Of individuals age 60 to 79, 72.6% of men and 71.9% of women have diagnosed cardiovascular disease. Of individuals 80 years and older, 80.1% of men and 86.7% of women have diagnosed heart disease. Cardiovascular disease is the leading cause of death for men and women in the United States, and there is an average of one death from this disease every 39 seconds (AHA, 2012).

Cardiovascular disease that affects the heart includes four major categories of illness: (a) coronary heart disease (CHD), (b) arrhythmia, (c) valve disease, and (d) congestive heart failure (CHF). Individuals with coronary heart disease may experience angina (chest pain), myocardial infarction (heart attack), or concomitant cardiac arrhythmias (AHA, 2012).

Coronary Heart Disease

Coronary Heart Disease is primarily caused by atherosclerosis, which results when fatty plaques develop in the arteries of the heart and interfere with the functioning of a blood vessel. There are three types of coronary heart disease: (a) unstable angina, which is a partial blocking of a coronary artery which is experienced as pressure or burning in the chest and often accompanied by shortness of breath; (b) non-ST segment elevation myocardial infarction (NSTEMI); and (c) ST segment elevation myocardial infarction (STEMI). In the last two types, the heart muscle beyond the obstruction may die and trigger a myocardial infarction, commonly known as a heart attack (Dornelas, 2008).

The primary changeable physiological risk factors for coronary heart disease are high cholesterol, cigarette smoking, high blood pressure, physical inactivity, obesity, and diabetes. The primary unchangeable risk factors are increasing age, male sex, and heredity. Other changeable risk factors include stress, alcohol use, and diet (AHA, 2012).

Arrhythmia

Disorders in the electrical system of the heart are collectively known as arrhythmias, the second major category of heart diseases. Arrhythmias can be caused by pre-existing damage from a heart attack, valve disease, cardiomyopathy, or congenital heart disease. Other causes are possible, including hypertension, overconsumption of caffeine and/or alcohol, low potassium, and stress (AHA, 2012).

There are three types of arrhythmias: (a) supraventricular arrhythmias, (b) ventricular arrhythmias, and (c) bradyarrhythmias (Cleveland Clinic, 2012). Atrial fibrillation, a type of supraventricular arrhythmia, occurs when electrical impulses fire from multiple parts of the heart simultaneously. Communication between the atria and ventricles of the heart is disrupted and the heart beats irregularly (Dornelas, 2008). Ventricular tachycardia, a type of ventricular arrhythmia, occurs when the heart rhythm is too fast. The symptoms of tachycardia include dizziness, faintness, heart palpitations, chest pain, or shortness of breath. Another type, ventricular fibrillation, can be fatal in minutes if the normal rhythm of the heart is not restored. This condition is known as sudden cardiac death or cardiac arrest. Incidences of ventricular fibrillation can be caused by obstructed coronary arteries, certain drugs, and/or extreme physical exertion in people with a genetic predisposition to the condition (Dornelas, 2008). The third type of arrhythmia is bradyarrhythmias, a heart rhythm that is too slow. The symptoms of bradyarrhythmia include dizziness and fatigue, which may result in fainting (Cleveland Clinic).

Valve Disease

The third major category of heart disease is valve disease. Valve disease occurs when the normal function of a valve is disrupted, e.g., the valve narrows, leaks, or stiffens. Valvular stenosis and mitral valve prolapse are two types of valve disease. In mitral valve prolapse, part of the valve extends into the atrium, causing blood to pass back into the left atrium rather than progressing to the left ventricle (Dornelas, 2008).

Congestive Heart Failure

Congestive heart failure, also known as heart failure or congestive heart disease, is caused by a disruption of the heart's ability to contract or relax sufficiently to send blood to the organs and extremities. These conditions are known as systolic heart failure and diastolic heart failure, respectively (Cleveland Clinic, 2012). The heart compensates for its compromised ability to pump by expanding its size through fluid retention. As a result of this fluid collection, fluid backs up into the lungs and the body. Causes of congestive heart failure include hypertension, excessive alcohol use, pregnancy, myocarditis, obesity, or diabetes, but any type of heart disease can progress to heart failure (Dornelas, 2008).

Cardiac Rehabilitation

Many individuals who have experienced a cardiac event or procedure participate in a four-phase cardiac rehabilitation program. These programs usually combine supervised exercise with health education in a social setting (AHA, 2012). Phase I occurs during hospitalization and involves an assessment of the patient's physical abilities and daily walking to improve strength after surgery. Upon release from the hospital, the patient enters phase II, which involves physical activities that are low-impact in nature, such as biking. This phase usually lasts up to 12 weeks. Phase III is designed to increase the individual's exercise intensity and duration. This phase may last from 8 to 12 weeks. Integrating lifestyle changes is the hallmark of phase IV. It is hoped that dietary changes and exercise habits will continue throughout the individual's life (AHA).

Needs and Resources

While cardiac rehabilitation programs address physical and dietary needs, individuals with coronary heart disease often experience other physiological symptoms, such as pain, and often under recognized psychological symptoms, including depressed mood, anxiety, and anger/hostility. The reader is referred to Chapter Three for a complete definition and description of music therapy interventions to address pain management in the medical care of adults. Definitions of selected psychological needs of adults with heart disease are drawn from the field of behavioral cardiology and presented here.

Depression

Depression has been identified in the literature as a changeable risk factor for heart disease. The symptoms of depression in individuals with CHD are similar to the symptoms of noncardiac patients and may include:

> [p]rolonged sadness and/or loss of interest in pleasure most of the day, nearly every day; significant weight loss or gain when not dieting; insomnia or hypersomnia; psychomotor agitation or retardation; fatigue or loss of energy; feelings of worthlessness or excessive guilt; diminished ability to think, concentrate, or make decisions; and recurrent thoughts of death, suicidal ideation, or suicide attempt. (Dornelas, 2008, p. 51)

Depression has been linked to the development of cardiac illness as well as to the long-term prognosis for an individual with CHD. Most of the literature in this area examines depressive symptoms rather than clinically diagnosed depression. Often the depression of an individual with CHD is less severe than that of noncardiac patients, but is still a major factor in morbidity and mortality particularly, as depressed patients may forget to take medications or stop practicing health-protective behaviors (Dornelas, 2008).

In a study to examine the frequency and severity of hopelessness and depression in people recovering from myocardial infarction, Dunn (2005) interviewed 351 patients approximately 14 days following discharge from the hospital. She then interviewed the participants again three months following discharge. She found that hopelessness and depression were frequent and moderate to severe for some participants at baseline and three months. While depression did decline from baseline to three months postincident, hopelessness remained statistically unchanged after three months, which included both inpatient and outpatient treatment. She concluded that it is important to assess and treat depression and hopelessness in this population as individuals with high hopelessness may choose not to start or may quit a cardiac rehabilitation program intended to reduce morbidity and mortality.

A review of studies on how anxiety and depression progress and the effects of interventions on them, have shown that anxiety and depression are common in patients with coronary heart disease (Herrmann-Lingen & Buss, 2007). They summarized that while symptoms of depression may decrease following inpatient treatment, depression often increases in the chronic phase of the disease when lifestyle changes need to be learned, practiced, and maintained. Because depression is a factor in prognosis, people with depression often have a poorer prognosis. The authors concluded that there are few studies about how depression can be successfully treated, so there is need for well-designed, multicenter studies with large numbers of participants in order to differentiate the effectiveness of psychological treatments.

Anxiety

Anxiety refers both to emotional states, e.g., nervousness, and physiological states, e.g., rapid heart rate, sweating, dry mouth, and vertigo. Anxiety can be conceptualized as both a personality trait and a response to stressful situations. In cardiac literature, it generally refers to the individual's response to the stress of cardiac diagnosis, illness, and/or procedures (Dornelas, 2008).

While anxiety often co-occurs with depression, particularly in the people with cardiac illness, the literature has shown only a weak link between anxiety and health outcomes, including mortality. Anxiety is more closely linked to the onset of cardiac illness than to the progression of the illness; however, it continues to be studied in the literature due to its link to stress and cardiac disease (Dornelas, 2008). It is thought that people with anxiety are more likely to be negatively affected by the stress of cardiac disease.

Several possibilities exist for relieving anxiety symptoms. Relaxation techniques, such as meditation, deep breathing, and progressive muscle relaxation, are suggested. Other approaches to address the physiological components of anxiety include biofeedback and exercise. Because anxiety is thought to relate to inner conflict, affect-focused therapy may be used to treat the anxiety by identifying and expressing the underlying emotion states (Dornelas, 2008).

Anger/Hostility

Anger manifests behaviorally as a range from minor irritation to rage. Aggression is an overt behavior and involves destructive or hurtful actions toward others. Hostility is the experience of anger toward others that manifests in a distrust of others and a wish to harm others. Individuals with hostility have underlying negative attitudes and beliefs and see others as a source of mistreatment or frustration (Smith, 1992, as cited in Sotile, 1996).

Investigators may use the terms anger, aggression, and hostility to describe this dependent variable. Anger manifests behaviorally as a range from minor irritation to rage. Aggression is an overt behavior and involves destructive or hurtful actions toward others. Hostility is the experience of anger toward others that manifests in a distrust of others and a wish to harm others. Individuals with hostility have underlying negative attitudes and beliefs and see others as a source of mistreatment or frustration (Smith, 1992, as cited in Sotile, 1996).

Individuals with hostility are often reluctant to engage in behavior change if they believe the change is needed for the benefit of other people (Sotile, 1996). They may feel that to deny their feelings of hostility toward others is to deny or suppress their true feelings. It may be beneficial to encourage modification of hostile behavior patterns to improve their own health rather than to improve their relationship with others. They may be more likely to try new behaviors if they anticipate a positive health outcome.

In many cases, individuals with hostility have a Type-A Behavior Pattern (TABP) personality. These individuals evidence signs of constantly striving to do more and more, perfectionism, feelings of hostility, time urgency, competitiveness, mistrust of others (Williams & Steele, 2005). Treatment for these individuals can be challenging, as they may need to feel in control of aspects of the treatment and have difficulty trusting the therapist. Sotile (1996) suggested identifying the individual's strengths and designing active interventions with this population such as relaxation practice logs, shared group decision-making, and options for choice in the sessions. In summary, the psychological aspects of heart disease such as stress perception, depression, anxiety, and anger/hostility play a role in the treatment and prevention of heart disease.

Stress

Stress is defined as a physiological and psychological response to external and internal stimuli. It is experienced as a result of personal and subjective responses to one's environment; no two people will experience the same events as stressful or to the same degree. Stress can be measured with both physiological and psychological measures (American Institute of Stress, 2011).

Chronic stress can cause prolonged activation of the fight-or-flight response system and the elevation of cortisol levels in the body through the HPA axis. The general adaptation syndrome model describes how high levels of stress hormones, such as cortisol, can increase blood pressure, triglyceride levels, low-density lipoprotein levels, and cholesterol levels (Dornelas, 2008). Stress and emotional distress can also increase inflammation, which increases the buildup of plaque in arteries. These are all risk factors from coronary heart disease.

While stress induces physiological changes in the body, there is a cognitive aspect to stress: specifically, how an individual perceives their stress. Even after risk factors were statistically controlled for in the study, the perception of stress, as measured by the Perceived Stress scale, was the strongest predictor of symptomatic cardiovascular disease in a sample of 10,432 women age 70–75 (Strodl, Kenardy, & Aroney, 2003), indicating the importance of addressing perceived stress to improve the coronary health of older women.

Social Support

Another changeable risk factor and need area cited in the literature is social support. While the health-protective mechanism of social support is less understood than stress and depression, it is still considered relevant to effective treatment of individuals with heart disease. In fact, risk of death is higher for people with fewer social support contacts (Dornelas, 2008). One possible explanation of the protective effect of social support is that it acts as a barrier to the detrimental effects of chronic stress, such as heart disease (Williams & Steele, 2005).

Family members, friends, health providers, and other patients can provide social support. It may take the form of having a social network, receiving tangible support, and/or receiving emotional support. According to Rhodes (2004), emotional support may be the most effective form of social support. It is important for practitioners to assess social support, since in some cases individuals such as family members may contribute to increased stress by having to cope with their own illnesses, becoming frustrated by caring for their family member, or contributing to a stressful home life through the development or continuation of abusive relationships. In these cases, family therapy may be warranted. While the mechanism of social support is unknown and is certainly complex, investigators in the field continue to recommend inclusion of measures of perceived social support and strategies for assisting individuals in identifying and accessing social support (Lett et al., 2005). Treatments that occur within a social setting, such as group therapy, are presumed to engage the health-protective mechanism of social support.

As indicated in the previous discussion, psychological distress may lead to increased disease symptomology followed by subsequent changes in quality of life; therefore, interventions, such as music therapy, are needed to reduce the symptoms of stress and anxiety while providing opportunities for emotional expression and processing within a supportive social setting.

Musical Background and Experience

While individuals in music therapy are not required to have musical training or experience to participate and benefit from music therapy, many individuals bring positive associations with music to the music therapy sessions. In Leist (2011), several group members reported participating in community music organizations such as bands and choirs. Two individuals reported a history of playing instruments and an interest in pursuing those interests again. Discussing musical interests became a way for the group to get to know each other and the therapist in order to share more intimate emotional information later in the session. The depth and breadth of the group's musical interests and experiences enriched the group process, as they offered suggestions for songs to sing and pieces to listen to during the sessions. Both before and after the sessions, participants were observed exchanging recordings and discussing upcoming community events involving music.

Referral and Assessment

Patients with cardiac needs may be referred to music therapy to address psychological and/or physiological needs. The referral source may be members of the hospital staff, a family member, the music therapist, or the patient. Hospital policies and procedures will dictate who may refer and what process will be used, for example, in some settings a physician's order may be required. In many cases, the music therapist will be able to devise the referral criteria for patients with cardiac care needs. Specific referral criteria may include pain, anxiety, mood, stress, coping, prolonged hospitalization, or isolation precautions. Following referral, the music therapist will assess the patient's strengths and needs to determine if music therapy is indicated, treatment goals, and preliminary estimates of the length of treatment.

Prior to seeing the patient for assessment, the music therapist is advised to determine any infection control precautions or activity status guidelines, e.g., preoperative or postoperative restrictions, in place for the patient and plan the assessment accordingly. Common preoperative restrictions include no food after midnight the night before surgery and cessation of smoking. Common postoperative restrictions are related to diet and physical activity. Calories, fat, sodium, and sugar are often restricted or modified after surgery. Physical activity restrictions after surgery include standing in one place for no longer than 15 minutes and sitting for no longer than one hour. Patients should also avoid activities that involve raising arms above shoulder level for long periods. Music therapists are advised to be mindful of these physical activity restrictions during assessment and treatment implementation (University of Southern California School of Medicine, 2012).

When conducting an initial assessment for treatment eligibility, the music therapist will collect demographic and diagnostic information of the patient along with information regarding the reason for referral to music therapy. Information about the patient's musical history, culture, preferences, and spiritual background is necessary to determine the music that will be used in sessions. For patients with cardiac needs, an imagery preferences inventory or checklist can be useful in planning music-assisted relaxation to reduce pain, discomfort, or anxiety. The music therapist could ask the patient to respond to a list of possible images to determine preferred, as well as distressing, images for the patient. The patient may also be invited to describe the sensory aspects of a relaxing place to be incorporated later into a music-assisted relaxation experience.

During the initial assessment and for ongoing treatment evaluation, there are three possible methods for assessing clients and evaluating the effectiveness of music therapy interventions: (a) observational methods, (b) self-report measures, and (c) physiological measures. See below for a summary of categories, outcome areas, and useful measures in music therapy treatment for adults with cardiac care needs.

- Observational Methods
  - Pain, comfort, and anxiety
  - Verbalizations and/or vocalizations
  - Facial expressions
  - Type and duration of body movements
- Self-report Measures
  - Pain, comfort, anxiety, and mood
    - Numerical rating scales
    - Picture Scales
    - Semantic Differential Scales
    - Visual Analogue Scales
  - Pain
    - Body Map
    - *McGill Pain Questionnaire* (Melzack & Torgerson, 1971)
  - Mood
    - *Profile of Mood States* (McNair, Lorr, & Droppleman, 1992)
  - Perceived Exertion During Task
    - *Borg Rating Scale of Perceived Exertion* (Borg, 1998)
- Physiological Measures
  - Heart rate
  - Blood pressure
  - Respiratory rate

When selecting an evaluation method, the music therapist is advised to consider several factors. First, the music therapist must select a tool or method that is a valid measure for the patient's goal area(s). A tool designed to measure pain would not be suitable to measure cardiac function. Second, the music therapist must consider the energy level of the client, as some self-report measures take more time and energy for the patient to complete than others. For example, the patient may need 5 to 30 seconds to make a mark on a visual analogue scale and 20 minutes to complete the *Profile of Mood States* (POMS; McNair, Lorr, & Droppleman, 1992); therefore, the visual analogue scale may be better suited for clinical practice, while the POMS could be used to evaluate a longer treatment time period or for research purposes. If possible, it is advised that the music therapist use at least two of the three method categories during assessment and evaluation in music therapy in order to gain a more complete view of the patient's progress. In most cases, the music therapist will assess the client prior to and after music therapy services to make conclusions about the effectiveness of the treatment.

For program evaluation and quality assurance purposes, the music therapist may routinely or periodically ask patients, family members, or hospital staff members to complete satisfaction surveys in order to evaluate the effectiveness of the music therapy program and implement enhancements to music therapy service delivery in the hospital (Hanson-Abromeit, 2010). See Appendix A for an example of a patient satisfaction survey for a community outpatient music therapy group (Leist, 2011). The reader is referred to Gerweck and Tan (2010) for an example of a survey designed to capture hospital staff perceptions of music therapy service delivery.

The remainder of the chapter will discuss seven examples of music therapy interventions used with this population presented within the framework of the following four music therapy method categories: (a) receptive, (b) improvisational, (c) re-creative, and (d) compositional.

Overview of Methods and Procedures

These methods and procedures have not been sequenced to reflect relative significance, effectiveness, or complexity.

Receptive Music Therapy

- Music-Assisted Relaxation: The application of receptive music listening to reduce anxiety and/or pain.
- Music Listening: Patient listening to music either alone or in the presence of the music therapist or other staff member.
- Music and Exercise: Music used in conjunction and/or coordinated with exercise routines.
- Guided Imagery and Music: Imaging to music in an expanded state of consciousness (Bruscia, 2002, p. xxi).

Improvisational Music Therapy

- Instrumental Improvisation: Any combination of pitches, rhythms, or sounds created with instruments.
- Vocal Improvisation: Any combination of lyrics, vocal sounds, toning, held pitches, or rhythmic use of voice, e.g., beat box.

Re-creative Music Therapy

- Expressive Singing: Selection and performance of songs that have meaning for the client or group.

Compositional Music Therapy

- Song Transformation: Modifying the lyrics of a precomposed song to support the strengths or meet the needs of the client group.
- Songwriting: Supporting the client in creating lyrics and/or instrumental music.

Guidelines for Receptive Music Therapy

Music-Assisted Relaxation (MAR)

Overview. Music-Assisted Relaxation (MAR) is the application of receptive music listening to reduce anxiety and/or pain in which the music therapist leads the individual or group through a relaxing scene, idea, or body response to the music. This intervention is indicated when the group or individual expresses or demonstrates a need for pain, stress, or anxiety management. This technique serves not only to decrease these areas in the moment, but also to teach the individual a way to use music as a self-regulation strategy. Music-assisted relaxation may also serve as a transition into the sessions from concerns of the outside world and prime the group for the music-based work that may follow the MAR. In terms of level of therapy, music-assisted relaxation would be classified as a Level Two Insight Music Therapy with Re-educative Goals intervention (Wheeler, 1987). Both classroom simulation experiences and implementation under the supervision of a board-certified music therapist are recommended before attempting music-assisted relaxation with a client.

For individuals who have had a near-death experience, perhaps while being resuscitated after a cardiac event, music-assisted relaxation experiences involving light or the sun may be contraindicated if the near-death experience was traumatic. For this reason, it is helpful to assess imagery preferences before engaging in MAR experiences. As noted in the previous section of this chapter, a simple checklist of images can be used for this purpose.

For individuals being treated as an inpatient following a cardiac surgical procedure or experiencing pain, it is contraindicated to engage them in progressive muscle relaxation (PMR), which will be described in the following section. The process of contracting and releasing muscles inherent in this type of MAR could cause pain or postoperative complications for these individuals. Image-based or autogenic inductions are better suited for these patients, as these require no movement on the part of the patient and may be effective in decreasing pain often experienced postsurgery.

Preparation. A recurrent theme in the literature regarding music therapy in cardiac health care is who should select the music to be used in the session and whether it should be individualized to each participant. Hanser and Mandel (2005) noted that none of the research studies conducted by medical professionals included music that was selected based upon participant's preferences. In many cases, the same music selection was used for all of the participants. They suggested that if music listening was effective for programs that were not individualized, then it is possible that music selected by the participant and administered by a qualified music therapist may have even greater benefit.

Consistent with the literature, music selections should have tempi of 60 to 70 beats per minute, be 3 to 8 minutes in length and instrumental only, and have consistent tempo, dynamics, and instrumentation (Grocke & Wigram, 2007; Leist, 2011; Mandel, 1996, 2007; Mandel et al., 2007; Schou, 2009). The music selections may be drawn from recordings or presented live by the music therapist. As the group or individual becomes more comfortable with music-assisted relaxation, the selections may gradually increase in length and complexity as the sessions progress. If the MAR is conducted across a series of sessions and is time-limited, the music therapist should be sure to end the treatment period with gradually shorter, less complex selections to prepare for termination (Leist, 2011).

Three types of music-assisted relaxation will be discussed in this chapter: (a) progressive muscle relaxation (PMR), (b) autogenic, and (c) image-based. The features of each technique are outlined below and organized according to the stability level needed within the musical elements. The music therapist is advised to select music that meets the guidelines discussed in the previous section.

- Progressive Muscle Relaxation (PMR)
    - Focus is on contraction and relaxation of muscle groups throughout the body
    - Script is repetitive and predictable
    - Selected music should be repetitive and predictable
- Autogenic
    - Focus is on one image or idea
    - Image or idea travels through the body
    - Script is repetitive and predictable
    - Selected music has elements of repetition and predictability

- Image-based
    - Focus is on a scene
    - Person travels through a scene
    - Script appeals to the senses
    - Music may have elements of increased complexity

In PMR, the music therapist guides the client in contracting and relaxing muscle groups systematically throughout the body. The process may begin from the head to the floor or vice versa (Grocke & Wigram, 2007). The words used to label the muscle groups should be drawn from everyday language rather than anatomical terms. If a client has to try to remember what "pecs" are, then he or she will be inhibited from experiencing the process to its fullest. The beginning music therapist is advised to plan what label will be used for the buttocks and practice saying the word aloud prior to implementing MAR. See Appendix B for an example of a PMR script (Leist, 2011).

In autogenic, the music therapist selects an image or quality that moves systematically through the body. Possible image choices include a ball of light, a color the client chooses, or a light breeze. Possible qualities include peace, relaxation, lightness, or healing (Grocke & Wigram, 2007). See Appendix C for an example of an autogenic script (Leist, 2011).

In image-based, the music therapist guides the client through a scene that is peaceful, safe, and relaxing. Possible scenes include a meadow, field, a park, a beach, a lake, or a mountain view. For both autogenic and image-based scripts, the music therapist must select images according to the preferences of the client (Grocke & Wigram, 2007). For example, some clients may find a woodland scene relaxing, while others may find it threatening. A client who is unable to swim may find an ocean or lake view uncomfortable. When crafting the script, the music therapist should consider what will be seen, heard, and felt by the client during the experience and use rich, sensory images accordingly. If possible, the beginning music therapist is advised to visit a place that is similar to the selected scene and record images and sensations to consider for inclusion in the script. See Appendix D for an example of an image-based script (Leist, 2011).

What to observe. In addition to using one or more methods of assessment and evaluation discussed earlier in the chapter, the music therapist must have enough familiarity with the script and music selection to be able to visually monitor the ongoing responses of the group or individual (Schou, 2009). In addition to signs of relaxation, the music therapist must also observe for signs of that may indicate distress, e.g., opening eyes, contracting muscles, sitting up if the client was in a prone position, vocal sounds, or verbalizations. Should an individual in a group show signs of distress, the music therapist may choose first to discreetly check in with the individual by asking members to give a sign if they wish to end the experience. In an individual setting, the process can be more direct since the concerns about privacy would not be present in a one-to-one treatment session. As discussed later, the music therapist will also check in at the end of the MAR.

Procedures. Prior to beginning MAR, the music therapist should prepare the room by lowering the lights, setting the volume level on the portable stereo, and posting a privacy sign on the door. For individuals with fast personal tempi, it can be helpful to relax with breathing, music, or calming thoughts prior to implementing relaxation experiences.

Music-assisted relaxation generally follows three phases: 1) opening conversation and transition to music, 2) music experience, and 3) the closing. Each will be described in detail below.

Music-assisted relaxation may be conducted with the client sitting or lying down on a mat. In medical settings, the clients will usually sit, as it can be difficult to get up and down from the floor, or stay reclined in their hospital bed or recliner. The procedure begins with the music therapist verifying the type of imagery and protocol to be used and then reminding about confidentiality and privacy if the MAR will be conducted in a group setting. The process will continue as she tells the group approximately how long the experience will last (Leist, 2011) and what might be experienced during the intervention. It is helpful to include a prompt that encourages mental focusing and offers a method for addressing any distracting thoughts that might surface during the experience. One way to address these distracting thoughts is to think of a neutral dismissing phrase, such as "Oh, well," and focus again on the protocol (Benson et al., 1975, as cited in Friedman et al., 1996). Participants should be given the opportunity to ask questions and invited to open their eyes at any time during the MAR. Next, participants are invited to get comfortable, close eyes, and focus on breathing for a few minutes. The music therapist should refrain from scripting the tempo of the breath, but should provide an auditory example of a deep, relaxing breath. Next, an initial image is given, with the suggestion to carry the suggested image into the music.

For all three types of MAR described earlier, the music therapist should strive to embody relaxation (or tension/release if using PMR) in her voice. The timbre and tempo of the speaking voice must be different from the everyday speaking voice, as those elements serve as a prompt for relaxation. Achieving this voice timbre and tempo may require some practice. Practicing with a friend or listening to a recording of oneself can be beneficial in achieving a relaxing voice.

At the close of the script, the music therapist should affirm that the individual(s) can return to their imagery at a later time should they wish to do so. To assist the participants in returning to an alert state, a suggestion is made to return their awareness to the room around them. Individuals should be encouraged to take as much time as needed to return to the present. Music therapists may choose from several options for processing the experience, i.e., verbal sharing, drawing images, creating mandalas, but only if the therapist has training in their use, or writing poems/phrases. Individuals should be encouraged to share, but not required to do so. The music therapist is advised to follow up with any individual who chooses not to share with the group to determine if he/she needs extra support.

Music Listening

Overview. This intervention entails the patient listening to music either alone or in the presence of the music therapist or other staff member. It is indicated when an individual expresses or demonstrates a need for pain, stress, anxiety, or insomnia management, either in addition to a course of music therapy treatment or as a stand-alone intervention. This technique serves not only to decrease these areas in the moment, but also to teach the individual a way to use music as a self-regulation strategy. This intervention is different from music-assisted relaxation in that the listener is not guided through a relaxation script or protocol.

Music listening is contraindicated when the individual is unable to indicate music preferences and/or unable to operate the music playback device, e.g., CD player or MP3 player. If music preferences are unknown, the music therapist or staff member may unwittingly select music that has a negative association for the individual or is based upon the staff member's music preferences. If the individual is unable to operate the music playback device, then he or she would be unable to stop the music listening intervention as needed due to fatigue or dislike of the selection.

Preparation. Medical facilities often collect CDs for a music listening library for patient use. Additionally, music therapists often have access to CD players or other digital music players with selections categorized by year and genre. Patients may like the room lights dimmed for the experience. Following completion of the music listening experience, the music therapist or staff member should sanitize any materials used in keeping with hospital policy.

What to observe. In addition to using one or more methods of assessment and evaluation discussed earlier in the chapter, the music therapist will visually monitor the ongoing responses of the group or individual (Leist, 2011).

Procedures. The music therapist or staff member will inquire if the patient would like to listen to some music. Following a discussion of music preferences, the staff member will select a CD or MP3 track(s) for the patient and explain the use of the device. If a music therapist is conducting or supervising the intervention, he or she may wish to discuss the patient's experience of listening to the music and seek input about future use of music listening in the hospital and postdischarge.

Music and Exercise

Overview. Music and exercise is defined here as music used in conjunction and/or coordinated with exercise protocols. Music and exercise serves to motivate movement in the moment and teach the individual a way to use music when they are exercising independently. It is indicated when a group or individual expresses or demonstrates a need for music to motivate during an exercise protocol. In terms of level of therapy, music and exercising would be classified as a Level One Music Therapy as Activity Therapy.

In order to effectively benefit from music and exercise, the patient must be cleared for activity by the medical team. If the music will be delivered individually, the client must be able to successfully operate the music playback device, whether it is a CD player or a digital music recorder. If the exercise will be occurring in a group setting such as cardiac rehabilitation, group members must collectively decide what artists or genres they would like to listen to as a group so the music serves as a motivator rather than a deterrent to exercise. Digital music recorders should be set with a maximum volume limit for hearing conservation purposes.

Preparation. Music selection is dependent upon the type of exercise that is to be done. Music for stretching, yoga, or Pilates could be selected with the same criteria as music-assisted relaxation, e.g., tempi of 60 to 70 beats per minute, instrumental only and consistent tempo, dynamics, and instrumentation (Grocke & Wigram, 2007; Leist, 2011; Mandel, 1996, 2007; Mandel et al., 2007; Schou, 2009). Music for aerobic or rhythmic exercises should have a tempo that encourages movement and be either emotionally neutral or positive in message. Music selections may be recorded or presented live by the music therapist. One advantage to live music is that the tempo may be adjusted in the moment according to the strengths and needs of the client.

What to observe. One or more of the methods of assessment and evaluation discussed earlier in the chapter may be used to evaluate the success of music and exercise protocols. The music therapist or staff member should periodically monitor the client to observe for responses that may indicate distress, and respond accordingly.

Procedures. After the room and music have been set up, the music therapist or staff member is responsible for adjusting the music selections and volume as needed. If treating solo, the music therapist should seek consultation from appropriate staff members regarding targeted movements and procedures. In many cases, the music therapist will serve as a consultant for music selection or will cotreat depending upon the specific needs of the individual or group. All facility procedures for infection control should be followed. Per client feedback, the music therapist may adjust the music selections as needed.

Guided Imagery and Music (GIM)

Guided Imagery and Music (GIM) is a receptive method involving imaging to music in an altered state of consciousness. According to Bruscia (2002), this method may include individual or group work and may be guided or unguided. It is briefly presented here in order to differentiate it from the earlier examples of music-assisted relaxation and music listening. Whereas the goals of music-assisted relaxation and music listening center on pain management, relaxation, and decreased anxiety, the goals of GIM are psychotherapeutic and reconstructive in nature. For an extensive discussion of GIM, the reader is referred to *Guided Imagery and Music: The Bonny Method and Beyond,* edited by Bruscia and Grocke (2002). This resource contains information about the history, music selection, and treatment process of GIM. For research specifically related to GIM in cardiac care, the reader is referred to Bonny (1983) and Short, Gibb, and Holmes (2011).

GUIDELINES FOR IMPROVISATIONAL MUSIC THERAPY

Instrumental Improvisation

Overview. Instrumental improvisation is defined here as any combination of pitches, rhythms, or sounds created by individuals with instruments. This type of intervention is indicated when the group or individual expresses or demonstrates a need to process feelings nonverbally. For this population, goals of this type of intervention include developing active listening skills, recognizing personal strengths, identifying coping skills, emotional identification, emotional expression, and celebrating accomplishments (Leist, 2011). Please see the previous chapter on pain for a discussion of improvisational music therapy for pain management. In terms of level of therapy, instrumental improvisation would be classified as a Level Two Insight Music Therapy with Re-educative Goals intervention (Wheeler, 1987). Both classroom simulation experiences and implementation under the supervision of a board-certified music therapist are recommended before attempting this technique with clients.

In order to fully benefit from instrumental improvisation, the patient must have the strength and energy to play instruments. The music therapist can assess this area and plan to use instruments that require less strength to play, e.g., chime tree.

Preparation. It is desirable to offer a variety of instruments that have a range of timbres for emotional expression purposes. The music therapist must verify that there are more than enough instruments for everyone in the group to have a choice. The following instruments may be considered for instrumental improvisation: tubanos or djembes with attached rubber feet, an ocean drum, maracas, frame drums and mallets, cabasas, claves, tambourines, chime tree, rain stick, and finger cymbals. The following keyed percussion instruments are useful as well: bass tone bars, xylophones, metallophones, and glockenspiels. The music therapist may choose to play piano, guitar, a percussion instrument, or a principal symphonic instrument to facilitate the intervention. Other instrumental choices should be considered, depending upon the strengths and needs of the group or individual.

What to observe. In addition to using one or more methods of assessment and evaluation discussed earlier in the chapter, the music therapist will visually monitor the ongoing responses of the group or individual (Leist, 2011). For improvisation-specific examples of assessment and evaluation, the reader is advised to consult *Improvisational Models of Music Therapy* (Bruscia, 1987).

Procedures. In a group setting, the music therapist must discuss confidentiality and privacy concerns with group members. After the explanation, it can be helpful for each individual to give a verbal confirmation at the beginning and end of the session that the privacy of their peers will be respected. Individuals may also wish to discuss their concerns in generalities while still focusing on feelings, e.g., "I felt angry when someone important to me walked away while I was talking." This technique keeps the group focus on feelings and helps protect the client's privacy.

Additionally, while many individuals do bring positive associations about music to music therapy, some may bring negative associations or a feeling of uncertainty to the sessions. Prior to the first treatment session in Leist (2011), one participant discussed her fear of making music in a group setting and cited her perceived inability to sing and play instruments as the reason for her fear. Situations such as this require sensitivity on the part of the music therapist. In this case, the music therapist validated her feelings, explained how the sessions would be structured for success, and invited the client to try just one session. The client agreed and attended every session during the treatment period.

The music therapist may choose to begin the session with a verbal check-in or by beginning the instrumental improvisation. Starting with a verbal check-in may help the music therapist to determine a presenting theme for the improvisation, while starting directly with improvisation may help the clients to become aware of their feelings in a way that words cannot. To structure instrumental improvisation, the music therapist may choose to begin the improvisation with a word, phrase, melodic motive, or ostinato drawn from the work of the group. For example, the music therapist might use instrumental improvisation to simulate a stressful situation, such as driving again following surgery, to facilitate the individual's awareness of what is happening in his or her body when thinking about a stressful situation. For a detailed discussion of the use of improvisation within psychotherapeutic models, the reader is advised to consult *Improvisational Models of Music Therapy* (Bruscia, 1987).

Adaptations. Vocal improvisation may be used separately or in conjunction with instrumental improvisation and may consist of any combination of lyrics, vocal sounds, toning, held pitches, or rhythmic use of voice, e.g., beat box. Some groups or individuals may need to experience success with instrumental improvisation before experiencing vocal improvisation, so the music therapist is advised to carefully assess the strengths and needs of the individual(s).

Guidelines for Re-creative Music Therapy

Expressive Singing

Overview. Expressive singing is the selection and performance of songs that have meaning for the client or group. Expressive singing is indicated when the group or individual expresses or demonstrates a need for growth in the following goal areas: developing active listening skills, recognizing personal strengths, identifying coping skills, emotional identification, emotional expression, and celebrating accomplishments (Leist, 2011; Mandel, 1996; Mandel et al., 2007). In terms of level of therapy, expressive singing would be classified as a Level Two Insight Music Therapy with Re-educative Goals intervention (Wheeler, 1987). Both classroom simulation experiences and implementation under the supervision of a board-certified music therapist are recommended before attempting this intervention with clients.

In order to fully benefit from expressive singing, the patient must have the strength and energy to sing; however, the patient could listen to the music therapist sing the songs and then participate in discussion.

Preparation. The music therapist will prepare for the session by considering the issues relevant to the group or population and the culture, age range, and music preferences of the group. Then, the music therapist will select songs that have relevance for the issues and background of the individual(s). Often, the music therapist will have a theme and songs selected in advance, but the experienced music therapist often will adjust the themes and song choices depending upon the presenting needs of the group. Preparing a songbook in advance can be helpful and provide the opportunity for clients to browse through the songs to make suggestions. In Leist (2011), as the clients developed group cohesion, the clients would often suggest songs for each other as gifts or in recognition of achievements. Generally, it is desirable to have handheld percussion instruments available should individual(s) choose to supplement the song with rhythm. Songbooks and instruments should be readily available. Clipboards can be useful if the music therapist invites each group member to mark lyrics that have meaning to them. The song may be used to literally express the topic, serve as a metaphor for the topic, or deepen or explore the topic.

What to observe. In addition to using one or more methods of assessment and evaluation discussed earlier in the chapter, the music therapist will visually monitor the ongoing responses of the group or individual (Leist, 2011). The music therapist also listens for themes or topics in the client's responses to the songs.

Procedures. In a group setting, the music therapist must discuss confidentiality and privacy concerns with group members. After the explanation, it can be helpful for each individual to give a verbal confirmation at the beginning and end of the session that the privacy of their peers will be respected. Individuals may also wish to discuss their concerns in generalities while still focusing on feelings, e.g., "The lyrics of this song remind me about when I felt sad when I separated from my loved one." This technique keeps the group focus on feelings and helps protect the client's privacy.

Because group members will often comment upon and relate to the responses of other group members, it can be helpful for the music therapist to set guidelines for participation. In Leist (2011), the acronym SAFE was used to represent four guidelines for the sessions. S represented *support similarities,* A represented *avoid advice,* F represented *focus on feelings,* and E represented *encouragement.* In this study, group members would often remind each other of the SAFE guidelines when a peer would offer unsolicited advice.

When facilitating expressive singing, the music therapist will usually begin with a verbal check-in, which will help the music therapist to select a song that relates to the information shared by the group or individual during the check-in. Another choice is for the music therapist to invite the individual(s) to select a song that has meaning for them or otherwise relates to them. In either case, verbal processing would follow the singing of the song. The music therapist should wait a few moments after the song has ended to allow space for clients to initiate a response to the song. Additionally, the music therapist should use open-ended questions to stimulate longer client responses. An exception to this might be a situation when the client has compromised energy or breath support for longer responses. The music therapist should allow opportunities for clients to relate to each other's comments and to link responses among group members to facilitate social support.

Guidelines for Compositional Music Therapy

Song Transformation

Overview. Song transformation is the process of modifying the lyrics of a precomposed song to support the strengths or meet the needs of the client group. It is indicated when the group or individual expresses or demonstrates a need for growth in the following goal areas: developing active listening skills, recognizing personal strengths, identifying coping skills, emotional identification, emotional expression, and celebrating accomplishments (Leist, 2011; Mandel, 1996; Mandel et al., 2007). In the Leist study, the song transformation experiences were used to process issues in the session and as reminders for the clients outside the session. For example, one client put her song about weight loss and self-love on her refrigerator as a helpful reminder during the week. In terms of level of therapy, expressive singing would be classified as a Level Two Insight Music Therapy with Re-educative Goals intervention (Wheeler, 1987). Both classroom simulation experiences and implementation under the supervision of a board-certified music therapist are recommended before attempting this technique with clients.

In order to fully benefit from song transformation, the patient must have some insight into their situation and the ability to think abstractly. The music therapist can adapt the song transformation to support the strengths and work within the skills of the client.

Preparation. The music therapist will prepare for the session by considering the issues relevant to the group or population and the culture, age range, and music preferences of the group. Then, the music therapist will select a song that can be modified by removing words or phrases from the song and leaving remaining lyrics as prompts. The intervention can be conducted as a group working on one song, or each individual can create their own song. The music therapist should consider the reading level of the group or individual when determining the materials to be used in the session. When preparing for the session, the music therapist should consider many possible responses to verify the functionality of the template. Additionally, lyrics and prompts should be modified for inclusion, e.g., changing the *girl I love* to the *one I love* or *he was standing there* to *you were standing there*. See Appendix E for a sample song transformation template. Clipboards can be useful if the music therapist invites each group member to create lyrics individually.

What to observe. During the intervention, the music therapist listens for themes in the client's responses to the songs and responds by furthering the client's exploration of the theme.

Procedures. In a group setting, the music therapist must discuss confidentiality and privacy concerns with group members. After the explanation, it can be helpful for each individual to give a verbal confirmation at the beginning and end of the session that the privacy of their peers will be respected. Individuals may also wish to discuss their concerns in generalities while still focusing on feelings, e.g., "The lyrics of this song remind me about when I felt sad when I separated from my loved one." This technique keeps the group focus on feelings and helps protect the client's privacy.

Frequently, the music therapist will present the intact song in order to familiarize the group with its style, mood, melody, and rhythmic flow. If the song has several blanks for the client to add personalized lyrics, the music therapist will usually invite the group members to fill in lyrics for a few blanks at a time. It can be helpful for the music therapist to hum the melody while the group members are creating their lyrics so that the musical qualities of the song remain clear. Volunteers can then offer to read or sing their lyrics aloud with the music therapist. Then, the next section of the song can be addressed. This process continues until the song is completed. While many group members will want to keep their transformed song, the music therapist could take a photo of the completed lyrics for assessment and documentation purposes. The photo should not contain information that would link the file to the group member.

Adaptations. When the individual or group is ready, the music therapist may facilitate songwriting. Generally, the process is collaborative, involving the music therapist and clients in the decision-making process. Usually, the theme is selected first, followed by musical elements such as style, accompaniment, key, and melody. Lyrics are then set to the chosen melodic line. At times, the lyrics may be generated first, perhaps as a poem, and then set to the melody. It is helpful for the music therapist to offer closed choices for musical elements such as accompaniment and key, e.g., playing a chord progression in a major key and another in a minor key for the individual(s) to choose between for the song. When songwriting, it is easy for the music therapist to spend too much time in verbal interaction about the song, so it is useful to frequently refer to the musical elements of the song, i.e., singing the melody on a neutral syllable when determining song lyrics or playing through the chord progression to keep the experience grounded in the selected musical style. Often the finished song will be recorded and the final product shared with loved ones.

RESEARCH

Receptive Music Therapy

Medical professionals have conducted most of the research involving music listening as the independent variable. The care given to the selection of the music used in these studies varies. In a study of the effectiveness of music listening on pain, anxiety, physiological parameters, and opioid consumption for patients recovering from cardiac surgery, Sendelbach, Halm, Doran, Miller, and Gaillard (2006) randomly assigned 50 participants to a music-listening protocol and 36 participants to a control condition of quiet, uninterrupted rest. The participants in the music group listened to 20 minutes of music two times a day on postoperative days 1 to 3. The investigators carefully selected music that had no dramatic changes, was consonant, was instrumental, and was between 60 and 70 beats per minute. Within these criteria, the participants could select from easy listening, classical, and jazz genres. Measures of the dependent variables were taken before and after each condition. No significant differences were found for systolic blood pressure, diastolic blood pressure, heart rate, and opioid use. Results indicated significant reductions in perceived pain (p = .009) and anxiety (p < .001) between groups. The investigators concluded that the psychological benefits of music listening after cardiac surgery may be of greatest benefit to patients (Sendelbach et al., 2006).

In an attempt to compare the possible differential effects of guided relaxation with music, music listening only, and control with rest, but no music, Schou (2009) implemented a study for patients after cardiac surgery. The 63 participants ranged in age from 40 to 80 years of age. The participants in the two music conditions selected from four styles: (1) easy listening, (2) classical, (3) music composed for relaxation, and (4) jazz. The music choices for the guided relaxation with music and the music listening groups were chosen by the investigator for stability and predictability of music elements and for the targeted tempo range of 60 to 70 beats per minute. Each participant in the two music groups listened to an excerpt of each choice and then selected the one to be played at each of their individual sessions. Sessions occurred once before surgery and three times after surgery. Measures included self-report of anxiety, pain, mood, and the importance of rest/relaxation, music, and the guiding procedures.

In her presentation, Schou (2009) indicated that, while there were no significant differences among the groups for each dependent variable, information regarding the music chosen for the sessions yielded important information for music therapists. Specifically, the investigator reported that 57% chose easy listening, 30% chose classical, 13% chose music specifically composed for relaxation, and none chose the jazz selection. She speculated that the low percentage of selection of the music for relaxation and the jazz selection might have been due to the contemporary nature of the choices and/or the age of the participants. Participants in the music groups were asked to rate the importance of musical elements to their experience of relaxation and chose the tempo as the most important musical element for their relaxation. They rated familiarity as a variable of less importance. She concluded that, in addition to knowing how to select music for relaxation purposes, the music therapist must be very familiar with the music selection in order to fit the verbal guiding to the music, including the phrasing and the length of the piece. She also stated that the music therapist must also be aware that, while many patients might enjoy the sessions, some may not like it at all, which would be contraindicated for the purposes of relaxation and stress management.

To synthesize the wide variety of interventions and protocols in the literature, Bradt and Dileo (2009) completed a Cochrane Review of music for individuals with coronary heart disease. They reviewed the findings of randomized controlled trials (N = 23) on the effect of music with this population, but most of these studies (N = 22) were classified as music-medicine studies using receptive music listening conducted by medical personnel for inpatients undergoing a medical procedure.

Based on their findings, Bradt and Dileo (2009) concluded that music listening may have a moderate effect on anxiety, but other areas of psychological distress were not shown to have strong evidence for the efficacy of music listening as an intervention. Physiological measures, including heart rate, respiratory rate, and blood pressure, may be affected by music and music may have a pain-reducing effect if two or more sessions are conducted. One consideration is that most of the studies used prerecorded, rather than live, music for the intervention. Additionally, some studies gave little information about the music used or the selection procedure. The authors indicated a need for further research and a need for research involving music therapy conducted by trained music therapists prepared to address the specialized emotional needs of this population.

Individuals with cardiac care needs often participate in cardiac rehabilitation programs. Mandel (1996) described a music therapy program for these individuals that included music-assisted relaxation and imagery (MARI). All patients participated in one educational program during their 12-week program using music for relaxation purposes. During this program, the patients discussed stress and were instructed in music-assisted relaxation and imagery (MARI). A physician, nurse, exercise physiologist, family member, music therapist, or patient could then make a referral to participate in individual sessions or a multiweek small-group music therapy program focusing on stress management, music-assisted relaxation, and social support. Six biweekly outpatient sessions were offered. Family members could participate in any part of the program and were encouraged to learn and practice the music-assisted relaxation techniques as well.

Several music therapy interventions were used in this program (Mandel, 1996). Both live and recorded music were used to support discussion and to explore feelings. Songs were selected to be relevant to an individual's situation or to general stressors of the population. Interventions included song lyric writing, interpretation of song lyrics, and selection of songs relevant to each person's experience. The investigator also recorded MARI scripts over recorded music for home practice. The author concluded that the program was beneficial to the participants (Mandel, 1996).

Using the music therapy protocol developed by Mandel (1996), Mandel, Hanser, Secic, and Davis (2007) designed a randomized controlled trial to determine the effectiveness of the music therapy intervention on physiological and psychological dependent variables. Sixty-eight people between the ages of 30 and 80 years old participated in this study. The participants were randomly assigned to the control group, which received the standard cardiac rehabilitation programming, or to the treatment group, which received standard care plus music therapy services. Physiological measures were diastolic and systolic blood pressure. Psychological measures were the State-Trait Anxiety Inventory (STAI-T), the Center for Epidemiologic Studies Depression Scale (CES-D), the Brief Symptom Inventory (BSI), the Medical Outcomes Study 36-item Short-Form Survey (SF-36), stress analogue scale, and anecdotal reports. Participants attended between four and six sessions every other week for 1.5 hours each session. The protocol consisted of several elements, including an opening song, a check-in, group work, active music-making, MARI practice, and reminder of homework assignment to practice MARI techniques at home.

In terms of the physiological hypotheses, the investigators noted that the music therapy group evidenced lower systolic blood pressure than the control group (p = .03). Regarding the psychological variables, the investigators retained the null hypotheses. Upon four-month follow-up, the music therapy group did evidence statistically significant improved functioning in anxiety, general health, and social functioning, although the investigators advised caution as some members of the wait-list control group were unavailable for comparison as they had already begun participating in music therapy. The groups were not statistically different from each other in terms of depression immediately after the study or at four-month follow-up. The authors concluded that a period of at least a month is needed to develop new stress management practices. The study did not control for the effect of the individual attention of the therapist. The investigators suggested assigning at least 75 participants to each condition and controlling for the individual attention of the therapist if the study is replicated (Mandel et al., 2007).

In a follow-up study to Mandel et al. (2007), Mandel (2007) designed a nonrandomized study to investigate the effect of MARI on blood pressure, anxiety, stress, depression, and health-related quality of life for patients (N = 15) participating in a cardiac rehabilitation program. The dependent variables and measures were similar to the previous study (Mandel et al., 2007) except that the BSI was not included. The data sources of behavioral observations during MARI and narratives of patient experiences were added. Another difference between the two studies was that the intervention was MARI-only without therapeutic intervention. In the previous study, the intervention included active music-making and therapeutic intervention of the music therapist.

Following the first MARI training session, significant differences were found for all variables except diastolic blood pressure, yet at the two-week and four-month follow-ups, no significant differences were found for any of the variables. Several questions were raised in the analysis section, including the clinical relevance of the significant findings after the initial session. Also, it is unclear if the nonsignificant blood pressure responses were due to the lack of therapeutic involvement, the variability of individual responses, or the small sample size. Another question was whether the significant results after the training session were due to the intervention or the presence of the therapist, even though she was instructed not to interact in a therapeutic manner. The author concluded that more research is needed about the effect of music therapy on this population, particularly since several of the participants could have benefitted from therapeutic involvement in the form of additional coaching, individualized recordings, preferred music, and emotional processing (Mandel, 2007).

In a study to determine if women graduate students could benefit from a music-assisted relaxation (MAR) program in terms of their stress level, anxiety, and mood state, Fu (2008) recruited 32 participants with an age range of 23 to 42 who were not currently taking medications for psychiatric conditions. Two 20-minute sessions were provided for each participant; one session was MAR, and the other was nonmusic. The measures were the STAI Y-1 for anxiety and the Profile of Mood States–Short Form (POMS-SF; McNair, Lorr, & Droppleman, 1992) for mood, blood pressure, and heart rate. Results indicated that there were significant differences between interventions for anxiety as measured by the STAI Y-1 and the tension-anxiety subscale of POMS-SF. Additionally, the results indicated that the MAR intervention increased the participants' vigor as measured by the vigor subscale of POMS-SF.

In order to further investigate the effect of music therapy on psychological risk factors of heart disease, Leist (2011) implemented a research study to examine the effect of a music therapy support group on depression, anxiety, anger/hostility, and stress of adults with coronary heart disease. Participants were randomly assigned to the music therapy experimental group or the wait-list comparison group. Depression, anxiety, anger/hostility, and total mood disturbance were measured with Profile of Mood States–Short Form (POMS-SF). Stress was measured with the intensity value of Hassles Scale (HS; Kanner, Coyne, Schaefer, & Lazarus, 1981). The measures were administered at pretest, posttest, and four-week follow-up. Seven women and six men (n = 13) with a mean age of 68 years completed the protocol through follow-up

Music therapy sessions were held weekly for six weeks and lasted for 1.5 hours. The purpose of the group was to improve participant functioning in the areas of identification and expression of the feelings. The sessions included active and receptive music therapy experiences consisting of an opening check-in, music-assisted relaxation (MAR), active music therapy interventions, and a closing. The active music therapy interventions included expressive singing, song lyric analysis, songwriting, and instrumental improvisation. The results indicated that there was no difference between groups at all data collection points for the depression, anger/hostility, and stress-dependent variables. For total mood disturbance, there was a marginally significant difference between groups. A post-hoc t-test between groups showed that there was a significant difference between groups at posttest, $t(1) = -2.41$, $p = .03$, that was not sustained at follow-up. For tension-anxiety, the repeated measures ANOVA indicated a group by time interaction that approached significance, $p = .06$. A simple effects analysis revealed that the participants in the experimental group reported a significant decrease in tension-anxiety at posttest, which was no longer present at follow-up. In an unanticipated finding, the experimental group reported a significant increase in vigor-activity at posttest that was not sustained at follow-up (Leist, 2011).

Individuals often listen to music while exercising, but does the music increase the effectiveness of the exercise, length of time spent exercising, or the individual's perception of the experience? The premise is that the more enjoyable the exercise, the more likely the person will be to continue exercising, which is of critical importance in cardiac care. To explore these ideas, MacNay (1995) investigated the effect of preferred music on perceived exertion, mood, and time estimation measures of four patients in a cardiac rehabilitation program. The treatment was listening to preferred music while exercising. The investigator concluded that the music listening did have a positive effect on all variables. Mood, as measured by a visual analogue scale, was identified as the most affected by the music.

In another study to determine the effect of music listening on perceived exertion and mood of individuals in cardiac rehabilitation following coronary bypass graft surgery, Murrock (2002) selected a classical music compilation CD because of its "upbeat tempo (128–160 bpm) and classical style of music, and because of the patients' ethnic backgrounds and ages" (p. 229). Thirty participants, 52 to 84 years old, were randomly assigned to the exercise with music group and the exercise without music group. Participants completed pretest and posttest measures of perceived exertion at each of 10 exercise sessions lasting 40 minutes each. While the music and exercise group did differ significantly in terms of perceived exertion, they did report significantly enhanced mood, whereas the exercise and no music group reported decreased mood.

In a study designed to determine secondary benefits of music listening while exercising, participants were asked to exercise on a treadmill while listening to music on headphones or without music (Emery, Hsiao, Hill, & Frid, 2003). The investigators were attempting to determine if exercising to music could be beneficial in enhancing cognitive performance by a verbal fluency task and mood functioning by POMS-SF in people in cardiac rehabilitation. Thirty-three participants, both male and female, completed the study. The investigators selected Vivaldi's "Four Seasons" for its moderate tempo and rhythmic features. The results indicated that verbal fluency was improved with the music condition and symptoms of depression were reduced in both conditions. The authors speculate that the exercise itself could have reduced the symptoms of depression since both groups experienced a reduction in symptoms without a significant difference between conditions.

In an article about the results of a survey of patients in a cardiac rehabilitation program regarding their uses of music for exercise, relaxation, and enjoyment, Metzger (2004) concluded that patients are open to using music and music therapy in their lives, but that few used music as a cue for exercise (i.e., matching the pace of walking to the beat of the music). The patients did indicate using music as a motivator for exercise, though. The author suggested that there is a need for more education about the possible uses of music for this population and that information about music preferences and uses of music by participants should be gathered prior to initiating a program (Metzger, 2004).

Improvisational Music Therapy

Currently, there is one study that used instrumental improvisation as part of the music therapy intervention for adults with cardiac care needs. The Leist (2011) study is described fully in the previous section about music-assisted relaxation. Instrumental improvisation was implemented weekly for six weeks as part of a support that also included music-assisted relaxation, expressive singing, and compositional music therapy. Participants reported benefitting from the use of instruments in the session (Leist, 2011).

Re-creative Music Therapy

Two music therapy studies include the use of expressive singing with patients with cardiac care needs (Leist, 2011; Mandel et al., 2007). Another article describes the use of expressive singing with an outpatient cardiac rehabilitation group (Mandel, 1996). All three sources are described in detail in the previous section about music-assisted relaxation. In each case, the songs were used to literally express the topic, serve as a metaphor for the topic, or deepen or explore the topic.

Compositional Music Therapy

Two music therapy studies include the use of compositional music therapy with patients with cardiac care needs (Leist, 2011; Mandel et al., 2007). Another article describes the use of compositional music therapy with an outpatient cardiac rehabilitation group (Mandel, 1996). All three sources are described in detail in the previous section about music-assisted relaxation. In each case, the compositions were used to literally express the topic, serve as a metaphor for the topic, or deepen or explore the topic.

Summary and Conclusions

While music therapy may implemented across all levels of music therapy and method categories for this population, music therapists most often work at the Insight Music Therapy with Re-educative Goals level (Wheeler, 1987) through mostly receptive (Leist, 2011; Mandel, 1996, 2007; Mandel et al., 2007; Schou, 2009), re-creative, and compositional methods (Leist, 2011; Mandel, 1996; Mandel et al., 2007). Only one study investigated instrumental improvisational music therapy for this population (Leist) and none addressed vocal improvisation specifically. Advanced training is required for Guided Imagery and Music, which is the only intervention in this chapter considered reconstructive in nature. See below for a visual summary of levels, method categories, and music therapy interventions presented in this chapter.

- Level I: Activity-Oriented
    - Receptive Music Therapy
        - Music Listening
        - Music and Exercise
- Level II: Insight-Oriented with Re-educative Goals
    - Receptive Music Therapy
        - Music-assisted Relaxation
    - Improvisational Music Therapy
        - Instrumental Improvisation
        - Vocal Improvisation
    - Recreative Music Therapy
        - Expressive Singing
    - Compositional
        - Song transformation
        - Songwriting
- Level III: Insight-Oriented with Reconstructive Goals
    - Receptive
        - Guided Imagery and Music

Certainly further research is needed to investigate the effects of music therapy for this population. Possible research areas include further investigation of the importance of therapeutic intervention in conjunction with music-assisted relaxation (Mandel, 2007). Also, research into the possible differential effects for men and women or for types of cardiac illness (Leist, 2011) is warranted. For music listening and music with exercise where music therapists often serve as consultants, research could be conducted to determine the most effective delivery of the music, the selection criteria, and the dosage needed for positive mood effects suggested in the literature (Murrock, 2002). Music listening and music with exercise will continue to be offered to patients so music therapists need to have input into its administration. In terms of improvisational, re-creative, and compositional interventions, these have been studied only as part of a music therapy protocol containing all four types of interventions (Leist, 2011; Mandel, 1996; Mandel et al., 2007). Perhaps music therapists could investigate the differential effects of each of the three methods to determine if any are more effective than others.

Since lifestyle change and enhancement are at the heart of current treatment for patients with cardiac illness (Billings et al., 1996) and the key to transformative life change is emotional functioning (Dornelas, 2008), then music therapy is indicated for this population. As more research is implemented and lives changed, then there will be more evidence for the short-term, and hopefully long-term, effects of music therapy.

References

American Heart Association. (2012). *Conditions*. Retrieved from http://www.heart.org

American Institute of Stress. (2011). *Definitions of stress*. Retrieved from http://www.stress.org

Billings, J. H., Scherwitz, L. W., Sullivan, R., Sparler, S., & Ornish, D. (1996). The lifestyle heart trial: Comprehensive treatment and group support therapy. In R. Allan & S. Scheidt (Eds.), *Heart and mind: the practice of cardiac psychology* (pp. 233–253). Washington, DC: American Psychological Association.

Bonny, H. (1983). Music listening for intensive coronary care units: A pilot project. *Music Therapy, 3,* 4–16.

Borg, G. (1998). *Borg's rating of perceived exertion and pain scales*. Champaign, IL: Human Kinetics.

Bradt, J., & Dileo, C. (2009). Music for stress and anxiety reduction in coronary heart disease patients. (Review). *Cochrane Database of Systematic Reviews 2009*(2), 1–77.

Bruscia, K. E. (1987). *Improvisational models of music therapy*. Springfield, IL: Charles C Thomas Publishers.

Bruscia, K. E. (2002). Preface: An opening metaphor. In K. E. Bruscia & D. E. Grocke (Eds.), *Guided imagery and music: The Bonny method and beyond* (pp. ix–xxiv). Gilsum, NH: Barcelona Publishers.

Bruscia, K. E., & Grocke, D. E. (2002). *Guided imagery and music: The Bonny method and beyond.* Gilsum, NH: Barcelona Publishers.

Cleveland Clinic (2012). *Diseases and conditions*. Retrieved from http://www.my.clevelandclinic.org

Dornelas, E. A. (2008). *Psychotherapy with cardiac patients: Behavioral cardiology in practice.* Washington, DC: American Psychological Association.

Dunn, S. L. (2005). Hopelessness and depression in myocardial infarction. Doctoral dissertation. Michigan State University. *Dissertation Abstracts International, 66,* 4724.

Friedman, R., Myers, P., Krass, S., & Benson, H. (1996). The relaxation response: Use with cardiac patients. In R. Allan & S. Scheidt (Eds.), *Heart and Mind: The Practice of Cardiac Psychology* (pp. 363–384). Washington, DC: American Psychological Association.

Fu, C. M. (2008). *Music therapy and women's health: Effects of music-assisted relaxation on women graduate students' stress and anxiety levels.* Unpublished master's thesis. Michigan State University, East Lansing, MI.

Gerweck, J. S., & Tan, X. (2010). Intensive care unit. In D. Hanson-Abromeit & C. Colwell (Eds.), *Medical music therapy for adults in hospital settings* (pp. 97–160). Silver Spring, MD: American Music Therapy Association.

Grocke, D., & Wigram, T. (2007). *Receptive methods in music therapy: Techniques and clinical applications for music therapy clinicians, educators, and students.* Philadelphia, PA: Jessica Kingsley Publishers.

Hanser, S. B., & Mandel, S. E. (2005). The effects of music therapy in cardiac healthcare. *Cardiology in Review, 13*(1), 18–23. DOI: 10.1097/01.crd.0000126085.76415.d7.

Hanson-Abromeit, D. (2010). Introduction to medical music therapy. In D. Hanson-Abromeit & C. Colwell (Eds.), *Medical music therapy for adults in hospital settings* (pp. 3–17). Silver Spring, MD: American Music Therapy Association.

Herrmann-Lingen, C., & Buss, U. (2007). Anxiety and depression in patients with coronary heart disease. In J. Jordan, B. Barde, & M. Zeiher (Eds.), *Contributions toward evidence-based psychocardiology: A systematic review of the literature* (pp. 125–157). Washington, DC: American Psychological Association.

Kanner, A. D., Coyne, J. C., Schaefer, C., & Lazarus, R. S. (1981). Comparison of two modes of stress measurement: Daily hassles and uplifts versus major life events. *Journal of Behavioral Medicine, 4*(1), 1–25.

Leist, C. P. (2011). *A music therapy support group to ameliorate psychological distress in adults with coronary heart disease in a rural community.* Unpublished doctoral dissertation. Michigan State University, E. Lansing, MI.

Lett, H. S., Blumental, J. A., Babyak, M. A., Strauman, T. J., Robins, C., & Sherwood, A. (2005). Social support and coronary heart disease: Epidemiologic evidence and implications for treatment. *Psychosomatic Medicine, 67*, 869–878.

MacNay, S. K. (1995). The influence of preferred music on the perceived exertion, mood, and time estimation scores of patients participating in a cardiac rehabilitation exercise program. *Music Therapy Perspectives, 13*(2), 91–96.

Mandel, S. E. (1996). Music for wellness: Music therapy for stress management in a rehabilitation program. *Music Therapy Perspectives, 14*(1), 38–43.

Mandel, S. E. (2007). Effects of music-assisted relaxation and imagery (MARI) on health-related outcomes in cardiac rehabilitation: Follow-up study. Doctoral dissertation. Union Institute and University, 2007. *Dissertation Abstracts International, 68*, 5179.

Mandel, S. E., Hanser, S. B., Secic, M., & Davis, B. A. (2007). Effects of music therapy on health-related outcomes in cardiac rehabilitation: A randomized controlled trial. *Journal of Music Therapy, 44* (3), 176–197.

McNair, D. M., Lorr, M. & Droppleman, L. F. (1992). Edits Manual: Profile of mood states. San Diego, CA: Educational and Industrial Testing Service.

Melzack, R., & Torgerson, W. S. (1971). On the language of pain. *Anesthesiology, 23*, 50.

Metzger, L. K. (2004). Assessment of use of music by patients participating in cardiac rehabilitation. *Journal of Music Therapy, 41*(1), 55–69.

Murrock, C. J. (2002). The effects of music on the rate of perceived exertion and general mood among coronary artery bypass graft patients enrolled in cardiac rehabilitation phase II. *Rehabilitation Nursing, 27*(6), 227–231.

Rhodes, J. E. (2004). Family, friends, and community: The role of social support in promoting health. In P. M. Camic & S. J. Knight (Eds.), *Clinical handbook of health psychology: A practical guide to effective interventions* (2nd rev., pp. 289–296). Cambridge, MA: Hogrefe & Huber Publishers.

Schou, K. (2009, May). *Music therapy for postoperative cardiac patients—with a special focus on the music.* Paper presented at the meeting of the Nordic Music Therapy Association, Aalborg, Denmark.

Sendelbach, S. E., Halm, M. A., Doran, K. A., Miller, E. H., & Gaillard, P. (2006). Effects of music therapy on physiological and psychological outcomes for patients undergoing cardiac surgery. *Journal of Cardiovascular Nursing, 21*(3), 194–200.

Short, A., Gibb, H., & Holmes, C. (2011). Integrating words, images, and text in BMGIM: Finding connections through semiotic intertextuality. *Nordic Journal of Music Therapy, 20*(1), 3–21.

Sotile, W. M. (1996). *Psychosocial interventions for cardiopulmonary patients*. Champaign, IL: Human Kinetics.

Strodl, E., Kenardy, J., & Aroney, C. (2003). Perceived stress as a predictor of the self-reported new diagnosis of symptomatic coronary heart disease in older women. *International Journal of Behavioral Medicine, 10*(3), 205–220. Retrieved from http://ehis.ebscohost.com/ehost/pdfviewer/pdfviewer?hid=14&sid=5240509a-6707-4522-bcfc-ca974b3a0e8a%40sessionmgr4&vid=6

University of Southern California School of Medicine. (2012). *Cardiothoracic surgery*. Retrieved from www.cts.usc.edu

Wheeler, B. L. (1987). Levels of therapy: The classification of music therapy goals. *Music Therapy, 6*, 39–49.

Williams, M. A., & Steele, M. G. (2005). Assessment and treatment of psychosocial issues with cardiac patients. In L. Vandecreek & J. B. Allen (Eds.), *Innovations in clinical practice: Focus on health and wellness* (pp. 85–104). Sarasota, FL: Professional Resource Press.

APPENDIX A

Dear participants: Please take a moment to complete this survey about the music therapy group. This survey will be anonymous. Please do not put your name or any identifying information on this survey. Thanks, Christine Leist

For items, 1–13, please circle ONE answer for each item.

1. How many music therapy groups did you attend? 1 2 3 4 5 6

2. The music and relaxation instruction and practice was helpful to me.

1	2	3	4	5
Strongly Disagree	Disagree	Neutral	Agree	Strongly Agree

3. I will use the music and relaxation process in the future to decrease stress.

1	2	3	4	5
Strongly Disagree	Disagree	Neutral	Agree	Strongly Agree

4. Music therapy helped me feel more comfortable expressing my feelings.

1	2	3	4	5
Strongly Disagree	Disagree	Neutral	Agree	Strongly Agree

5. Music therapy helped me feel more comfortable listening to and supporting the feelings of others.

1	2	3	4	5
Strongly Disagree	Disagree	Neutral	Agree	Strongly Agree

6. The music therapist listened to me and supported my work in the group.

1	2	3	4	5
Strongly Disagree	Disagree	Neutral	Agree	Strongly Agree

7. Singing songs about feelings and issues was helpful to me.

1	2	3	4	5
Strongly Disagree	Disagree	Neutral	Agree	Strongly Agree

8. Discussing songs about feelings and issues was helpful to me.

1	2	3	4	5
Strongly Disagree	Disagree	Neutral	Agree	Strongly Agree

9. Writing songs about feelings and issues was helpful to me.

1	2	3	4	5
Strongly Disagree	Disagree	Neutral	Agree	Strongly Agree

10. Engaging in music improvisation with instruments and voice was helpful to me.

1	2	3	4	5
Strongly Disagree	Disagree	Neutral	Agree	Strongly Agree

11. I would recommend this group to other individuals with heart-related medical conditions.

1	2	3	4	5
Strongly Disagree	Disagree	Neutral	Agree	Strongly Agree

12. Please evaluate the hour and a half session length by choosing one choice below.

1	2	3
Too Short	Just Right	Too Long

13. Please evaluate the six-week length of time for the music therapy sessions by choosing one choice below.

1	2	3
Too Short	Just Right	Too Long

14. What was the <u>most beneficial</u> part of the music therapy group?

15. What was the <u>least beneficial</u> part of the music therapy group?

16. Other comments:

Appendix B

Example of Progressive Muscle Relaxation

Album: *The Segovia Collection,* Vol. 1; Andres Segovia, Guitar, track 10
J. S. Bach, Suite No. 3 (for solo cello; arranged by Duarte), IV. Sarabande. (4:22)

Preparation:
Check-in about the choice of image, can open eyes, dismiss unwelcome thoughts ...
Will last approximately ...
Close eyes and comfortable position ...
Breathing ... relaxation to body, center, back, hips, legs, calves, feet, shoulders, neck, face, hands, fingers, continues to relax you.

Music:
Focus on muscles of feet ... tense ... tighter ... tighter ... release and feel relaxation
Tense muscles of right leg ... up to hip ... tense ... tighter ... tighter ... release and feel relaxation
Tense muscles of left leg ... up to hip ... tighter ... tighter ... release and feel relaxation
Tense muscles of pelvis through lower back ... tense ... tighter ... tighter ... release and feel relaxation
Tense muscles of stomach and chest ... tense ... tighter ... tighter ... (continue)
Tense muscles of shoulders by pulling them up to your ears ...
Tense muscles of arms ...
Tense muscles of hands ...
Tense muscles of face ...
Be aware of how the body feels ... Feel your body fully relaxed.

Bringing the client back to an "alert" state:
Music has ended for now ... Turn awareness back ... aware of breath... Own pace ... open eyes ...
Take some quiet time to reflect ...

APPENDIX C

EXAMPLE OF AUTOGENIC MUSIC-ASSISTED RELAXATION

Image: Healing Light (contraindicated for people with near-death experience)
Antarctica Echoes (Vangelis, 1983, track 2). (5:54)

Preparation:
Check-in about the choice of image, can open eyes, dismiss unwelcome thoughts ...
Will last approximately ...
Close eyes and comfortable position ...
Breathing ... relaxation to body, center, back, hips, legs, calves, feet, shoulders, neck, face, hands, fingers, continues to relax you.
Let your breath ... A ball of healing light ... notice its form and texture ... bring with you into the music.

Music:
Time:

0:00	Feet ... Draw in and fill ...
0:39	Both legs ... draw in and fill ... (1:00) knees, upper part of legs ... hips ... bringing what your body needs
1:36	Lower back ... draw in and fill ... to stomach ... as much as it needs ...
2:15	Chest ... draw in and fill ... to shoulders ... arms ... fingers ... bringing what your body needs
3:05	Gently through neck ... draw in and fill ... jaw ... cheeks ... eyes ... as much as it needs
3:50	Entire body ... area needs more color ... take it there ... Entire body ... what it needs ...
5:00	(time to imagine)

Bringing the client back to an "alert" state:
Music has ended for now ... Turn awareness back ... aware of breath ... Own pace ... open eyes ...
Take some quiet time to reflect ...

APPENDIX D

EXAMPLE OF IMAGE-BASED MUSIC-ASSISTED RELAXATION

Image: Sunrise
The Swan (Saint-Saens, 2007, track 8). (3:00)

Preparation:
Check-in about the choice of image, can open eyes, dismiss unwelcome thoughts ...
Will last approximately ...
Close eyes and comfortable position ...
Breathing ... relaxation to body, center, back, hips, legs, calves, feet, shoulders, neck, face, hands. Find yourself in a comfortable, safe place to enjoy the sunrise.

Music:
Look around you ...See the drops of dew on the grass
See the leaves on the trees move in the gentle breeze
Breathe in the clean air of sunrise
Listen to the birds in the trees
Feel the calm and peace of this moment
Notice the rays of the sun peaking through the clouds
The light is gold and pink with the energy of the sunrise
Feel the slight warmth of the sun of your skin
2:00 Enjoy this moment with the sunrise
2:40 Let its warmth bring you energy for your day

Bringing the client back to an "alert" state:
Music has ended for now ... Turn awareness back ... aware of breath ... Own pace ... open eyes ... Take some quiet time to reflect ...

Appendix E

Song Transformation Example: "Kansas City Blues" by Lieber & Stoller, 1958.

I'm going to ____.
(a goal you would like to accomplish)

That's what I'm gonna do.

I'm going to ____.
(same goal as first blank)

That's what I'm gonna do.

I've got ______________________ and _________________________
(a strength or skill you have) (another strength or skill you have)

I'm goin' ____.
(a benefit of working toward your goal)

Well, it might take____.
(a strategy needed for working toward your goal)

And it might take ____.
(a strategy needed for working toward your goal)

If I have to ____,
(something you might not want to do, but may have to do)

I'm goin' to get there just the same!

I'm going to ____.
(same goal as first blank)

That's what I'm gonna do.

I'm going to ____.
(same goal as first blank)

That's what I'm gonna do!

Chapter 6

Adults with Stroke

Simon Gilbertson

Stroke is one of the many diseases that can suddenly and dramatically affect the health of a human being. The changes to the structures and functions of the arteries and veins of our bodies caused by a stroke highlight the fragility and complexity of the human predicament. When the channels of our blood, and with them the essential nutrition of oxygen and nutrients, become blocked or ruptured, our lives become at risk. We become at risk of losing life completely or losing the lives that we have lived up to those traumatic moments of cellular failure. It is from this fragility that survivors of a stroke move forward in their lives. This chapter focuses on how music has been used in diverse ways in therapy to support these patients on their path of recovery.

Diagnostic Information

The brain connects within itself and within the body via a combination of single cells and neurons, which are grouped together; these groups are referred to as axons. Axons are organized in the form of tracts that connect the brain via the spinal cord, the peripheral nervous system, and the environment (Widmaier, Raff, & Strang, 2006). The communication of information within the central nervous system is performed by way of intercellular electrochemical activity, a process that requires nutrition to generate energy and to operate successfully. It is here that the role of unimpaired blood flow is important. It is the integrity of the arterial structures and function that is essential for the continuance of life both at singular cellular level and as an organism as a whole. As Widmaier, Riff, and Strang (2006) describe,

> [u]nder normal conditions, glucose is the only substrate metabolized by the brain to supply its energy requirements, and most of the energy from the oxidative breakdown of glucose is transferred to ATP. Since the brain's glucogen stores are negligible, it depends on a continuous blood supply of glucose and oxygen. In fact, the most common form of brain damage is caused by a decreased blood supply to a region of the brain. When neurons in the region are without a blood supply and deprived of the nutrients and oxygen for even a few minutes, they cease to function and die. This neuronal death, when it results from vascular disease, is called stroke. (p. 205)

The term "stroke" is an umbrella term which refers to a large group of diseases and illnesses and has been described as having "more than 150 known causes" (Amarenco et al., 2009, p. 493). Over the past decades, the classifications and subgroups of stroke have changed and evolved mainly in reflection of diagnostic technology and the diagnostic procedures that have been developed by large agencies, including the World Health Organization (WHO, 1978), the National Institutes of Health (NIH, 2012), and the National Institute of Neurological Disorders and Stroke (NINDS, 2009). A recent review of diverse classifications of stroke (Amarenco et al., 2009) identified the core subtypes of stroke:

- *Ischemic stroke:* blockages restricting or prohibiting the flow of blood. This can be caused by arteriosclerosis, where the arteries are narrowed, or by the arteries becoming blocked by a blood clot (embolic stroke).
- *Hemorrhagic stroke:* leakage of blood into and between the structures of the brain caused by the rupturing of arteries.
- *Subarachnoid hemorrhage:* leakage of blood from core arteries within the brain.
- *Cerebral venous thrombosis:* leakage of blood into the channels within the dura mater, layers which cover the brain.
- *Spinal cord stroke:* blockage of blood flow to, or within, the spinal cord. (Amarenco et al., 2009)

The various causes of a stroke are listed in the 2010 International Statistical Classification of Diseases and Related Health Problems in the section of cerebrovascular diseases under the classifications I61–I64 (WHO, 2010). In accord with these classifications, traumatic brain injuries, which include the severance of arteries of the brain, are also causes of hemorrhagic and subarachnoid hemorrhage. This leads to an overlap in some of the literature on effects and symptoms of both stroke and traumatic brain injury and rehabilitation. However, there are distinct differences in recovery and rehabilitation. Some of the treatment procedures and rationales for stroke and traumatic brain injury are shared, and it is advisable to consult these two areas of the literature when exploring treatment possibilities. Although not included in this review on stroke, examples of this aspect include the publication on Modified Melodic Intonation Therapy by Baker (2011), Magee and Wheeler's (2006) chapter on traumatic brain injury, and Schaefer, Murray, Magee, and Wheeler's (2006) chapter on melodic intonation therapy with brain-injured patients, which all hold valuable information and resources that are also relevant for patients following stroke.

In the same way that stroke shares some conceptualization with other diseases/injuries, it is also important to consider that stroke is a global phenomenon. It affects individuals in all regions and countries of the world. Though the factors of risk of stroke are considerably different throughout the world, a focus in the literature—in particular, the music therapy literature—has evolved from particular parts or places in the world. Much of the research and clinical literature pertaining to the treatment of stroke with music originates from a small number of countries, including, but not exclusive to, the USA and UK, Germany, South Korea, and Australia. Much of the internationally available literature on stroke focuses on the work of the World Health Organization in relation to epidemiological data on stroke and on national guidelines created in the USA and UK (WHO, 2002). In terms of the diagnosis of stroke, this bias is also evident, and these countries provide the sources cited in this chapter on the topics of treatment and diagnosis.

The American National Stroke Association, through the promotion of the abbreviation F.A.S.T., has highlighted immediate suspicion of possible stroke occurrence. This acronym refers to changes to a person's ability to smile and whether one side of the face ("F") drops. The letter "A" is used to refer to testing whether one arm drifts downward when the potential victim is asked to lift both arms. "S" is used to assess any changes in speech when asked to repeat a simple sentence. "T" is to remind the observer to call the emergency services at 9-1-1 immediately and write down the time when the symptoms were first noticed (National Stroke Association, 2012).

After the transfer of a patient to emergency services, there are a variety of techniques that are used to diagnose stroke accurately. This includes a behavioral assessment of speech and movement patterns, an assessment of common risk factors (including lack of exercise, increased intake of fatty foods, cigarette smoking, family history of vascular disease), and medical examinations, including blood tests and technology-supported examinations such as viewing the integrity of the arteries of the head and brain using computer tomography, angiography, and magnetic resonance imaging (Amarenco et al., 2009).

One of the major concerns following the initial occurrence is stroke reoccurrence (Fullerton, Sidney, & Johnston, 2007). This is common for both adults and children, for whom the reoccurrence rate lies between 6 and 20 percent for arterial ischemic stroke and over 60 percent for sickle-cell disease (Royal College of Physicians, 2004). This is related to the underlying causes for the initial stroke and highlights the necessity for extensive diagnostic examinations following the initial stroke occurrence. A very useful guide to stroke and stroke recovery can be found in the National Institute for Neurological Disorders and Stroke booklet titled *Stroke: Challenges, Progress, and Promise* (NINDS, 2009).

Epidemiology

The World Health Organization (Murray & Lopez, 1996) has estimated that stroke accounts for approximately 30 percent of the annual total of deaths worldwide, and one study (Wolfe, 2000) has shown that there is a one in four to five chance that a 45-year-old will have a stroke if they live to be 85 years of age. Stroke is a global phenomenon, and the WHO estimated that there were around 20.5 million strokes in 2001 over the whole globe (WHO, 2002).

Although there is a large focus in the literature on the occurrence of stroke in adult age, some authors are pointing out the significance of pediatric stroke as a cause of death and disability (Lopez-Vicente et al., 2010) and noting that "it is among the top 10 causes of child mortality, and the incidences reported in several studies are as high as those for brain tumors" (Simma & Lütschg, 2010, p. 245). In slight contrast to adult stroke, it is important to note that pediatric stroke is caused by a wider diversity of diseases, such as sickle-cell disease and other underlying diseases that provoke the stroke (Royal College of Physicians, 2004). Pediatric strokes can occur during all stages of childhood, including the perinatal period and infant and child phases, with outcomes generally being worse for children under one year of age (NINDS, 2009). It has also been suggested that the estimated cost for the treatment of pediatric stroke was $42 million in 2003 in the United States and that though the overall costs of stroke per patient during the acute phase are similar between adults and children, "the lifetime cost of stroke care may have greater financial impact given the longer life expectancy for a child ... [t]he cost to the family and the larger society can be used as one measure of the effects of current treatments" (Perkins, Stephens, Xiang, & Lo, 2009, pp. 2825–2826). Whereas the focus of many of the authors of literature referred to in this chapter is upon stroke with adult onset, music therapists should not forget that pediatric stroke affects the whole lives of those individuals and that adults presenting to music therapy may in fact have experienced a stroke in childhood. With the increase in survivors of pediatric stroke, this is an important future theme that demands attention.

Needs and Resources

Stroke can cause damage to almost any area of the brain and spinal cord. Because of the nature of the localization of functional and cognitive ability within the brain, the site of damage is directly related to the effects of stroke and the resulting symptoms and disorders. In children and adults, the most common disorders include changes in the areas of movement, speech and language, perception, cognition, and emotion. Essentially, as humans are social beings and these domains are highly utilized in the lives of all humans, these may also be considered as social disorders. In turn, these changes may negatively influence the developmental progression of the patient at a multitude of individual and social layers. In essence, it is important for the therapist and researcher to remember that stroke does not lead to individual symptoms or disorders, but to a set of interrelated symptoms, a symptom matrix.

In addition to focusing on the stroke patient, consideration must be given to the caregivers of those who have experienced a stroke. Because stroke affects communication, independence, and the ability to participate in work and leisure activities and because it is characterized by a change in identity, it is not only the person with the stroke who is affected, but also their families, friends, and acquaintances. Some studies have shown that caregivers of those with a stroke are at increased risk of developing depression, and, contrastingly, for some, caregiving leads to positive changes within the relationship with the individual who had experienced a stroke (Han & Haley, 1999). In this light, it continues to be important to explore therapy and care options for stroke caregivers in the future.

To provide for the needs and wishes of patients following a stroke and their caregivers, a multidisciplinary approach is required. Treatment team members for patients following stroke may include experts in the following areas: physiotherapy, occupational therapy, speech and language therapy, rehabilitation medicine, neuroimaging consultation, neuropsychology, neurosurgical consultation, balneotherapy, sports therapy, art therapy, psychotherapy, music therapy, rehabilitative nursing, and therapeutic gardening (Gilbertson & Ischebeck, 2001).

To achieve successful multidisciplinary therapy for the patient following stroke, much effort must be made on the part of all involved to become familiar with the terminology, procedures, assessment and outcome measurement, documentation, and techniques of those working in a team. Commonly, a lack of time to exchange this information can lead to misunderstandings based on insufficient levels of knowledge of the various therapies. Unequal distribution of power within hierarchical team structures also leads to shifts in treatment concepts, with the prioritization of therapeutic goals becoming based on quantitative aspects of therapy cost and availability and the simple factor of familiarity. Though reading relevant literature and engaging in conversations with team members provides some knowledge of the work of others, direct observation and participation in therapy processes is the best way in which to gain a functional understanding of the work of the therapeutic team. An example of multidisciplinary collaboration can be seen in Knight and Wiese's (2011) discussion of how music can be considered within the field of nursing in poststroke rehabilitation and how disciplines can collaborate and devise a way of considering music and the therapeutic use of music within and between different professions. The patient with stroke profits enormously from collaborative and multidisciplinary therapy, and it is advisable for multidisciplinary teams to invest time and effort in becoming knowledgeable about the possibilities for the patient with stroke.

In terms of resources, patients following stroke have attracted the attention of both music therapists and neuroscientists alike (for an excellent introduction to cognitive neurosciences and music, see Levitin & Tirovolas, 2009). Where neuroscience is increasingly identifying the human brain's capacity to change and develop by means of neuroplasticity, stroke recovery specialists are looking to the neurosciences for rationale for the potential of accessing neuroplastic processes during therapeutic music-making, music listening, and music-supported activities (Baker & Roth, 2004). In essence, it is the patient's resource of neuroplasticity that lies at the foundation of many therapeutic endeavors within music-based practices, which also highlights points of contact between disciplinary boundaries as represented in many significant studies in music therapy (Altenmüller, Marco-Pallares, Münte, & Schneider, 2009; Fujioka et al., 2012; Koelsch, 2009; Rodrigez-Fornells et al., 2009; Rojo et al., 2011; Särkämö et al., 2010; Schlaug, 2009; Schlaug, Marchina, & Notron, 2009; Thaut, 2010).

Music is an ultimately human phenomenon, which

> places unique demands on the nervous system, leading to a strong coupling of perception and action mediated by sensory, motor, and multimodal integrative regions distributed throughout the brain. Furthermore, listening to music and

> making music ("musicking") provokes motions and emotions, improves and increases between-subject communication and interaction, and is considered to be and is experienced as a joyous and rewarding activity. (Schlaug, 2009, p. 372)

From this description of music, it is clear to see that there is a multilayered spectrum of facets of music and music-making which may hold potential for rehabilitative music practices. When considering the rehabilitative potential of music, Schlaug (2009) goes on to state:

> Music is a strong multimodal stimulus that simultaneously transmits visual, auditory, and motoric information to a specialized brain network consisting of fronto-temporal-parietal regions whose components are also part of the putative human mirror-neuron system. Among other functions, this system might support the coupling between perceptual events (visual or auditory) and motor actions (leg, arm/hand, or vocal/articulatory actions). Music might be a special vehicle to engage components of this mirror-neuron system. Furthermore, music might also provide an alternative entry point into a "broken" brain system to remediate impaired neural processes or neural connections by engaging and linking up brain centers that would otherwise not be engaged or linked with each other. (p. 372)

Referral and Assessment

Referral and assessment procedures vary widely within institutions, reflecting local and national practices, guidelines, and regulations. Some models of referral and assessment are based on the team structure itself, where each profession will contribute to an overall assessment of the patient. In some institutions, the medical doctor of the unit is responsible for generating referrals to all therapy modalities. In other situations, case managers are allocated to be responsible for the care of individual patients, whereby the choice of the team member for this is made on a pragmatic basis in relation to the main needs of the patient and the expertise of each team member.

At a national level, the National Institutes for Health have developed the NIH Stroke Scale (NIH, 2011) for the assessment of patients following stroke. The scale covers levels of consciousness, gaze, visual activity, facial palsy, motor activity in the upper and lower extremities, sensory perception, language ability, dysarthria, and visual/spatial neglect and anosognosia (lack of awareness of illness). Other standardized assessment tools in the field of neurorehabilitation include the Glasgow Coma Scale (Teasdale & Jeanette, 1974), Glasgow Outcome Scale (Jeanette & Bond, 1975), Rancho Los Amigos Levels of Cognitive Functioning Scale (Hagen, Malkmus, & Durham, 1987), or Rappaport Disability Rating Scale (Rappaport et al., 1982).

Following many years of clinical and research experience gathered by a team of music therapy clinicians and researchers at the Royal Hospital for Neurodisability in London, the Music Therapy Assessment Tool for Low Awareness States Scale (MATLAS) has been developed for the assessment of patients in neurorehabilitation (Magee, 2007). The scale has been validated and "contains 14 items covering the five behavioral domains consistently included in other assessment formats: motor, communication, arousal, auditory, and visual responsiveness. Each item is categorized hierarchically into levels of observed behavioral responses with a numerical grading. Each level specifies an observable behavior, with definitions of behaviors provided in an accompanying instruction manual" (Magee, 2007, p. 321). The scale is currently (2012) undergoing a change of name from MATLAS to MATDOC to reflect a change in conventional terminology use from "low awareness states" to "disorders of consciousness." The MATDOC assessment scale is uniquely important in the field of music therapy in neurorehabilitation and makes a significant contribution to the multidisciplinary assessment of patients with disorders of consciousness. The use of this scale should be included as a standard procedure in the assessment of patients with disorders of consciousness in neurorehabilitation. Specialist training is available in the application of the scale to ensure the best possible quality of assessment for the patient with a disorder of consciousness.

Though in many instances there may be a multidisciplinary assessment of the initial and primary needs of the patient at time of admission, the referral process may not be systematic in all institutions. Often there are many more patients with symptoms that have been shown to be responsive to music therapy interventions through research for whom there are simply not enough music therapy resources. As David Aldridge pointed out when writing about the development of links and bridges between research and practice within a multidisciplinary field in the mid-1990s, "Some bridges can bring too much activity and overload the inhabitants. My music therapy colleagues have been so successful in their work with postcomatose patients in neurological rehabilitation that they simply cannot provide enough music therapists for the hospital positions. [...] Need has outstripped our training capabilities since the bridge of credibility has been constructed" (Aldridge, 1996, p. 273). In these situations, the assessment and referral process becomes in jeopardy of losing its integrity within the treatment situation. Waiting lists during acute phases of rehabilitation following stroke are not a preferred mechanism, as some research shows that timely and intense intervention leads to most positive results (Hu, Hsu, Yip, Jeng, & Wang, 2010). It is important in this light also to point out that in addition to a focus on acute phase rehabilitation, research has also shown significant benefits from music therapy provision after many years poststroke (Hough, 2010; Jungblut & Aldridge, 2004).

Assessment and referral to music therapy following stroke very much reflects the changing and developing expertise and research results of innovative emerging studies. As a result, the area of assessment and referral to these new interventions may need more attention in research than has been given in the past.

Overview of Methods and Procedures

In many health contexts, a dynamic exists between the promotion of guidelines solely based on research evidence which is of an accepted and particular type and practices that have evolved eclectically in a pioneering fashion. In some instances, treatment has been based on the evidence-based medicine and practice models that evolved during the 1990s (Sackett, Rosenberg, Gray, Haynes, & Richardson, 1996) that coincided with early pioneering work in music therapy and neurorehabilitation (for examples, see Erdonmez, 1991; Gilbertson, 1998; McMaster, 1991; Purdie & Baldwin, 1994, 1995; Purdie, Hamilton, & Baldwin, 1997; Thaut, McIntosh, Prassas, & Rice, 1992; Thaut, Kenyon, Schauer, & McIntosh, 1999). With a significant emphasis on patient safety and the integrity of treatment standards, the influence of evidence-based medicine on the area of the subject of this chapter, namely stroke, reflects many of the values and categorizations of the medical model of treatment (Barnes, 2000) and medical model in neurological rehabilitation (Hömberg, 2005).

In the field of music therapy and acquired brain injury, there is a wide diversity in the levels of evidence for methods and techniques. As discussed in the later section on efficacy studies, only a small number of methods have been researched at all, and even a smaller, but highly significant, number of methods have received the research attention sufficient to propose their use based on an acceptable body of evidence. There are some exceptions, and Michael Thaut's (2008) core publication, titled *Rhythm, Music and the Brain,* is an excellent example of how research can be designed and carried out in a way that facilitates the development of accepted clinical methods and at the same time generates rationales for practice and research that can reach far into the future. In their core reference publication titled *Music Therapy Methods in Neurorehabilitation: A Clinician's Manual* (2006), Felicity Baker and Jeanette Tamplin have also made an excellent contribution in which they describe how

> [m]ost of the techniques have emerged from our clinical work—looking at which techniques have worked consistently, what did not work, and how we explained these outcomes to the treatment team. It is important to remember when considering these interventions that many have not yet been tested through rigorous research. While we are actively contributing to the research base with this population, data collection is time-consuming, and we felt a sense of urgency to get some of our clinical methods "out there." Although some interventions presented in this manual have not been tested through rigorous research, it must be remembered that very few music therapy techniques have been standardized and yet are practiced widely. (Baker & Tamplin, 2006, p. 16)

While the increase in knowledge about music and the brain has provided unique insights into therapeutic possibilities, it has also pointed to the need for a consideration of the professional aspects of the use of music therapeutically. As in all health care strategies, safe practice is of utmost importance. Concurrent with the discovery of new findings about how the brain and music influence each other, many questions have been raised during the past decade in relation to professional issues such as, "Who is qualified to use music in poststroke rehabilitation treatment?," "What training backgrounds and qualifications are required?," and "Who has the right to treat?" The core questions about education and training in the use of music in poststroke rehabilitation are reflecting a change in how rationales for the provision of therapy services have leaned toward an evidence-based practice model in which contemporary neuroscience has played an essential role.

In their succinct and inspired perspective on the role of music therapy in physical rehabilitation following stroke, Weller and Baker's (2011) recent systematic review highlights the importance and challenges of considering such issues. Increasingly, neuroscientific models of therapeutic change are taking the lead in creating evidence and rationale for the mechanisms of change in poststroke rehabilitation and thus forming the therapeutic use of music in this area. As the focus upon the use of controlled stimuli in research increases, the musical dynamic elements of music are removed to make way for experimental stimuli that fulfill the needs of specific research paradigms. In short, the music in music therapy is diverse, ranging from metronomes to advanced improvisation.

Significantly in this light, the authors of the Cochrane Review of music therapy for acquired brain injury (Bradt et al., 2010) stated,

> It is important to distinguish music therapy interventions from the administration of music to patients by medical personnel. Music therapists have specific clinical training in assessing [an] individual patient's needs. Clinical practice is underpinned by music therapy theory. Treatment involves selecting from a range of music-based interventions, using both music and the therapist-patient relationship as agents of change. (p. 3)

This statement suggests that there are clear implications for the development of the field of music therapy as a profession and also for the use of music in therapeutic strategies carried out by non–music therapy specialists. The aspect of the professional background of the person responsible for the use of music in poststroke rehabilitation creates an interesting dilemma—there are a small number of music therapists educated or experienced in neuroscientific research, and there are a small number of neuroscientists educated or experienced in music therapy. Obviously, all of these individuals and their activities are very important for the patient following stroke, and any discussion of the relevance of the professional backgrounds of those helping them should be carried out with the patient in the foreground.

Thus, the literature related to music, music therapy, and stroke presents a complex range of recommendations that are built on a wide range of forms of substantiation, both qualitatively and quantitatively. The remaining parts of this chapter present a selection of the ways in which music has been applied and researched in relation to stroke rehabilitation.

Receptive Music Therapy

- Music Listening: Patient listens to self-selected music.

Improvisational Music Therapy

- Vocal Improvisation: Therapist improvises, synchronized with the breathing timing, timbre, and rhythm of the patient.

Re-creative Music Therapy

- Singing Familiar Songs: Therapist engages the patient in singing familiar songs with the original text.
- Breathing into Single-Syllable Sounds: The process of generating single-syllable sounds.
- Musically Assisted Speech: Conversational phrases are associated with musical melodies for patients with nonfluent aphasia.
- Dynamically Cued Singing: Enhancing the dynamic qualities of a known song.
- Rhythmic Speech Cuing: Patient is guided to clap or tap on the drum the speech rhythm to the phrase that is being exercised.
- Oral Motor Exercises: The therapist presents a short portion of a familiar song, exaggerating mouth and tongue movements. The patient is asked to closely watch and follow the therapist's facial and oral movements.
- Vocal Intonation: Intentional variations of the intonation of daily speech phrases are introduced to help the patient better convey different meanings in speech.
- Melodic Intonation Therapy: Melodic structures are imposed onto phrases of everyday language through a systematic progression of vocal and verbal exercises.
- SIPARI®: Music-supported treatment incorporating music and speech elements of language for patients with chronic aphasia.
- Music Therapy Protocol for Nonfluent Aphasia: Specifically designed protocol of singing familiar songs, breathing into single-syllable sounds, musically assisted speech, dynamically cued singing, rhythmic speech cuing, oral motor exercises, and vocal intonation for treatment of nonfluent aphasia.
- Vocal Intervention for Ataxia of Speech and Dysarthria: Song-based singing and rhythm-based voicework and respiratory voicework for patients with ataxia of speech and dysarthria.

- Speech-Music Therapy for Aphasia (SMTA): An individualized approach that fuses speech language pathology and music therapy to create a concurrent treatment for patients with aphasia and apraxia of speech. It focuses on sound, word, and sentence levels.

GUIDELINES FOR RECEPTIVE MUSIC THERAPY

Music Listening

Overview. Listening to self-selected music, particularly during the first six months poststroke, is gradually being established as a recommended use of music in the rehabilitation process. Participation and motivation are crucial prerequirements of a successful rehabilitation process, and music listening is proving to be an effective activity in this regard. Though the use of music listening in everyday life can be self-directed and administered, there may or may not be the need for the professional involvement of a music therapist during the process. In some instances, the topic of self-directed music listening may be a subject that leads to interdisciplinary collaboration and exchange between colleagues and, most importantly, with the patient and their family members. Please refer to the later section on efficacy research below for more detail about the effects and use of music listening in everyday life for people with stroke and their caregivers.

GUIDELINES FOR IMPROVISATIONAL MUSIC THERAPY

Vocal Improvisation

Overview. This method is orientated by a frame of reference which aims to recontextualize the relationship with the patient from that of someone who needs to be treated and stimulated, to the therapist offering themselves as a spontaneous communicative partner who follows and is led by the patient's movements, breathing, vocalization, and any early attempts at contact. The vocal improvisation of the therapist is synchronized with the breathing timing, timbre, and rhythm of the patient. The improvised melodies should use the techniques of matching and mirroring of improvisational music therapy. The vocal improvisation is without words and should construct simple, identifiable, and repeatable melodic structures. The authors suggest that the selection of musical genre and style should be made on the basis of the therapist's overall impression of the patient's breathing. It is suggested that all sounds and movements made by the patient be integrated into the vocal improvisation. The authors state that instruments are seen to be obtrusive and negatively affect the possibility for direct communicative contact. The goals of the use of vocal improvisation are to provide an opportunity for emergent direct interpersonal contact based on the dynamic interaction in the elements of breathing and the voice.

Vocal improvisation with patients in coma continues until the patient is able to generate identifiable communicative gestures or vocalizations and is able to enter into a conventional form of interpersonal interaction.

When considering this method, it is important to note that it has not been validated by way of efficacy research or controlled trial, but researched by means of multiple case study and expert opinion (see Gustorff & Hannich, 2000). At the time of this writing, there is no advanced training offered in this method. Working with patients in coma is not to be considered as an entry-level type of music therapy provision. Usually, advanced clinical training is considered to be a minimum requirement, alongside appropriate education in regard to the multidisciplinary intensive care context.

Vocal improvisation is contraindicated in patients who show signs of overstimulation or who are physiologically instable. Consultation with nursing and medical staff is essential at all times during the treatment process to ensure safe practice for the patient and staff.

Preparation. It is important to create as calm and quiet an atmosphere as possible and to arrange a period of undisturbed time before, during, and following the music therapy session. As it is essential for nursing and medical staff to have access to the patient at all times of need, the music therapist must remain flexible and calm even if the session needs to be paused or interrupted. It is also important to be considerate of other patients and family members who may be in a shared room, and the music therapist must be observant of any effects on additional patients if they are in the room.

When working with a patient for the first time, it is imperative that the music therapist inform them about all sensorimotor activity which has been observed previously and enquire about any reduction or loss of hearing prestroke.

What to observe. The ways in which patients who are in and emerging from coma change are at times minute and difficult to perceive. Where appropriate according to the ethical procedures of the treatment institution, audio and video recording of the music therapy sessions can provide a wealth of information about the actions of both the therapist and the patient. The primary modes of interrelated actions that should be observed are changes in breathing and vocalizations, physical movements, and facial expressions and any physiological monitoring such as heart rate or oxygen saturation of the blood. During the music therapy process, any changes in medication should be noted and considered.

Procedures. The patient should be positioned according to their physiological needs and if possible have both ears free from pillows or at least one ear free of obstructions. The therapist needs to be able to see the patient's face and chest. Using the approach described above, the authors suggest that the session should not exceed 10 minutes, after which, if possible, the patient should be in the company of a relative or other member of staff, as delayed responses to the music-making may be observed during that time.

As an integral part of the conducting the session, a detailed log of the session is created directly thereafter; preferably, a descriptive microanalysis of the audio/video recordings should be made (Wosch & Wigram, 2007). Each moment of the session should be captured in a time-indexed log that also provides material for preparing for the next session. Depending on the logistics of the therapist's employment and general practices of the institution, music therapy sessions are offered daily.

Guidelines for Re-creative Music Therapy

The voice is a significant domain in the field of stroke rehabilitation and many other fields of music therapy application (Baker & Uhlig, 2011). In relation to stroke rehabilitation, this is determined by two factors. First, the voice is commonly negatively affected by stroke; it is a human capacity which spans many elements of the central and peripheral nervous systems. Second, as a social organ, the voice is also a core aspect of human communicative interaction. Though studies have provided a certain level of evidence of the positive effects of the use of music in the rehabilitation of speech and language function, there are many questions that remain in relation to the mechanism of rehabilitation; a recent comprehensive, systematic review concluded that more research is needed to clarify the exact role of musical elements in therapeutic change (Hurkmans et al., 2012). Before going on to describe specific therapeutic strategies that appear in the literature, there are many common aspects in relation to preparing the session and environment and possible contraindications that require consideration.

Preparation. If practical, an undisturbed quiet environment is beneficial for voicework. It may be necessary and useful to consult with family members about the patient's known vocal habits and any song preferences and known repertoire. This will make it possible for the therapist to search and retrieve the songs, practice until fluent, and prepare any written materials that will be used for the session. The timing of sessions may be an important factor when considering the rhythms of daily life. Also, the placement of the music therapy session before or after other therapy sessions may be important. As an example, music therapy sessions that focus on facilitating vocalization and use of the voice may well be placed before speech and language therapy. Similarly, music therapy sessions that follow physiotherapy may help the patient mobilize their physical coordination and use trunk control and other positional exercises from physiotherapy. Finally, the patient may in some instances prefer privacy from family members when taking initial experimental steps while regaining vocal capacity. Conversely, some patients may be encouraged and inspired by the presence of their loved ones. A sensitive and flexible awareness of these differences will aid in making informed decisions in each individual case.

Contraindications: As the voice is related to basal functions, including breathing and swallowing, it is essential to closely observe and monitor any changes in the patient's behavior and actions in relation to the intervention. Some interventions may require a heightened awareness of related challenges that the patient may be experiencing. Singing familiar songs, for example, is compromised by depression, a lack of interest in the activity of singing, and confusion about the purpose and reason for singing. In some instances, the singing of familiar songs can emphasize the patient's sense of the magnitude of their speech and language disorder and can result in resignation and withdrawal from the therapy. This must be carefully monitored, and, where necessary, a reconsideration of the selected intervention may be required. In some instances, this developing awareness of the actual life situation, if not retraumatizing or leading to an increase in withdrawal, may provide the patient with opportunities for addressing the theme of loss during their rehabilitation process.

Singing Familiar Songs

Overview. Many patients with nonfluent aphasia experience the capacity to sing familiar songs with the original text at times when their spontaneous speech is limited as enjoyable, surprising, and uplifting. This is a useful way of beginning music therapy sessions with patients with nonfluent aphasia. It is important to select songs that are most familiar to the patient to ensure the best possible level of involvement and attention. The goals of singing familiar songs are to engage the patient at the outset of the therapy in a positive manner and to improve the rate and flow of speech and support the development of breath support, intonation, and articulation.

What to observe. It is important to observe whether the familiarity of the consequent verses of familiar songs are consistently familiar, or whether the patient does not know the text of the second and subsequent verses of a song. It has been observed that the familiarity of different sections of songs is inconsistent, which in turn has negative effects of the level of involvement and focus on the activity.

It is also important to observe the patient while exploring extended ranges of changes in dynamic and temporal qualities of the song-singing. By halving the tempo of a familiar song, the patient with nonfluent aphasia may become able to become fluent in their singing; the temporal aspects of song-singing need to be explored and observed carefully.

Adaptations. The addition of tapping along with a hand or being responsible for the strumming of a guitar held by the therapist may assist the patient in increasing the fluidity of their singing. Clear rhythmic cuing will be need from the therapist to support this additional feature. In addition, Kim and Tomaino (2008) have suggested the use of hand gestures to indicate and cue the pitch of melody, and this may help the patient develop their range of pitch while singing familiar songs.

Breathing into Single-Syllable Sounds

Overview. The process of generating single-syllable sounds is an important initial step for many patients following stroke and is particularly, but not exclusively, recommended for patients with nonfluent aphasia. The goal of this method is to assist the patient in generating the basic functions underlying speech and singing as an initial step in speech and language recovery.

What to observe. It is important to observe any challenges the patient may be experiencing in relation to increased production of saliva, an aspect of vocalization with which it can be very difficult for patients with disorders of swallowing to cope. As with all therapeutic interventions with patients following stroke, it is important to observe levels of involvement and fatigue. In the early phases of therapy, energy levels may be depleted due to many reasons and the therapist must be prepared to end the session and to return to the process at a later time.

Procedures. Kim and Tomaino (2008) suggest a progressive procedure for the generation of single-syllable sounds as follows: Focus on spontaneous breathing (rhythm and quality) and natural vocal responses (such as yawning), then progress to sighing on selected vowels, then move on to the singing of single syllables. The vocalizations are to be carried out while exhaling in a slow and pronounced exhalation.

Adaptations. To support the rhythmicity of the breathing and single syllables, it is possible to use visual or instrumental cuing using hand gestures or guitar-playing.

Musically Assisted Speech

Overview. Musically assisted speech has been specifically conceived for use with patients with nonfluent aphasia, wherein conversational phrases are associated with musical melodies that are familiar to the patient. These musically assisted phrases are exercised in themselves as well as played out in the imaginary contexts the patient would encounter in his or her daily life (Kim & Tomaino, 2008).

What to observe. When introducing musically assisted speech, it is important to observe the patient's process of transitioning from the original text to the overlaid new daily speech phrase. Often patients manage the transition if the melody is sung with the original text first before moving on to the new text. Preparing the patient for the phrase with counting in and guitar accompaniment has also been very useful to some patients. It will be important to find a balance between waiting for the patient's tempo of singing and maintaining a general sense of the flow of the music. If this cannot be facilitated, changing the underlying rhythmical division of a guitar accompaniment may facilitate a greater sense of rhythmic flow for the patient and therapist.

Procedures. When introducing phrases from daily life, it is important to consult with the speech and language therapist about any choice of targeted phrases for use in the session. If the associative potential of the melody is to be accessed, it is important that the level of potential confusion of target phrases or original texts and melodies be avoided as much as possible. Finger-tapping or drum-beating may assist the facilitation of flowing rhythmic text production when using the musically assisted speech method.

Dynamically Cued Singing

Overview. This is the "the intentional use of musical dynamics in singing a familiar song to create a strong sense of anticipation for a certain part of the song to facilitate interpersonal interaction and emotional expression" (Kim & Tomaino, 2008, p. 563). Dynamically cued singing has been developed for patients with speech and language disorders, including nonfluent aphasia, and has been described as enhancing the dynamic qualities of a known song and the patient's sense of anticipation. The ability to generate tension-and-release has been described to also aid in the development and rehabilitation of the timing of spontaneous speech. Through this method, it is possible to focus on the dynamic interpersonal factors that are usually embedded and hidden from everyday perception of the emotional and expressive elements of speech.

What to observe. Changes in the temporal aspects of repeated and spontaneous speech can be observed if the patient is maintaining attention and the dynamic elements of the therapist's vocalizations are not so exaggerated that they become redundant for the patient's understanding of the interaction. It will be important to observe the reciprocity of eye contact, as this is a primary indicator of attention, a prerequisite for the continuation of the dynamic flow of the expressions. Clear visual cuing with facial gestures is useful for the patient, but the therapist should be observant of any negative responses as shown by distraction or fatigue.

Procedures. When working with dynamically cued singing, it is useful to prepare and select the song material based on known patient preferences. Kim and Tomaino (2008) have warned about the use of improvised vocalization on the therapist's behalf possibly due "to the lack of consistency in such improvisational musical patterns and its consequent failure in providing strongly engraving perceptual structures" (p. 564). The addition of guitar accompaniment may be considered when using dynamically cued singing, although the therapist should monitor any negative effects of this adaptation due to a lack of or confusion over the dynamic properties of their voice and the guitar.

Rhythmic Speech Cuing

Overview. In rhythmic speech cuing, "the patient is guided to clap or tap on the drum the speech rhythm to the phrase that is being exercised. The therapist may use lyric phrases, daily conversational phrases, or phrases that are related to the immediate context. The rhythmic cues include (a) slow, steady beats that are gauged to the patient's speech tempo; (b) prosodic rhythms of the speech phrases; and (c) musical phrase rhythms for the song lyrics" (Kim & Tomaino, 2008, p. 558). The goals of this method are to improve the rhythmicity and temporal organization of syllable organization and therefore the overall clarity of speech. This can be further improved if the patient experiences a sense of success that in turn supports an increase in rhythmic prosody of their singing and their speech output.

What to observe. Some patients may experience difficulties in actually tapping the rhythmic speech cues, and it may be helpful to explore alternative motor patterns such as sliding and reaching between two defined positions. Also, it may be beneficial to explore whether the patients find it more useful to tap or have contact with their own body or on a different object, such as a drum or tabletop.

Procedures. When beginning the use of rhythmic speech cuing, the therapist should first introduce short and distinct phrases and then progress to longer, more complex phrases once each developmental step has been reached. It is important to monitor general signs of fatigue and lack of focus when assessing the suitability of the selected target phrases.

By dynamically varying the rhythmic speech cues, Kim and Tomaino (2008) have described a significant increase in attention and prolonged eye contact. Care must be taken not to overextend the dynamic nature of the presentation of the cues so as to flood the perceptual capacities of the patient, which may lead to a loss of contact and attention in the moments critical to the exercise.

Oral Motor Exercises

Overview. For patients with nonfluent aphasia having problems with motor control and stamina, oral motor exercises have been conceived "to help the patient improve oral motor formations. The therapist presents a short portion of a familiar song in an exaggerated manner of mouthing and tongue movements. The patient is asked to closely watch and follow the therapist's facial and oral movements" (Kim & Tomaino, 2008, p. 558).

What to observe. Positive changes elicited by oral motor exercises can be observed in direct mimicry and "improvement in speech articulation and vocal quality" (Kim & Tomaino, 2008, p. 565). As with many exercises described here, it is important to monitor the patient's level of contact, as a steady stream of eye contact is relative to the success of the method. This is important due to the need for the patient to visually perceive the therapist's actions concurrently with the aural perception of the same actions.

Procedures. A progressive approach should be taken when using oral motor exercises with patients with nonfluent aphasia. Beginning with short, clear, and distinct phrases, the therapist should move on to longer phrases only once the patient has demonstrated the ability to mimic the oral motor pattern either by mimicry or repetition.

Vocal Intonation

Overview. This is a method for nonfluent aphasia in which "intentional variations of the intonation of daily speech phrases are introduced to help the patient better convey different meanings in speech. The intonations are exaggerated. Visual cues such as head movement or hand conducting may be added to assist the patient's perception of intonation contours and to enhance contextual meanings" (Kim & Tomaino, 2008, p. 558). The goals and outcomes of vocal intonation include many of the core facets shared by singing and speech. As Kim and Tomaino (2008) describe in their qualitative assessment of the method with patients with nonfluent aphasia, "the use of intoned phrases helped the patients improve the melodic aspect of speech prosody. Through the repeated exercise of intoned phrases over time, the patients regained some of the ability to differentiate inflection, pitch, and intensity in their speech that approximated that of normal conversational prosody" (Kim & Tomaino, 2008, p. 565).

What to observe. It has been described that positive change elicited by the use of this method can be identified when the patient relaxes, particularly when being more involved in the conversational aspects of speech than the more mechanical production of successful speech. Paradoxically, this form of therapeutic method benefits from a reduction in the level of concentration on the therapeutic "work" and by focusing more on the dialogical content of a relevant and interesting conversation.

Procedures. It is important to note that the use of this method is planned to build on the previous use of oral motor exercise, rhythmic speech cuing, dynamically cued singing, musically assisted speech, breathing into single-syllable sounds, and singing familiar songs.

Melodic Intonation Therapy and Modified Melodic Intonation Therapy

Overview. The formalization of the method Melodic Intonation Therapy (MIT) is commonly associated with the work of Sparks, Helm, and Albert (1974) and Sparks and Holland (1976), wherein melodic structures were imposed onto phrases of everyday language through a systematic progression of vocal and verbal exercises. The method requires specialist training and will be only mentioned here, rather than provided with limited guidelines for this extensive method. It is, however, a significant part of the repertoire of the use of music and musical elements in the rehabilitation of aphasia and continues to be important in contemporary rehabilitation. The way in which expertise and experience in the use of singing and vocalization exercises were extended during the 1990s can be seen in the publications by Cohen and Ford (Cohen 1992, 1995; Cohen & Ford, 1995). More recently, significant research is being carried out on the effects of melodic intonation therapy as captured using neuroimaging and electrophysiological data on neural plasticity as exemplified by the research group around Gottfried Schlaug (Norton, Zipse, Marchina, & Schlaug, 2009).

SIPARI®

Overview. The SIPARI® approach has been developed specifically for the treatment of patients with Broca's or global aphasia many years after stroke (Jungblut, 2005). This method has been researched in a controlled trial. For details regarding the research base of this method, please refer to the section below on Research Evidence. Training in this method is offered as an independent advanced training for qualified music therapists (see www.sipari.com).

The goals of the SIPARI® method are to activate the compensatory neural mechanisms which can be accessed via a combination of "resource-orientated and training-centred music therapy interventions" (Jungblut, 2005, p. 195). The method includes "Singing, Intonation, Prosody, Breathing [German: Atmung], Rhythm, and Improvisation as essential elements" and the goals of the method "include improving linguistic, motor, and cognitive functions and thereby supporting speech-motor processes and those speech-systematic processes that encourage planning and sequencing performance" (www.sipari.com).

Music Therapy Protocol for Nonfluent Aphasia

Overview. Kim and Tomaino (2008) have created and researched a music therapy protocol for the treatment of nonfluent aphasia as a result of stroke. The protocol has been based on many years of clinical experience supported by existing literature. The elements and order of the protocol are singing familiar songs, breathing into single-syllable sounds, musically assisted speech, dynamically cued singing, rhythmic speech cuing, oral motor exercises, and vocal intonation. In their qualitative assessment of the protocol, Kim and Tomaino (2008) have identified the importance of each of the elements individually and also the overall significance of the role of the therapist's sensitivity to the patient in terms of levels of attention, involvement, timing, dynamic qualities of nonverbal interaction, the therapist's ability to engage with the patient at a personal level, and the therapist's sound knowledge and understanding of the protocol itself.

Vocal Intervention for Ataxia of Speech and Dysarthria

Overview. The vocal interventions developed by Felicity Baker and Jeanette Tamplin have been created for patients with two common symptoms following stroke, ataxia of speech (AOS) and dysarthria (Baker & Tamplin, 2011; Tamplin, 2008). The authors have developed three approaches for these groups: 1) song-based singing, 2) rhythm-based voicework, and 3) respiratory voicework. The authors distinguish the two diagnoses as follows: "Patients with AOS have difficulty sequencing movements together to articulate various sounds correctly. In contrast, patients with dysarthria have difficulty articulating speech because of muscle weakness or paralysis resulting from neurological damage" (Baker & Tamplin, 2011, p. 195). The goals of this approach are to increase the patient's ability to sequence speech movement patterns (AOS) and to increase muscle strength and the use of residual ability to generate the words and melody of familiar songs to extend the accuracy of timing, breathing, and oral motor control.

Speech-Music Therapy for Aphasia (SMTA)

Overview. Speech-Music Therapy for Aphasia has been specifically developed based on the shared dynamic elements of music and speech aimed at improving expressive speech. In contrast to Melodic Intonation Therapy, SMTA is a result of a fusion of therapeutic strategies found in speech and language therapy and music therapy and is performed in a collaborative process by a speech and language therapist and a music therapist. This approach refrains from targeting set phrases as in MIT, but aims at assisting the patient to be able to generate spontaneous expressive speech in everyday life situations. The SMTA process rests on a series of speech and language therapy exercises which are set to music. It is suggested that sessions should be 30 minutes long, twice a week, for between three and six months (de Bruijn, Hurkmans, & Zielman, 2011). Cohesion for the speech and language therapy and music therapy elements is provided by a basic conceptualization of all exercises in terms of "sound-level exercises," "word-level exercises," and "sentence-level exercises" (de Bruijn, Hurkmans, & Zielman, 2011, pp. 213–218). As an integrated element of the treatment of patients with aphasia in many health care centers in the author's country, the Netherlands, SMTA has shown positive results; at the time of the writing of this chapter, an efficacy study into SMTA is in progress.

COMPOSITIONAL MUSIC THERAPY

Compositional music therapy is not represented in the methods identified in the literature in relation to the treatment of stroke. This may have many causes, which could include the health systems, which have demanded research and clinical evidence; the personal training and clinical expertise of therapists and researchers working the area of stroke rehabilitation; and, finally, the nature of stroke and stroke rehabilitation itself. It will be interesting to see whether this area of the use of music in stroke rehabilitation receives attention in the future as more knowledge and expertise is gained in the treatment of patients with stroke.

RESEARCH EVIDENCE

The theme "music and the brain" has attracted worldwide interest for many decades. Recently, there has been a marked increase in the amount and scope of research into the use of music in therapy with individuals who have experienced a stroke. As stroke and the resulting damage to the brain can potentially affect many areas of human development and capabilities, music can be used in diverse ways for the therapeutic purposes. The four major categories of methods used in music therapy are receptive, improvisational, re-creative, and compositional. The literature can be classified according to whether the authors have identified the treatment to have been carried out by a qualified music therapist or a member of another profession and also according to the types of study, which include meta-analyses, controlled randomized trials, and case studies and reports.

For the purposes of the first section of this chapter, only studies have been included in the following section on efficacy studies of music therapy and stroke according to the inclusion criteria as applied in the Cochrane Review on music therapy and acquired brain injury (Bradt et al., 2010). In a later section, a selection of efficacy research on music in stroke rehabilitation that was not included in the Cochrane Review will be presented.

The studies included in the Cochrane Review (Bradt et al., 2010) were: Baker (2001), on the effect of live and recorded music on agitation and orientation in cases of post-traumatic amnesia; Jungblut (2004), on singing for the treatment of chronic aphasia; Kim (2005), on the effects of music on pain perception during upper-extremity exercises; Paul and Ramsey (1998), on electronic music-making for improving upper-extremity range of motion; Thaut (1997), on rhythmic facilitation of gait training; Thaut (2002), on rhythmic entrainment of paretic arm movements; and Thaut (2007), on rhythmic auditory stimulation on gait training against NDT/Bobath training in near-ambulatory patients.

Receptive Methods

Baker (2001) carried out a study of the effect of music on listening to live and recorded music on the levels of agitation and orientation in 22 people who were experiencing post-traumatic amnesia as a result of severe head injury. There were three experimental conditions of listening to live or recorded songs suggested by the participant's family as belonging to the participant's musical preference and no music in random order two times over a period of six days. The results of the study showed a statistically significant effect of music listening on levels of orientation and agitation in comparison to the no-music condition. Though there was a slightly larger effect when listening to live music in comparison to recorded music, this was not statistically significant. The measures were carried out using the Westmead Post-Traumatic Amnesia scale for orientation and the Agitation Behaviour scale for agitation.

The effects on pain perception of prerecorded music listening vs. no-music listening during upper-extremity joint exercises for hand, wrist, arm, and shoulder over eight weeks have been studied by Kim and Koh (2005). The study did not find any statistically significant differences between the music listening and no-music conditions; however, important findings were made in relation to increased overall motivation in the rehabilitation process and positive feelings during the music-assisted exercises. Importantly, Kim and Koh (2005) highlighted the significant role that motivation has in determining commitment and immersion in the rehabilitation process and the way in which the music-supported exercises have been able to contribute to this important factor.

Whitall and colleagues (2000) studied the effects of auditory cues on bilateral arm movement in a pilot study with 14 participants. The study identified that three 20 minute sessions over six weeks led to significant improvements in relation to individual elements of upper-extremity ability, including hand, elbow ,and shoulder flexion and extension. Altenmüller and colleagues (2009) have carried out significant research into the effects of music-supported therapy upon motor dysfunction following stroke in terms of neural reorganization as captured in electrophysiological change in areas of the brain responsible for motor function. This study built on Altenmüller's earlier research which identified the positive effects of musical instrument–playing, including drumming and piano-playing for patients following stroke (Schneider, Schönle, Altenmüller, and Munte, 2007). The method of using piano-playing as therapy with music in motor coordination of arm and finger movements has been taken up in a study by Moon (2008) which added evidence of the positive and significant effects of the use of piano-playing as a therapeutic strategy.

In one further study on upper-extremity function, Thaut and colleagues (2002) studied the effects of rhythmic auditory stimulation (RAS) vs. no RAS on upper-extremity function of patients with hemiplegia between 4 and 19 months after experiencing hemispheric stroke. The 21 study participants were required to move their hand between two sensors that were placed on a table surface with and without rhythmic auditory stimulation. The authors describe the stimulation and trial paradigm as follows: "The auditory rhythm consisted of a metronome-like 1,000 Hz square wave tone with a 50 ms plateau time produced by a computerized MIDI-sequencing sound software (Logic 2.5). During rhythmic trials, patients were asked to move their arm in time with the rhythm by touching the sensors on the beat"

(Thaut et al., 2002, p. 1075). Movement data was captured via the sensors and through three-dimensional motion analysis for both conditions. This study is unique in providing evidence of the positive effects of RAS on arm movements of paretic poststroke patients. In particular, significant changes were measured in relation to an increased elbow extension angle that was statistically significant against no RAS, and the variability of timing, enhanced timing of movement, and trajectory of wrist, elbow, and shoulder, which showed a significant effect of the RAS on upper-extremity performance.

Thaut, McIntosh, and Rice (1997) investigated the effect of rhythmic auditory stimulation (RAS) vs. conventional physiotherapy for gait training within three months of stroke. With 10 participants in the experimental and control groups, both groups received two 30-minute training sessions five days a week for six weeks by trained physiotherapists. The experimental group trained with a metronome or prepared music tapes. The authors described the auditory stimulation as follows: "To control for motivational-emotional factors in the music to enhance gait performance, the same music was used for a patient's training period. Repetitive use of music of relatively low complexity has been shown to provide redundancy in music perception, which strongly reduces affective arousal related to motivational states (Berlyne, 1971)" (Thaut, McIntosh, & Rice, 1997, p. 211). The experimental group demonstrated statistically and clinically significant positive results in stride length, but no statistical significance was found in the measures of symmetry, step cadence, or velocity improvement. EMG measurements of the medial gastrocnemius (calf muscle) highlighted a reduction of amplitude variability in the experimental group that was found to be statistically significant and highly significant in the treatment of gait for stroke patients.

In 2007, Thaut and colleagues studied the effect of rhythmic auditory stimulation vs. neurodevelopmental training/Bobath therapy to train gait in near-ambulatory patients within three weeks of stroke (Thaut et al., 2007). In this study, 78 participants in two centers in Germany and the United States were allocated to the control or experimental group randomly. Both groups received one 30-minute training session per day, five days a week, for three weeks and the experimental group received RAS training as established in an earlier study (Thaut, McIntosh, & Rice, 1997). In the experimental group, significant effects were observed in velocity, stride length, cadence, and symmetry when compared to the control group. The study also showed that the reduction in overall duration of treatment from six weeks in a previous study (Thaut, McIntosh, & Rice, 1997) to three weeks in the 2007 study highlights the importance of exploring the effects of the duration of this significant therapeutic modality in the improvement of gait in this group of near-ambulatory acute stroke patients.

A series of related studies exploring the effects of music listening in everyday life as compared to listening to audio books has elicited significant findings in favor of listening to music in everyday life following stroke (Forsblom, Laitinen, & Särkämö, 2009; Forsblom, Särkämö, Laitinen, & Tervaniemi, 2010; Särkämö et al., 2008). Collectively, these studies, through gathering qualitative data from the patient perspective and nurses' perspectives alongside data via standardized neuropsychological assessments, have identified how listening to self-selected and self-directed music during the first half a year following stroke can significantly positively affect the patients' cognitive recovery process, improve verbal memory, reduce depression, and increase positive mood. Although studies on neuroplastic change during phases of music listening in daily life await, the authors suggest that contemporary models of neuroplastic change (see Janssen et al., 2010; Pekna, Pekny, & Nilsson, 2012) may be tentatively proposed to explain the effects of music listening in their studies (Särkämö et al., 2008).

Re-creative Methods

Jungblut (2004) carried out a study of the effects of a music therapy method she created called SIPARI®, which is a program of a combination of methods which mostly focus on vocal exercises but also include instrumental exercises and music improvisation. The program aims at improving the speech production abilities of patients with chronic aphasia of global or Broca's type. The average time between stroke and treatment of the participants in the study was 11.5 years. The combination of methods was provided to the experimental group in a series of 20 group sessions and 10 individual sessions during seven months. The results of the study showed statistically and clinically significant effects overall as measured by the Aachen Aphasia Test and in particular on articulation, prosody, speech repetition, and speech comprehension. This study is unique in demonstrating the effectiveness of music therapy many years poststroke beyond the conventional understanding of the time frame of recovery. Although not included in the Cochrane Review, Jungblut and colleagues (2009) provided an excellent overview of the SIPARI® method which is supported by a single case description in a later publication.

Paul and Ramsey (1998) carried out an investigation into the use of music-making to improve sensorimotor ability of shoulder flexion and elbow extension. The authors describe the experimental condition as being "a form of occupational embedded exercise" (p. 223) that was used in a controlled trial with 10 participants in the treatment and control groups. The study premises are based on findings in the literature suggesting that enhanced outcome through purposeful activities such as making music as opposed to isolated movement patterns void of naturally occurring purposefulness. Thus the aspects of intervention were blended—activities known to music therapy practices blended into occupational therapy processes and shared aims. Though the study did not identify any statistical significance of the effect of embedded music-making, a clinically significant increase in the range of shoulder and elbow range was found. The authors summarize that the study results "support the occupational therapy principle of preventing disability, improving human performance, and maintaining health through meaningful occupation" (Paul & Ramsey, 1997, p. 237).

Research Evidence on Music Therapy and Acquired Brain Injury (Not Included in the Cochrane Review)

Receptive Methods

Särkämö and colleagues (2008) explored the effect of music listening vs. audiobook and no listening in a randomized trial with 60 participants who had experienced an acute ischemic middle cerebral artery stroke. Over a period of two months of self-administered listening to one to two hours of self-selected music or audiobook recordings, the participants were in constant contact with a music therapist to encourage and support the listening activities, provide new listening material, and aid with the equipment use. The results of the study were highly significant and demonstrated both statistical and clinical significance of the effects of the music listening in improving focused attention and verbal memory and also effecting less depression and less confused mood.

Phipps, Carroll, and Tsiantoulas (2010) studied the effects of music listening on a convenience sample of 56 patients treated in an inpatient neuroscience unit. Although the study included only six patients with stroke, it does demonstrate statistically significant reductions in anxiety and depression using standardized scales for those patients. For the purposes of this chapter, it is of interest to note the way in which the authors frame the concept of music and music therapy in their discussion of the implications of their findings:

> Music as an intervention to create a therapeutic and healing environment appears to be a successful strategy for the neuroscience patient. Integrating music within the clinical environment requires the essential equipment of music, a CD player or other type of music player, and headphones as needed.

> Implementation of music therapy could provide diversion during the stressful experience of hospitalization for a neuroscience condition. This type of diversion has the potential to promote relaxation during this period of uncertainty and turmoil and reduce the altered physiological and psychological responses for neuroscience patients. (Phipps, Carroll, & Tsiantoulas, 2010, p. 141)

What is striking in this description is the absence of professional responsibility for the administration of the music selection and reception and monitoring of any negative signs of music reception. In addition, it will be interesting to see how music and neuroscience research responds to the scenario of music reception via headphones during acute phases of neural reorganization and unstable phases of hemodynamics and intracranial pressure that are common for patients in the neuroscience unit.

Although the application of rhythmic auditory stimulation (RAS) in the treatment of movement disorders has received a large amount of attention and demonstrated significant positive change in a number of studies as summarized in a recent review (Thaut & Abiru, 2010), questions remain as to the role of musical elements existing in the form of external or internal stimuli as discussed by Schauer and Mauritz (2003). In their study of musical motor feedback (MMF), Schauer and Mauritz (2003) noted that their participants, rather than responding positively to an external auditory timekeeper, were able to improve core aspects of their gait through self-generated auditory stimuli generated from sensors placed in the heels of their shoes and also from internal song recall from memory. Although the results of contrasting studies demonstrate clinically and statistically positive change in the rehabilitation of gait, it is important to note that there may in fact be more to explore in the future in relation to the inner processes of perception, cognition, and motor control within a model of external and internal multimodal sensorimotor loops.

Re-creative Methods

Kim (2010) carried out a pilot study and an efficacy study of the effects of a music therapy protocol to attend to a common disorder of swallowing following stroke, also known as dysphagia, with eight participants in the experimental study. Dysphagia is a serious disorder that, as it has the potential to obstruct the patient's breath, can represent a risk to the patient's life. Any strategies that lead to improvements in the individual elements of the swallowing process can contribute significantly to the reduction of risk and increase in quality of life following stroke. The music therapy protocol in Kim's study (2010) is based on vocalization exercises involving oral motor exercises and breathing exercises. The research protocol is described as a music-enhanced swallowing treatment (Kim, 2010, p. 110) and consists of a warm-up; song-singing; breathing exercises to music; vocalization exercises that emphasized muscular development necessary in swallowing; and a closing repetition of the song used in the warm-up section. The results of the study identified statistically significant positive change in the regions of pitch control in the midway assessment and in the reduction of dribbling and improvement of breathing at rest and during singing and, importantly, in laryngeal elevation. These two final findings are particularly significant, as they demonstrate statistically significant positive change in two of the most important aspects of the swallowing function, thus showing how music therapy contributes to the amelioration of dysphagia following stroke.

Combined Methods

Often research studies include a combination of music therapy methods within the research protocol. This reflects common therapy practice wherein many methods and techniques are selected by the therapist to match the individual needs and resources of the patients. One example of this is the study carried out by Kim and colleagues (2011) in which the music therapy intervention for patients following stroke included a wide range of activities structured as a "40-minute patient performing treatment method" (p. 980). The session "consisted of a hello song and sharing of events in their lives (5 minutes); planned musical activities (30 minutes), including respiration and phonation, improvised play, hand bell play, singing, songwriting, and expression in tune with music; and the sharing of feelings and a good-bye song (5 minutes). Keyboards, hand bells, percussion instruments, flutes, and other tools such as picture cards, flowers, and fruit scents were used in accordance with the planned activities. Patients were encouraged to improvise, depending on their feelings, and sing children's and folk songs" (p. 978). Although the study included a small number of patients, it was successful in creating evidence about how music therapy can contribute to the rehabilitation of patients following stroke by reducing depressed mood and have positive effects on mood. Both the Beck Depression Inventory (BDI) and Beck Anxiety Inventory (BAI) were used to assess change. Though no statistical significant change was registered using the Beck Anxiety Inventory, statistically significant change was reported in BDI for the music group (p = 0.048), as opposed to the control group. The study also added information on the perceived positive emotional change after music therapy, increase in motivation, and usefulness in rehabilitation through questionnaires completed by patients and caregivers.

Another example of research using a mixture of music therapy elements is the study carried out by Nayak, Wheeler, Shiflett, and Agostinelli (2000) into the effect of music therapy on mood and social interaction with patients with traumatic brain injury and stroke. The results of the study highlighted the positive effects on measurements of social and behavioral outcomes, and some clinically but not statistically significant trends in relation to the patient's mood. What is interesting about this study is the music therapy treatment condition that the authors described in detail: "Ten participants in this group met two or three times a week for the duration of their stay in the hospital and received up to a maximum of 10 treatment sessions in addition to their standard rehabilitation (M = 5.9, SD = 1.73; range: 4–10). A variety of music therapy procedures were used to enhance mood and social interaction. The specific music activities used, and their selection, were based on the needs of the group and are typical of music therapy practice.

In this study, each session began with an opening song or activity designed to set the mood and to help participants become involved in the session. This was frequently some type of instrumental improvisation in which participants used simple percussion and melodic instruments along with the therapist. In some sessions, participants were asked to play together in a manner that expressed how they were feeling at that time. This was accomplished by having each group member select a simple percussive instrument from among a collection. A number of sessions involved simple pitched instruments (bells or chimes); each participant was assigned several pitched instruments and played his or her pitch when cued. Instruments included drums, tambourines, maracas, xylophones, and tone bars (each bar is an individual note, beaten with a stick to produce the sound). The therapist would then structure the improvisation by asking participants to play their instruments to express how they were feeling or first asking a participant to describe how he or she was feeling and then asking that member and the rest to play their instruments in a manner reflecting their mood. Both of these approaches were followed by a brief discussion of how well the musical improvisation reflected and supported the feelings being experienced. In other sessions, participants were asked to simply play together and then were later cued verbally to listen to one another as they played or took turns playing musical leadership or supportive roles.

One or two additional music therapy activities, such as singing, composing, playing instruments, improvising, performing, and listening formed the core of each group. The specific musical activities were chosen on the basis of the interests and abilities of the participants, and consideration was given as to whether the activity could be used to address the goals of enhancing mood and social interaction. The music therapist provided physical cues, or participants read from a color- or letter-coded chart. Another activity that was used frequently was composition, accomplished by substituting words of participants' choice for the normal words of a song. These compositions helped participants to express how they were feeling or what they were thinking. Singing was frequently incorporated. Each group of people had favorite songs, most of which were on song sheets or charts. All activities involved verbal processing, including some focus on mood. The amount and quality of verbal processing varied, depending on the abilities and needs of the participants" (Nayak et al., 2000, p. 278).

The music therapy treatment, described in this study as "typical of music therapy practice" (Nayak, Wheeler, Shiflett, & Agostinelli, 2000, p. 278), is a very good example of the common complexity of conventional music therapy practices when compared with the treatment condition described in other efficacy studies on motor ability or speech and language ability. The study clearly documents the significance of music therapy practice and provides an essential view of conventional multiperspective music therapy practice that contrasts the therapeutic use of musical elements in motor function rehabilitation.

Doğan, Tur, Dilek, and Küçükdeveci (2011) carried out a study into the effects of a single music therapy on anxiety with patients with stroke. Thirty-one patients with stroke and 53 healthy volunteers received 35 minutes of listening to classical music, followed by five minutes of rhythmic respiratory exercises, and concluded with 15 minutes of conversation regarding their emotions and thoughts. Levels of anxiety were measured using the State-Trait Anxiety Inventory. Though only minimal detail is given with regard to the results of the study, the investigators noted a similarly significant reduction in anxiety in both the experimental and control group, without any significant differences between the two groups. In this study, it seems that the selected relaxation strategy was similarly effective for all participants regardless of whether they had experienced a stroke.

Dunham's study (2010) examined the efficacy of music therapy in combination with conventional treatments of aphasia and apraxia of speech. Apraxia of speech was addressed as far back as 1975 by Keith and Aronson (1975), when they presented the use of singing in a single case description. In Dunham's study (2010), two patients presenting aphasia, ataxia of speech, and hemiparesis following a stroke completed three treatment sessions each week for three blocks of three weeks, alternating between conventional speech and language therapy and conventional speech and language therapy plus music therapy, and then returning to conventional speech and language therapy. The speech and language therapy consisted of 45 minutes of cuing hierarchy therapy approach, followed by a word modeling and repetition speech therapy technique. The combined sessions shared 30 minutes for speech and language therapy and 30 minutes for the music therapy section. The music therapy protocol included singing familiar songs, breathing exercises to single-syllable sounds, musically assisted speech, dynamically cued singing, rhythmic speech cuing, and oral motor exercises (Dunham, 2010). Whereas both participants demonstrated positive effects of both the experimental conditions, both participants demonstrated the largest treatment effect during the combined conventional speech and language therapy and music therapy. The results suggest that a combination of conventional speech and language therapy and music therapy could lead to better results for the patients. In addition, it is suggested that this may also be responsible for the continuation of therapeutic progression in conventional speech and language therapy even after the music therapy elements was removed. Thus, the implications for the study in terms of the significance of further researching the timing, dosage, and combination of therapies is of utmost importance in the development of the provision of music therapy for patients experiencing aphasia and ataxia of speech following stroke.

Kim and Tomaino (2008) investigated the effectiveness of a music therapy protocol comprising "seven structured musically assisted speech exercises" (p. 556) with seven nonfluent aphasic patients following stroke. The music therapy protocol included singing familiar songs, breathing into single-syllable sounds, musically assisted speech, dynamically cued singing, rhythmic speech cuing, oral motor exercises, and vocal intonation (Kim & Tomaino, 2008, pp. 557–558). The report of the study is highly significant, as it is unique in providing insight into the researchers' reflections on the elements of therapists' provision of the seven exercises and recommendations on adaptation and flexibility in relation to the individual patients, which is one of the essential elements of successful patient-led rehabilitation.

The use of improvisation is an aspect of music therapy practice in the rehabilitation of people following stroke that has become established in pockets of the world. Though there have not been a large number of publications, research on the use of improvisation with patients with stroke has spread over the past two-and-half decades. McMaster (1991) published one of the earliest treatises on the use of improvisation with patients with stroke. In her detailed and highly descriptive case study, McMaster highlighted the way in which spontaneous interaction through music co-improvisation made possible a process of gaining orientation to oneself and each other, which consequently led to the re-emergence of a new identity for the patient that was an expression of and incorporation of her current self. The case study is particularly revealing of how, by keeping a detailed focus on the music-centered interaction, important stages of recovery and discovery of new capacities were possible. Now, over 20 years after McMaster's publication, the need for interpersonal and socially directed care strategies in stroke rehabilitation is ever increasing (Satink, 2013).

One further example is Tamplin's (2000) paper on improvisational music therapy in relation to coma arousal following neurological insult including stroke. In that paper, Tamplin (2000) described how improvisational music therapy could be used to work on integration of rhythms of the body's physiology and sensory stimulation and awareness.

Another example of improvisational music therapy was published in 1998 and described elements of improvising with an adult patient who had experienced a subarachnoid and intracerebral hemorrhage resulting in global aphasia and early signs of social isolation (Gilbertson, 1998):

> In one particular session, through the use of pointing, he chose a set of five woodblocks from a selection of melodic and percussive instruments to play with the therapist at the piano. Out of the stillness of reflection, he began to carefully try out the five tones of the woodblocks. During his initial phase, he only looked down at his instrument while playing. Each tone was repeated once or twice, and then he moved to the next tone. By imitating the quiet, short, staccato nature of his playing and the number of times each note was struck, the therapist reflected his playing in her playing at the piano. After a short time, perhaps half a minute, he looked up from the woodblocks, entered into eye contact with the therapist, and grinned. He had, perhaps, recognized the intention behind the music coming from the therapist and recognized a relationship between his playing and the therapist's playing. Suddenly, the two players became almost simultaneously louder and faster, and a sense of rhythmic organization for the exchange of rhythmic patterns developed. The improvisation continued with exchanges of rhythmic motives, mood qualities, and a wide range of stylistic forms which both players could recognize and respond to. [...] Mr. D's initiative toward self-expression through music and the modulation of expressive qualities in his playing enabled the development of a

> relationship with the therapist. He could enter into musical interaction with another person, which was not possible in verbal communication [...] the use of music as a therapeutic medium [was] aimed not only at encouraging interactive experience within the music therapy setting but also at providing Mr. D with positive experiences, increasing his confidence to enter into other communicative situations in daily life and within other forms of therapy" (pp. 236–237).

As discussed in other areas of music therapy applications, music co-improvisation provides the therapist and patient with a process of real-time interaction based on dynamic forms of movement, imitation, intentionality, and learning. Though models of social cognition (Menary, 2006) and embodied interpersonal neural action (Shapiro, 2011) have only gradually emerged during recent years, these will certainly provide a great deal of impetus in the research and practice of co-improvisation in music therapy. In addition, it may inform the importance of music therapy with individuals with stroke and their caregivers, identifying interpersonal cognitive processes needed for interpersonal communication and emotional expression. Not only might this development support the application of music improvisation in rehabilitation following stroke, but also it will demonstrate how an understanding of the process of change and interpersonal relating may be conceived in many areas of music therapy application.

One of the most significant pieces of work being carried out in relation to the use of music improvisation in the rehabilitation processes of individuals who had experienced stroke is a randomized controlled crossover trial of active music therapy (Ala-Ruona, 2009). This groundbreaking study examines the effects of improvisation in active music therapy on mood, experienced quality of life, motor function, awareness of deficit, rhythmic motor performance, and neural activity in music-related perception exercises.

Jeong and Kim (2007) carried out a study into the effects of a music and movement program for people with stroke in a community setting. This significant study was based on the methods of rhythmic auditory stimulation. The authors focused on a wide range of outcome measures, including physical capacity of shoulder, arm, and ankle movement of the affected side; mood states; interpersonal relationships; and quality of life. These are in fact a combination of many of the dominant outcome measures commonly used individually in earlier studies. The music-based intervention took place in a community center, making the study unique in relation to the combination of the treatment intervention, the extensive range of outcome measures, and the nonclinical community setting. The authors identified statistically and clinically significant positive change in all areas of the outcome measures and emphasized the need for the provision of music-based therapy during all poststroke stages, the significance of rhythmic elements of music-making, and the importance of community-situated rehabilitation strategies.

This review of research concludes with a consideration of the unpublished doctoral thesis by David Ramsey (2002). In his thesis, Ramsey considers the role of music therapy for people with nonfluent aphasia. He includes people with traumatic brain injury and stroke and finds that alongside improvements in speech and language capacity, the music therapy group provided the potential for "communal experiences" (p. 114), a form of "essential human experiences" (p. 125) from which this patient group conventionally becomes excluded. Ramsey also uncovered the three levels of knowledge from his research data and identified them as the surface structure of the familiar song; the midstructures of essential human experiences—competency, frustration, humor, camaraderie, self-assertion, and community; and the deep structures of time management and interpersonal realization (pp. 139–141). It becomes obvious through Ramsey's text that the work with people with nonfluent aphasia holds the potential to change the therapist and their perspective on human interaction if they can open themselves to change: "The study influenced my observations of the conversational act, and helped me see beyond the exterior context of words exchanged. I caught a glimpse of the personal exchange, a transaction dependent upon a spiritual bonding that needed no words. I came to view the human exchange as a dance of souls combining rather than passing pieces of information from one separate mind to another separate mind" (Ramsey, 2002, p. 144).

In his reflections on music therapy with people with aphasia related to stroke and traumatic brain injury, Ramsey (2002) concludes,

> In my experience as a clinician who works under a rehabilitation, medical model of treatment, it is important to remain aware of clinical benefits that are not easily measured. It is my hope that this research will validate the improvement of the quality of life obtained by providing expressive, communal experiences for patients who are deprived of such encounters due to their loss of speech. In this document, I present my key concept, principles and the guidelines to my work with aphasic patients. These findings are in the context of a small group format, and most of the findings are related to the restoration of essential human experiences in a communal milieu. Since there is very little published in the field of music therapy in regard to this population, it is my hope that some of the principles and techniques will be used by other music therapists. As others incorporate such techniques, it may become clearer to the music therapy profession which are of value and which are not. (pp. 147–148).

For those who would like to gain a comprehensive and balanced perspective of the culture of care for people who have experienced stroke that has emerged during the past two decades, Ramsey's thesis should be added to their list of compulsory reading.

Summary and Conclusions

Movement, emotion, and speech are common areas affected by stroke, and it is to these human qualities that neuroscientists and music therapists have responded, although not all clinicians who use music therapeutically with patients with stroke are music therapists, nor are all neuroscientists researching the relationship between music and stroke trained as music therapists. The development seen in clinical work and research clearly reflects the process of this overlap, however, and the future of music therapy and neuroscience promises to be very bright. This chapter has aimed to present the ways in which music has been and can be used in therapy with people with stroke, although there is much work that remains to be done.

It is important that in the future music therapists consider the diverse effects of stroke at various levels of severity. In the literature, there is a tendency more toward targeting the less serious degrees of disorders rather than the more serious extremes that the symptoms and symptom complexes of stroke can cause.

In the future, it will be important to consider the potential uses of music therapy during the entire life span of the patient affected by a stroke and not only in the acute and continuing rehabilitation phase. Though many research studies look at the use of music during inpatient contexts, future research may be developed to support the practice of music therapy in the everyday lives of those affected by stroke.

References

Ala-Ruona, E. (2009). Active music therapy for post-stroke recovery. *ISRCTN Trial Register*. DOI: 10.1186/ISRCTN03493594.

Aldridge, D. (1996). *Music therapy research and practice in medicine: From out of the silence.* London: Jessica Kingsley Publishers.

Altenmüller, E., Marco-Pallares, J., Münte, T. F., & Schneider, S. (2009). Neural reorganization underlies improvement in stroke-induced motor dysfunction by music-supported therapy. *Annals of the New York Academy of Sciences, 1169,* 395–405.

Amarenco, P., Bogousslavsky, J., Caplan, L.R., Donnan, G.A., & Hennerici, M.G. (2009). Classification of stroke types. *Cerebrovascular Disease, 27,* 493-501.

Baker, F. (2001). The effects of live, taped, and no music on people experiencing posttraumatic amnesia. *Journal of Music Therapy, 38*(3), 170–192.

Baker, F. (2011). Facilitating neurological reorganization through music therapy: A case of modified melodic intonation therapy in the treatment of a person with aphasia. In: A. Meadows (Ed.), *Developments in music therapy practice: Case study perspectives* (pp.280-296). Gilsum, NH: Barcelona Publishers.

Baker, F., & Roth, E. (2004). Neuroplasticity and functional recovery: Training models and compensatory strategies in music therapy. *Nordic Journal of Music Therapy, 13*(1), 20–32.

Baker, F., & Tamplin, J. (2006). *Music therapy methods in neurorehabilitation: A clinician's manual.* Philadelphia, PA: Jessica Kingsley Publishers.

Baker, F., & Tamplin, J. (2011). Coordinating respiration, vocalization, and articulation: Rehabilitating apraxic and dysarthric voices of people with neurological damage. In F. Baker & S. Uhlig (Eds.), *Voicework in music therapy: Research and practice* (pp. 189–205). Philadelphia, PA: Jessica Kingsley Publishers.

Baker, F., & Uhlig, S. (Eds.). (2011). *Voicework in music therapy: research and practice.* Philadelphia, PA: Jessica Kingsley Publishers.

Barnes, M. (2000). Concepts of rehabilitation. In M. Barnes & A. Ward, *Textbook of rehabilitation medicine* (pp. 1–23). New York: Oxford University Press.

Berlyne, D.E. (1971). Aesthetics and psychobiology. New York: Appleton-Century-Crofts.

Bradt, J., Magee, W. L., Dileo, C., Wheeler, B. L., & McGilloway, E. (2010). Music therapy for acquired brain injury. *Cochrane Database of Systematic Reviews, Jul 7*(7), CD006787.

Cohen, N. S. (1992). The effect of singing instruction on the speech production of neurologically impaired persons. *Journal of Music Therapy, 29*(2), 87–102.

Cohen, N. S. (1995). The effect of vocal instruction and Visi-pitch feedback on the speech of persons with neurogenic communication disorders: Two case studies. *Music Therapy Perspectives, 13*(2), 70–75.

Cohen, N. S., & Ford, J. (1995). The effect of musical cues on the nonpurposive speech of persons with aphasia. *Journal of Music Therapy, 32*(1), 46–57.

de Bruijn, M., Hurkmans, J., & Zielman, T. (2011). Speech-Music Therapy for Aphasia (SMTA): An interdisciplinary treatment of speech-language therapy and music therapy for clients with aphasia and/or apraxia of speech. In F. Baker & S. Uhlig (Eds.), *Voicework in music therapy: Research and practice* (pp. 206–227). Philadelphia, PA: Jessica Kingsley Publishers.

Doğan, Ş.. K.., Tur, B. S., Dilek, L., & Küçükdeveci, A. (2011). Single music therapy session reduces anxiety in patients with stroke. *Journal of Physical Medicine and Rehabilitation Sciences, 14,* 12–15.

Dunham, D.J.A. (2010). Efficacy of using music therapy combined with traditional aphasia and apraxia of speech treatments. Unpublished master thesis: Department of Communication Sciences and Disorders: University of Western Carolina.

Erdonmez, D. (1991). Rehabilitation of piano performance skills following a left cerebral vascular accident. In K. E. Bruscia (Ed.), *Case studies in music therapy* (pp. 561–570). Gilsum, NH: Barcelona Publishers.

Forsblom, A., Laiteinen, S., Särkämö, T., & Tervaniemi, M. (2009). Therapeutic role of music listening in stroke rehabilitation. *Annals of New York Academy of Sciences, 1169,* 426–430.

Forsblom, A., Särkämö, T., Laiteinen, S., & Tervaniemi, M. (2010). The effect of music and audiobook listening on people recovering from stroke: The patient's point of view. *Music and Medicine, 2*(4), 229–234.

Fujioka, T., Ween, J. E., Jamali, S., Stuss, D. T., & Ross, B. (2012). Changes in neuromagnetic beta-band oscillation after music-supported stroke rehabilitation. *Annals of the New York Academy of Sciences, 1252,* 294–304.

Fullerton, H. J., Wu, Y. W., Sidney, S., & Claiborne Johnston, S. (2007). Risk of recurrent childhood arterial ischemic stroke in a population-based cohort: The importance of cerebrovascular imaging. *Pediatrics, 119*(3), 495–501.

Gilbertson, S. (1998). Music therapy in neurosurgical rehabilitation. In T. Wigram & J. De Backer (Eds.), *Clinical applications of music therapy in developmental disability, paediatrics and neurology* (pp. 224–245). Philadelphia, PA: Jessica Kingsley Publishers.

Gilbertson, S. (2009). A reference standard bibliography: Music therapy with children who have experienced traumatic brain injury. *Music and Medicine, 1*(2), 129–139.

Gilbertson, S., & Ischebeck, W. (2001). Merging pathways: Music therapy in neurosurgical rehabilitation. *Acta Neurochirurgica, Suppl., 79,* 41–42.

Gustorff, D., & Hannich, H.-J. (2000). Jenseits des Wortes: Musiktherapie mit komatösen Patienten auf der Intensivstation (SG1). [*Beyond words: Music therapy with comatose patients on the intensive care ward*]. Bern: Verlag Hans Huber.

Hagen C., Malkmus, D., & Durham, E. (1979). Rehabilitation of the head-injured adult: Comprehensive physical management. Downey, CA: Professional Staff of Rancho Los Amigos Hospital.

Han, B., & Haley, W. E. (1999). Family caregiving for patient with stroke: Review and analysis. *Stroke, 30,* 1478–1485.

Hömberg, V. (2005). Evidence-based medicine in neurological rehabilitation—A critical review. *Acta Neurochirurgica, 93,* 3–14.

Hough, M. S. (2010). Melodic Intonation Therapy and aphasia: Another variation on a theme. *Aphasiology, 24*(6–8), 775–786.

Hu, M.-H., Hsu, S.-S., Yip, P.-K., Jeng, J.-S., & Wang, Y.-H. (2010). Early and intensive rehabilitation predicts good functional outcomes in patients admitted to the stroke intensive care unit. *Disability and Rehabilitation, 32*(15), 1251–1259.

Hurkmans, J., de Bruijn, M., Boonstra, A. M., Jonkers, R., Bastiaanse, R., Arendzen, H., & Reinders-Messelink, H. A. (2012). Music in the treatment of neurological language and speech disorders: A systematic review. *Aphasiology, 26*(1), 1–19.

Hyde, K., Zatorre, R., & Peretz, I. (2011). Functional MRI evidence of an abnormal neural network for pitch processing in congenital amusia. *Cerebral Cortex, 21,* 292–299.

Janssen, H., Bernhardt, J., Collier, J. M., Sena, E. S., McElduff, P., Attia, J., et al. (2010). An enriched environment improves sensorimotor function post-ischemic stroke. *Neurorehabilitation and Neural Repair, 24,* 802–813.

Jennett, B., & Bond, M. (1975). Assessment of outcome after severe brain damage. *Lancet, 1,* 480–484.

Jeong, S., & Kim, M. T. (2007). Effects of a theory-driven music and movement program for stroke survivors in a community setting. *Applied Nursing Research, 20*(3), 125–131.

Jungblut, M. (2005). Music therapy and chronic aphasia: A controlled study. In D. Aldridge (Ed.), *Music therapy and neurological rehabilitation: Performing health* (pp. 189–209). Philadelphia, PA: Jessica Kingsley Publishers.

Jungblut, M., & Aldridge, D. (2004). Musik als Brücke zur Sprache—die musik-therapeutische Behandlungsmethode SIPARI® bei Langzeitaphasikern [Music as a bridge to speech—the music therapeutic treatment method SIPARI® with chronic aphasics]. *Neurologie und Rehabilitation, 10*(2), 69–78.

Jungblut, M., Suchanek, M., & Gerhard, H. (2009) Long-term recovery from chronic global aphasia: A case report. *Music and Medicine, 1*(1), 61–69.

Keith, R. L., & Aronson, A. E. (1975). Singing as therapy for apraxia of speech and aphasia: Report of a case. *Brain and Language, 2,* 438–488.

Kennelly, J. (2006). Music therapy in paediatric rehabilitation. In F. Baker & J. Tamplin (Eds.), *Music therapy methods in neurorehabilitation* (pp. 219–233). Philadelphia, PA: Jessica Kingsley Publishers.

Kim, D. S., Park, Y. G., Choi, J. H., Im, S-H., Jung, K. J., Cha, Y. A., ... Yoon, K. J. (2011). Effects of music therapy mood in stroke patients. *Yonsei Medical Journal, 53*(6), 977–981.

Kim, M., & Tomaino, C. M. (2008). Protocol evaluation for effective music therapy for persons with nonfluent aphasia. *Topics in Stroke Rehabilitation, 15*(6), 555–569.

Kim, S. J., & Koh, I. (2005). The effects of music on pain perception of stroke patients during upper-extremity joint exercises. *Journal of Music Therapy, 42*(1), 81–92.

Knight, A. J., & Wiese, N. (2011). Therapeutic music and nursing in poststroke rehabilitation. *Rehabilitation Nursing, 36*(5), 200–204.

Koelsch, S. (2009). A neuroscientific perspective on music therapy. *The Neurosciences and Music III – Disorders and Plasticity*: *Annals of the New York Academy of the Sciences, 1169*, 374-384.

Levitin, D. J., & Torovolas, A. K. (2009). Current advances in the cognitive neuroscience of music. *Annals of New York Academy of Sciences, 1156,* 221–231.

Lopez-Vicente, M., Ortega-Gutierrez, S., Amlie-Lefond, C., & Torbey, M. (2010). Diagnosis and management of pediatric arterial ischemic stroke. *Journal of Stroke and Cerebrovascular Diseases, 19*(3), 175–183.

Magee, W. (2007). Development of a music therapy assessment tool for patients in low awareness states. *NeuroRehabilitation, 22*(4), 319–324.

Magee, W., & Wheeler, B. (2006). Music therapy for patients with traumatic brain injury. In G. J. Murray (Ed.), *Alternate therapies in the treatment of brain injury and neurobehavioral disorders* (pp. 51–74). London: The Hawthorn Press.

McMaster, N. (1991). Reclaiming a positive identity: Music therapy in the aftermath of a stroke. In K. Bruscia (Ed.), *Case studies in music therapy* (pp. 547–560). Gilsum, NH: Barcelona Publishers.

Menary, R. (Ed.). (2010). *The Extended Mind*. London: MIT Press.

Moon, S.Y. (2008). The effects of piano-playing music therapy on motor coordination of stroke patients using MIDI-based computer analysis. *Neurorehabilitation and Neural Repair, 22*(5), 593.

Murray, C. L., & Lopez, A. D. (Eds.) (1996). *The global burden of disease: A comprehensive assessment of mortality and disability from disease, injuries, and risk factors in 1990 and projected to 2020.* Boston: Harvard University Press.

National Institutes of Health (NIH). (2012). *NIH Stroke Scale*. Retrieved from http://www.ninds.nih.gov/doctors/NIH_Stroke_Scale.pdf. Accessed on April 4, 2012.

National Institute of Neurological Disorders and Stroke (NINDS). (2009). *Stroke: Challenges, progress, and promise*. Retrieved from http://stroke.nih.gov/documents/NINDS_StrokeChallenge_Brochure.pdf. Accessed on December 14, 2011.

National Stroke Association. (2012). *F.A.S.T. Warning signs of stroke*. Internet site available at www.stroke.org. Last accessed May 10, 2012.

Nayak, S., Wheeler, B. L., Shiflett, S. C., & Agostinelli, S. (2000). Effect of music therapy on mood and social interaction among individuals with acute traumatic brain injury and stroke. *Rehabilitation Psychology, 45*(3), 274–283.

Norton, A., Zipse, L., Marchina, S., & Schlaug, G. (2009). Melodic Intonation Therapy: Shared insights on how it is done and why it might help. *Annals of the New York Academy of Sciences, Jul, 1169,* 431–436. DOI: 10.1111/j.1749-6632.2009.04859.x.

Paul, S., & Ramsey, D. (1998). The effects of electronic music-making as a therapeutic activity for improving upper-extremity active range of motion. *Occupational Therapy International, 5*(3), 223–237.

Pekna, M., Pekny, M., & Nilsson, M. (2012). Modulation of neural plasticity as a basis for stroke rehabilitation. *Stroke, 43,* 2819–2828.

Perkins, E., Stephens, J., Xiang, H., & Lo, W. (2009). The cost of pediatric stroke acute care in the Uniter States. *Stroke, 40*, 2820-2827.

Phillips-Silver, J., Toiviainen, P., Gosselin, N., Piché, O., Nozaradan, S., Palmer, C., & Peretz, I. (2011). Born to dance but beat deaf: A new form of congenital amusia. *Neuropsychologia, 495,* 961–969.

Phipps, M.A., Carroll, D.L. & Tsiantoulas, A. (2010). Music as a therapeutic intervention on an inpatient neuroscience unit. Complementary Therapies in Clinical Practice, *16*, 138-142.

Purdie, H., & Baldwin, S. (1994). Music therapy: Challenging low self-esteem in people with a stroke. *British Journal of Music Therapy, 8*(2), 19–24.

Purdie, H., & Baldwin, S. (1995). Models of music therapy intervention in stroke rehabilitation. *International Journal of Rehabilitation Research, 18*(4), 341–350.

Purdie, H., Hamilton, S., & Baldwin, S. (1997). Music therapy: Facilitating behavioral and psychological change in people with stroke: A pilot study. *International Journal of Rehabilitation Research, 20,* 325–327.

Ramsey, D. W. (2002). *The restoration of communal experience during the music therapy process with the non-fluent aphasic patients.* Unpublished doctoral dissertation. New York City: New York University.

Rappaport, M., Hall, K. M., Hopkins, H. K., Belleza, T., & Cope, D. N. (1982). Disability rating scale for severe head trauma: Coma to community. *Archives Physical Medicine and Rehabilitation, 63,* 118–123.

Rodriguez-Fornells, A., Rojo, N., Amenguel, J. L., Ripollis, P., Altenmüller, E., & Monte, T. F. (2012). The involvement of audio-motor coupling in the music-supported therapy applied to stroke patients. *Annals of the New York Academy of Sciences, 1252,* 282–293.

Rojo, N., Amengual, J., Juncadella, M., Rubio, F., Camara, E., & Marco-Pallares, J. (2011). Music supported therapy induces plasticity in the sensorimotor cortex in chronic stroke: A single-case study using multimodal imaging (fMRI-TMS). *Brain Injury, 25*(7–8), 787–793.

Royal College of Physicians. (2004). *Stroke in childhood: Clinical guidelines for diagnosis, management and rehabilitation.* Available from http://bookshop.rcplondon.ac.uk/contents/f98c6540-a541-4bed-837d-ef293ac458bf.pdf. Last accessed on June 1, 2012.

Royal College of Physicians. (2008). *Stroke: National clinical guideline for diagnosis and initial management of acute stroke and transient ischaemic attack (TIA).* Retrieved from http://www.nice.org.uk/guidance/index.jsp?action=download&o=41363. Last accessed January 8, 2012.

Sackett, D. L., Rosenberg, W., Gray, J. A. M., Haynes, R. B., & Richardson, W. S. (1996). Evidence-based medicine: What it is and what it isn't. *British Medical Journal, 312,* 71–72.

Särkämö, T., Tervaniemi, M., Laitinen, S., Forsblom, A., Soinila, S., Mikkonen, M. ... Hietanen, M. (2008). Music listening enhances cognitive recovery and mood after middle cerebral artery stroke. *Brain, 131*(3), 866–876.

Särkämö, T., Tervaniemi, M., Soinila, S., Autti, T., Silvennoinen, H. M., Laine, M., Hietanen, M., & Pihko, E. (2010). Auditory and cognitive deficits associated with acquired amusia after stroke: A magnetoencephalography and neuropsychological follow-up study. *PLoS One, 5*(12), e15157.

Satink, T., Cup, E. H., Ilott, I., Prins, J., de Swart, B. J., & Nijhuis-van der Sanden, M. W. (2013). Patients' views on the impact of stroke on their roles and self: A thematic synthesis of qualitative studies. *Archives of Physical Medicine and Rehabilitation*. DOI: 10.1016/j.apmr.2013.01.011.

Schaefer, S., Murray, M. A., Magee, W., & Wheeler, B. (2006). Melodic Intonation Therapy with brain-injured patients. In Murray, G. J. (Ed.), *Alternate therapies in the treatment of brain injury and neurobehavioral disorders* (pp. 51–74). London: The Hawthorn Press.

Schauer, M., & Mauritz, K. H. (2003). Musical motor feedback (MMF) in walking hemiparetic stroke patients: Randomized trials of gait improvement. *Clinical Rehabilitation, 17*(7), 713–722.

Schlaug, G. (2009). Listening to and making music facilitates brain recovery processes. *The Neurosciences and Music III: Disorders and Plasticity: Annals of the New York Academy of Sciences,* 1169: 372–373.

Schlaug, G., Marchina, S. & Norton, A. (2009). Evidence for plasticity in white-matter tracts of patients with chronic Broca's aphasia undergoing intense intonation-based speech therapy. The Neurosciences and Music III: Disorders and Plasticity: Annals of the New York Academy of Sciences, 1169: 385-394.

Schneider, S., Schönle, P. W., Altenmüller, E., & Munte, T. F. (2007). Using musical instruments to improve motor skill recovery following a stroke. *Journal of Neurology, 254*(10), 1339–1346.

Shapiro, L. (2011*). Embodied Cognition*. London: Routledge Publishers.

Simma, B., & Lütschg, J. (2010). Epidemiology and etiology of pediatric stroke. *Journal of Pediatric Neurology, 8,* 245–249.

Sparks, R., Helm, N., & Albert, M. (1974). Aphasia rehabilitation resulting from Melodic Intonation Therapy. *Cortex, 10,* 303–316.

Sparks, R., & Holland, A. L. (1976). Method: Melodic Intonation Therapy for aphasia. *Journal of Speech and Hearing Disorders, 41,* 287–297.

Tamplin, J. (2000). Improvisational music therapy approached to coma arousal. *Australian Journal of Music Therapy, 11,* 38–51.

Tamplin, J. (2008). A pilot study into the effects of vocal exercises and singing on dysarthric speech. *NeuroRehabilitation, 23*(3), 207–216.

Teasdale, G., & Jennet, B. (1974). Assessment of come and impaired consciousness. *The Lancet, 2,* 81–84.

Thaut, M. H. (2008). *Rhythm, music, and the brain: Scientific foundations and clinical applications.* New York: Taylor and Francis.

Thaut, M. H. (2010). Neurologic Music Therapy in cognitive rehabilitation. *Music Perception, 27*(4), 281–285.

Thaut, M. H., & Abiru, M. (2010). Rhythmic auditory stimulation in rehabilitation of movement disorders: A review of current research. *Music Perception, 27*(4), 263–269.

Thaut, M. H., Kenyon, G. P., Hurt, C. P., McIntosh, G. C., & Hoemberg, V. (2002). Kinematic optimization of spatiotemporal patterns in paretic arm training with stroke patients. *Neuropsychologia, 40*(7), 1073–1081.

Thaut, M. H., Kenyon, G. P., Schauer, M. L., & McIntosh, G. C. (1999). The connection between rhythmicity and brain function. *IEEE Engineering in Medicine and Biology, 3,* 101–108.

Thaut, M. H., Leins, A. K., Rice, R., Argtatter, H., Kenyon, G. P., McIntosh, G. C. ... Fetter, M. (2007). Rhythmic auditory stimulation improves gait more than NDT/Bobath training in near-ambulatory patients early poststroke: A single-blind randomized trial. *Neurorehabilitation and Neural Repair, 21*(5), 455–459.

Thaut, M. H., McIntosh, G. C., Prassas, S., & Rice, R. (1992). Effects of auditory rhythmic pacing on normal gait and gait in stroke, cerebellar disorder, and transverse myelitis. *International Symposium on Postural and Gait Research, 2,* 437–440.

Thaut, M. H., Rice, R. R., & McIntosh, G. C. (1997). Rhythmic facilitation of gait training in hemiparetic stroke rehabilitation. *Journal of Neurological Sciences, 151,* 7–12.

Weller, C. M., & Baker, F. A. (2011). The role of music therapy in physical rehabilitation: A systematic literature review. *Nordic Journal of Music Therapy, 20*(1), 43–61.

Wheeler, B. L., Shiflett, S. C., & Nayak, S. (2009). Effects of number of sessions and group or individual music therapy on the mood and behavior of people who have had strokes or traumatic brain injuries. *Rehabilitation Psychology, 45*(3), 274–283.

Whitall, J., McCombe, A., Waller, S., Silver, K. H., & Macko, R. F. (2000). Repetitive bilateral arm training with rhythmic auditory cuing improves motor function in chronic hemiparetic stroke. *Stroke, 31*(10), 2390–2395.

Widmaier, E. P., Raff, H., & Strang, K. T. (2006). *Vander's human physiology: The mechanisms of body function, 10th Edition.* New York: McGraw Hill.

Wolfe, C. (2000). The impact of stroke. *British Medical Bulletin, 56,* 275–286.

World Health Organization. (1978). *Cerebrovascular disorders: A clinical and research classification.* Geneva: World Health Organization.

World Health Organization. (2002). *The World Health Report 2002: Reducing risks, promoting healthy life.* Geneva: World Health Organization.

World Health Organization. (2010). *International Statistical Classification of Diseases and Related Health Problems Internet Application.* Retrieved from http://apps.who.int/classifications/icd10/browse/2010/en#/I61. Last accessed February 12, 2012.

Wosch, T., & Wigram, T. (Eds.). (2007). *Microanalysis in music therapy: Methods, techniques and application for clinicians, researchers, educators, and students.* Philadelphia, PA: Jessica Kingsley Publishers.

Chapter 7

Adults with Traumatic Brain Injury

Victoria Policastro Vega

In a time of fast cars, high-risk sports, escalating violent crimes, and the aging of our society, 1.7 million people in the United States sustain a brain injury each year. Of those individuals, approximately 275,000 require hospitalization and 99,000 exhibit a lifelong debilitating loss of function. It is estimated that Traumatic Brain Injury (TBI) is responsible for over 52,000 deaths in the United States each year and is the number one cause of death and disability for those ages 1 to 44 (Faul, Xu, Wald, & Coronado, 2010).

Diagnostic Information

Several associations have defined Traumatic Brain Injury. The Brain Injury Association of America (BIAA) defines TBI as "an alteration in brain function, or other evidence of brain pathology, caused by an external force" (BIAA, 2011). The Centers for Disease Control (CDC) define traumatic brain injury as "an occurrence of injury to the head (arising from blunt or penetrating trauma or from acceleration-deceleration forces) that is associated with any of the following symptoms or signs attributable to the injury: decreased level of consciousness, amnesia, other neurologic or neuropsychologic abnormalities, skull fracture, diagnosed intracranial lesions, or death" (CDC, 2012). Finally, the National Brain Injury Foundation (NBIF) defines TBI as "damage to living brain tissue caused by an external, mechanical force. It is usually characterized by a period of altered consciousness due to coma or amnesia and can be as brief as a few minutes or exceedingly long (months/indefinitely). The resulting tissue damage impairs an individual's physical, mental, and/or psychosocial abilities" (NBIF, 2012). Traumatic brain injuries are classified as mild, moderate, severe, or catastrophic, as follows.

Mild: A mild brain injury accounts for 75%–90% of all TBIs (CDC, 2003). Individuals with a mild TBI may have a confused, vacant stare directly after the insult, but have not had a loss of consciousness for more than 15 minutes. Neurological testing as well as CT and MRIs fall within the normal range. However, individuals may suffer from headaches, dizziness, and/or nausea along with periods of disorientation and inconsistent memory. The individual's speech may be inarticulate and verbal and motor responses to questions may be delayed. Other physical symptoms may include blurred vision, being easily fatigued, and having sensitivity to light and noise. Cognitive symptoms associated with mild TBI include distractibility, difficulty concentrating, poor problem-solving skills, and difficulty with reading and language comprehension. Emotionally, the individual with a mild TBI may suffer from depression, mood shifts, anxiousness, insomnia, irritability, and loss of libido. Over 50% of individuals with a mild TBI return to work within two weeks, while one-third are unable to return to work 3–6 months after injury. Lastly, as many as 15% of individuals with a mild TBI continue to experience periods of depression, irritable behavior, and headaches throughout their life (CDC, 2003). Concussions are one example of a mild TBI.

Moderate: A person who has sustained a moderate TBI may be unconscious from 15 minutes up to 24 hours. Moderate brain injuries can result in hospitalization for several weeks. Many cognitive deficits are present at this level, such as memory deficits and poor safety/judgment and problem-solving skills. Communication skills are severely impaired, as the person with a moderate TBI will have both expressive and receptive language problems. Motor skills are impaired, which often results in ataxia movements, impaired coordination, perceptual difficulties, balance issues, and even paralysis. All of these deficits lead to a low frustration threshold and behavioral issues. To compound these problems, the individual with a moderate TBI displays impulsiveness, making them at risk for further injury due to their poor safety and judgment skills. Not surprisingly, as many as two-thirds of these individuals are unable to return to work.

Severe: A severe head injury is categorized at the bottom of the Glasgow Coma Scale (GCS) with a score of 3 to 8 (Dawodu, 2012). A person with a severe TBI has deep and widespread brain damage and will exhibit all of the aforementioned challenges listed under moderate brain injury. Cognitively, these individuals have short attention spans and impaired short- and long-term memory. The person with a severe TBI will have severe communication deficits and may communicate only through yes/no gestures. In addition, these individuals will have very limited or absent active motor skills and display poor balance and trunk control. Individuals with severe TBI have a very small probability of returning to a work environment, even in a reduced capacity (CDC, 2012).

Catastrophic: A catastrophic brain injury in characterized by the individual being in a deep coma anywhere from a few months to maintaining a chronic persistent vegetative state. These individuals may exhibit sleep and wakeful cycles without any true awareness. They display poor responses to their environment and are unable to communicate their wants and needs. Furthermore, they are usually wheelchair-bound, fed through a gastronomy tube, and require 24-hour nursing care. These individuals are unable to communicate even with gestures and have no purposeful motor skills.

In addition to the medical severity, TBI can be classified by the nature of the injury itself. The following are terms and definitions related to this classification system:

- *Closed Head Injury (CHI)* is an injury to the brain that occurs due to the violent shearing (tears) of the brain inside the skull (CDC, 2012).
- *Penetrating Head Injury* occurs when a foreign object enters the skull and strikes the brain (CDC, 2012).
- *Anoxic brain injury* occurs from lack of oxygen.
- *Hypoxic brain injury* occurs when there is insufficient oxygen to the brain.

In addition to classifications of brain injury types, a variety of other medical terms and conditions are associated with traumatic brain injury. The most common of these are listed below.

- *Coma* is an altered state of consciousness where even powerful stimulation cannot arouse the patient.
- *Vegetative comatose state* is when an individual returns to a state of wakefulness but without cognitive functioning. They may open their eyes and even exhibit a sleep-wake cycle, but they do not respond to environmental stimulus.
- *Persistent vegetative comatose state* is characterized by no responses to the environment for a month or more (BIAA, 2011).

- *Post-Traumatic Amnesia (PTA)* may also be a factor and is defined as the loss of the ability to remember day-to-day events after the traumatic event. The longer the TBI displays signs of PTA, the less the likelihood of a good recovery.
- *Recurrent traumatic brain injury* may occur when the individual with a mild TBI doesn't show signs of the initial brain injury and sustains a second impact to the brain that can cause "muscle spasms, increased muscle tone, rapidly changing emotions, hallucinations, and difficulty thinking and learning" (CDC, 2012).
- *Continuous memory* is the length of time between the traumatic incident and when the individual can recall day-to-day events.
- *Seizure, absence,* also known as *petit mal seizure,* is defined as "a sudden interruption of conscious physical and mental activities and a short period of unconsciousness" (Medical-Dictionary, 2012).
- *Seizure, complex partial,* is a "seizure stemming from a localized part of the brain indicated by the presence of a state similar to a trance, varying degrees of awareness, and the manifestation of purposeless behaviors or motions. The seizure may be followed by an indeterminate period of confusion, garbled speech, poor mood, and an inability to recall the events of the episode" (Medical-Dictionary, 2012).
- *Seizure, generalized,* also known as *grand mal seizure,* is a "convulsive spell that has a simultaneous effect on the entire brain" (Medical-Dictionary, 2012).

Needs and Resources

The brain is a complex highway of nerves that coordinates the body's ability to function. It is the master organ that enables each of us to be unique individuals, which is why no two individuals with a TBI are alike. When this three-pound spongy tissue is impaired, our ability to communicate, move, and think is impacted. The individual's characteristics before the TBI occurred, such as age, intellectual and physical levels, general health, and personality characteristics such as motivation, can influence the person's recovery. Younger brains still developing have an increased chance of developing other areas of the brain to compensate for damaged areas. Initial indicators of recovery post injury include the area and extent of the injury, length of coma, the period of time since the traumatic insult, and whether the person experienced post-traumatic amnesia. Finally, how quickly and to what extent treatment was given and the support of loved ones is an important factor in the recovery of a TBI (National Institute of Neurological Disorder & Stroke, [NINDS], 2012).

The individual recovering from a TBI is usually struggling with issues relating to more than one area of functioning. Cognition is the most affected area, as the person may have difficulty in any of these areas: alertness level; attention span; orientation to person, place, and time; short-term memory; and sequential memory. Motor skills may be severely impacted, as the individual may have difficulty with fine and gross motor skills, eye-hand coordination, ambulation, and overall motor strength and endurance. Communication deficits may include receptive and expressive language impairments as well as deficits in articulation. Finally, the individual may display difficulties expressing their emotions and/or navigating social situations.

The music therapist gains information about the individual's needs by having knowledge about the right and/or left hemisphere damage and the resulting symptomology. These are described in more detail below.

Right Hemisphere Damage

An individual with right hemisphere damage may exhibit physical deficits in several areas. The most common physical deficit is left hemiplegia that results in the person having partial or total paralysis. This may be further complicated with left-sided neglect, where the individual doesn't consider their left side when completing motor or visual tasks. Further complications may include overestimation of their abilities, decreased performance on visual tasks, and poor safety-judgment skills, all of which put the individual at risk for falls and further injury.

Cognitively, the patient with TBI with right hemisphere damage has a shortened attention span that can be as little as a few seconds or minutes. This makes the process of building on past information to learn new information almost impossible. Consequently, individuals may display concrete-thinking and have a decreased appreciation for subtleties.

Behaviorally, individuals with right hemisphere damage may display a lack of inhibition or impulse control This can result in verbal outbursts and social inappropriateness, as they will state whatever is on their mind. The inability to filter and control impulses may lead to a great strain on relationships with family and friends.

Left Hemisphere Damage

An individual with left hemisphere damage will exhibit the same motor deficits as the person with the right hemisphere damage but on the opposite side of the body. Hemiplegia with partial or total paralysis and neglect may occur on the right side. To further complicate matters, the individual with left hemispheric damage may have difficulty distinguishing their left from right. The person with left hemispheric damage may have decreased performance on mathematics intelligence tests. Using simple math to navigate day-to-day living, such as negotiating money, may be difficult.

Perhaps the largest issue with a survivor of TBI with left hemispheric damage is impairments in language and communication skills. The most common disorders are defined below.

- *Aphasia* is a speech disorder due to brain damage and can seriously impact receptive and expressive language (Taylor, 1989, p. 169). Specifically, an individual with aphasia will have difficulties in naming objects, impaired verbal learning, and word-finding problems that leave the person unable to express the simplest of daily needs.
- *Apraxia* is characterized by an inability to verbally express oneself due to lack of oral-motor and articulation skills (Taylor, 1997, p. 92).
- *Dysarthria* is defined as the inability to control movements required for speech, which causes abnormal prosody (rate of speech) and intelligibility issues (Taylor, 1997, p. 92).
- *Alexia* and *Agraphia* are when an individual is unable to make sense of reading and writing, respectively (Medical-Dictionary, 2012).

With both expressive and receptive language issues, the individual may be easily frustrated, and the inability to express themselves and understand others may lead to depression.

Referral and Assessment

The journey to recovery for the individual who has sustained a TBI can be long and encompass several medical settings. Initially, the individual will be treated in an inpatient medical facility until their medical status is stable. Once medically stable, they will be moved to an inpatient rehabilitation center. Inpatient rehabilitation centers focus on treatment that will lead to individuals gaining independence in the areas of cognition, motor, communication, social, and emotional skills. Upon discharge from inpatient rehabilitation, the patient may move to outpatient rehabilitation or a group home.

There are several standardized assessment tools used by medical facilities to assess the individual's alertness level and cognitive functioning. Each is discussed below.

Glasgow Coma Scale (GCS). The GCS is the most frequently used diagnostic tool to evaluate the level of coma and impaired consciousness following the initial traumatic incident (Teasdale & Jennett, 1974). This scale ranges from 3–15 and has three categories: eye opening, motor response to pain stimulus or command, best verbal. Each category has subscales, and a point is counted if the patient who has sustained a TBI is able to execute the desired response. The overall score is used to determine the severity of the TBI client and is as follows: Severe (1–8), Moderate (9–12) and Mild (13–15) (Dawodu, 2012). See Appendix A.

Ranchos Los Amigos Scale of Cognitive Functioning (RLA). The *RLA Scale of Cognitive Functioning* is an assessment tool that is used throughout the rehabilitation of an individual who has sustained a TBI. The first three levels state that the individual needs total assistance with all Activities of Daily Living (ADL). These levels are: Level I—no response, Level II—generalized response, and Level III—localized response. The next two levels state that the individual requires maximum assistance. These levels are; Level IV—confused/agitated, and Level V—confused, inappropriate non-agitated. Level VII—automatic, appropriate only—states that the individual receives minimal assistance for ADLs. Level VIII—purposeful, appropriate—states that the individual requires standby assistance, and Level IX—purposeful, appropriate—is standby assistance upon request from the patient. Finally, Level X—purposeful, appropriate—is modified independent. See Appendix B.

Claeys, Miller, Dalloul-Rampersad, and Kollar (1989) suggest using the *RLA Scale of Cognitive Functioning* to aid in determining music therapy treatment with patients who have sustained a TBI. They further suggest a transdisciplinary approach that focuses on the patient's physical, emotional, and spiritual needs. When the patient is within RLA levels I–III, the focus is on increasing consistent responses to presented stimuli, electing vocalizations, and facial movements. The foci of patients on the Ranchos IV and V levels are to increase motor and communication goals. For the person with an RLA VI- and VII-level TBI, music therapy treatment focuses on continuing to work on previously stated goal areas in addition to emotional expression and socialization skills. It should be noted that at the time of this study the RLA contained only eight levels, whereas the revised scale contains ten levels.

Disability Rating Scale. The *Disability Rating Scale (DRS)* is used to accurately describe the functioning level of a survivor of a severe TBI. A total Disability Rating Score (DR Score) is calculated and based upon nine levels of disability, from no disability to extreme vegetative state (Rappaport et al., 1982). Subscales assess the survivor of a TBI in the five categories of arousal (score 0–3), cognition for ADLs (score 0–4), dependence on others (score 0–5), and psychosocial adaptability (score 0–3). See Appendix C.

Music Therapy

Individuals who have survived a TBI are often referred to music therapy to address their inability to consistently respond to their environment and loved ones. Often, music has played an important role in an individual's life. Initially, reaching them through music during low awareness states is the paramount reason why the individual is referred to music therapy. As the individual becomes more alert, music therapy may aid in orientation, attention to task, and memory. When the individual with TBI becomes overwhelmed and agitated, music therapy relaxation techniques can calm and provide respite. The active playing of music instruments can restore motor and coordination skills. The singing of songs and playing of wind instruments can facilitate communication. Self-expression may be facilitated through lyric analysis, song composition, or music improvisation. Group music therapy sessions can provide a venue to engage in socialization. Finally, survivors of TBI may be referred to music therapy to gain support from peers who have experienced similar tragedies.

Wilson (1990) states music therapists might assume a major responsibility in three modalities of medical practice. He suggests that physical, cognitive, and emotional areas of patients with neurological impairments be targeted during rehabilitation. Similarly, Thompson and Murray (1990) state that music therapy assessment requires several sessions and should encompass each of the following domain areas: cognitive, communication, motor, social, and visual. The music therapist, in working with the interdisciplinary team, can ensure maximum rehabilitation benefits for the patient and a more comprehensive treatment program by addressing domains suggested.

To assess the patient's environmental alertness, the music therapist may play live, patient-preferred music. The music therapist may present the music both aurally and tactilely to one side of the patient to elicit consistent sound localization skills. The patient's cognitive status is also assessed through the medium of music. For example, when evaluating the patient's sequential memory, the therapist may play rhythm instruments in a sequence and ask the client to repeat what was presented. The patient's physical functioning may be assessed through instrument play. For example, to assess the areas of fine and gross motor function, the music therapist may provide opportunities for the patient to manipulate and play various music instruments. The area of communication may be assessed through participation in song and call-and-response music interventions. The social/emotional domain may be assessed through the patient's overall participation level in individual and group music therapy sessions. The patient's level of functioning determines to what extent each modality will be assessed. For instance, if a patient is in a deep coma, only the area of environmental alertness will be actively addressed. Since each patient has their own individual strengths and weaknesses, no two patients can be assessed using the same techniques.

The most important part of music therapy assessment with the patient who has sustained a TBI is the determination of the patient's music preferences. Often, the individual has severe cognitive deficits and is unable to provide this information. The music therapist may begin by interviewing family members and friends to obtain information about the patient's personal music listening preferences. The music preferences of this clinical population have more to do with the patient's age group than as a function of their diagnosis. Therefore, the music therapist can consult the music therapy literature for music preference studies with regard to the age group of each individual.

Daveson (2008) introduced the Meta-Model of Music Therapy in Neuro-Disability (MIND) as a five-step process in assessing the rehabilitation needs of individuals with neurodisabilities. The first step is providing the rationale for music therapy treatment with regard to motor, communication, cognitive, social/emotional, behavioral and occupational needs. The second step is determining restorative, compensatory, and/or psycho-social-emotional treatment approaches. In step three, the initial assessment is completed and treatment focus is identified. In step four, measurable goals and objectives are formulated. Finally, in step five, appropriate music therapy models are identified to aid the individual in attaining treatment goals.

Overview of Methods and Procedures

The following methods and procedures are most commonly used with individuals who have sustained a TBI. These have not been sequenced to reflect relative significance, effectiveness, or complexity.

Receptive Music Therapy

- Music Listening for Sensory Stimulation: The therapist presents age-appropriate, patient-preferred music, either live or recorded, to enhance environmental stimulation.
- Music to Increase Attention Span: The therapist presents vocal and/or instrumental music, either live or recorded, to engage the patient musically.
- Songs for Receptive Language Skills: The therapist presents songs that tell a story, and the patient is asked to relay the story back in proper sequence.
- Emotional Expression Songs: Lyrics of a popular song are discussed and a meaning or central theme is pinpointed in relation to the patient's current emotional state.
- Music Relaxation: The therapist designs a relaxation experience with music.
- Music for Gait Training: Patient-preferred music is used to retrain an individual to walk.
- Music for Range of Motion: Songs are used to increase upper- and lower-extremity range of motion and endurance.

Improvisational Music Therapy

- Music Instrument Improvisation: Music co-created in the moment by the therapist and patient for nonverbal means of expression.
- Story Improvisation: The patient chooses music instruments, vocalizations, and or/body percussion to depict a story based on feelings and emotions related to the rehabilitation process.

Re-creative Music Therapy

- Song Orientation: The use of songs to prompt and reinforce knowledge of temporal, spatial, and personal information.
- Activities of Daily Living Songs: The use of simple melodic lines to increase sequential memory.
- Song Communication: Using vocalization and singing techniques to improve verbal communication.
- Songs for Speech Production: The use of songs with simple or repetitive melodic lines to increase vocal articulation, volume, and prosody.
- Melodic Intonation Therapy: Words, short phrases, and sentences are coupled with melodic and rhythmic components.
- Musical Instrument Instruction: The therapist teaches the patient to play a selected instrument.

Compositional Music Therapy

- Songwriting: The therapist-assisted process of creating music and lyrics to communicate thoughts and feelings.

GUIDELINES FOR RECEPTIVE MUSIC THERAPY

Music Listening for Sensory Stimulation

Overview. With this technique, the therapist presents age-appropriate, patient-preferred music, either live or recorded, to enhance environmental awareness. Music sensory stimulation has been shown to be effective in increasing consciousness of the patient by stimulating the neural pathways that are responsible for arousal (Meyer et. al., 2010). The three senses of tactile, auditory, and visual stimulation should be targeted. Patients who do not consistently respond to traditional therapies often demonstrate sound localization skills and visual tracking skills through presentation of a variety of music instruments and through commands given in music.

Treatment goals for the patient with a TBI greatly depend on the individual's cognitive functioning and level of alertness. At the most basic responsiveness level, treatment goals will focus on increasing consistent environmental responses. This may include changes in vital signs, eye opening, visual gazing and tracking, and motor and verbal skills.

To ensure that the patient who has sustained a TBI is indeed responding to the music stimulus, only one sense should be stimulated at a time. For example, when providing tactile stimulation through music instruments, do so by presenting just vibrations, without adding stimulation such as singing. Consequently, other environmental noises should be held to a minimum whenever possible. This will help to ensure that the individual is putting the music stimulus to the forefront and not responding to a conglomerate of noises. Providing hand-over-hand assistance may be required when handheld music instruments are presented or when the patient requires assistance in placing a hand on an instrument (e.g., guitar or piano) for vibratory stimulation..

The individual who is in a coma displays very limited and inconsistent responses to their environment. Delayed responses to presented stimuli will be the norm, not the exception; therefore, the music therapist must be patient and allow time for responses. The individual with a TBI may exhibit some responses to music stimuli in the morning on one day and in the afternoon on the next. What should be consistent is the time of day and length of the music therapy session. This will provide more accurate information about the individual's alertness level. It is more advantageous to present stimuli twice a day for shorter intervals such as 10–15 minutes than once a day for 30 minutes, as the patient is actively healing and fatigue may be an issue.

Preparation. The therapist will need to be prepared to offer age-appropriate, patient-preferred music, both live and recorded.

What to observe. The music therapist working with a patient in a coma must be a master observer. Many times, the patient with a neurological impairment is being electronically monitored, and the music therapist can watch these monitors for changes in blood pressure, respiration, and heart rate. Other behavioral indications in response to music are the patient's outward physical changes, such as facial pallor, grimacing, teeth grinding, extremity movement, startle response, vocalizations, and/or diaphoresis, which is excessive sweating due to the body's inability to regulate its temperature. The individual may also move toward or away from the presented stimulus. If the patient's vital signs drastically change, this may be a sign of overstimulation; therefore, the music therapist will stop the music stimulation and wait until the patient's vital signs return to a more homeostatic state.

The patient may exhibit tactile defensiveness, defined as "a sensory integrative dysfunction characterized by tactile sensations that cause excessive emotional reactions, hyperactivity, or other behavior problems" (*Mosby's Medical Dictionary,* 2012). Often, the only time when they are being touched is to aid them in ADLs or for invasive medical procedures. Other times, it may just be due to the patient's internal psychomotor agitation. Tactile stimulation should be presented gradually, verbally telling the patient what you will be presenting before it is presented and by stimulating only one sense at a time.

Procedures. The therapist should begin by introducing themselves to the patient, informing the patient who they are and what they are going to do. Short, simple statements are best and will be repeated prior to the presentation of any tactile, auditory, and visual stimulation. The therapist should always speak directly to the patient, in a normal tone of voice, and frequently using the individual's name. Often, the patient may seem unresponsive, but they may comprehend more than they can verbally or physically act upon.

Choose each stimulus according to the patient's current behavioral level. If the patient who has sustained a TBI is calm and alert, exhibited by eye opening, begin with visual stimuli such as bright, shiny music instruments. Present the visual stimulus at the patient's midline. Individuals with a TBI typically display visual tracking of objects horizontally before they are successful doing so vertically. Move the stimulus slowly to the patient's right and left horizontally. Then repeat the same movement by moving the stimulus vertically. The music therapist should observe the patient's eye movements to determine if they are visually tracking the stimulus. This includes whether the patient moves his or her head to continually track the stimulus when the object moves out of their field of vision.

Music instruments provide a variety of tactile stimulation through vibrations. Instruments such as the guitar and drums are presented first on one side of the patient's body and then on the other. Observe the individual for a startle response such as an eye blink or if they look and/or turn toward the sound source. Provide a variety of high- and low-pitched sounds, as the individual may respond more readily to drastic changes more than to subtle ones.

If the individual with a TBI appears lysergic, begin with auditory stimuli such as singing. Again, present the auditory stimulus first on one side of the individual and then on the other. Songs with a strong beat in the patient's preferred genre will be more effective, as more emphatic changes will gain the individual's attention. Song lyrics can also be substituted for commands such as "make your eyes blink" and can be incorporated into a song to elicit a response.

Adaptations. When the patient is in a coma, psychomotor agitation sometimes occurs. Sedative music may or may not have an impact on decreasing this restlessness, as it may be the result of internal agitation rather than external environmental factors. When the patient responds favorably to quiet, then the music therapist will provide a listening/quiet schedule for the patient in an effort to provide periods of rest.

Music to Increase Attention Span

Overview. With this technique, the therapist engages the patient through vocal or instrumental music to increase the length, frequency, and duration of his/her attention. The patient who has sustained a TBI and is emerging from a coma will display inconsistent alertness levels. The attention span of a patient may be as short as just a few seconds to a minute.

Preparation. Minimizing environmental distractions is always a must with this clinical population. To initially enhance the patient's focus, use brightly colored objects that will move the visual stimulus to the forefront. When presenting written words or symbols, be sure to enlarge the print and use color contrasts so that the words or symbols are in the foreground. Whenever possible, close the patient's room door to block out hallway distractions, use the curtain often found in hospital rooms between patients, and use the window curtain or face the patient away from the window. These small steps will help to ensure that the patient has a more successful session.

What to observe. The music therapist must intently observe the individual for this slightest response. Often, the patient's responses are delayed, so the music therapist must be patient. Responses might come in the form of an eye and/or head turn toward the sound source. They may physically turn away from or toward the sound source. Other responses include reaching for a musical instrument or increased vocalizations.

Survivors of a TBI are at risk for seizures, so it is imperative that sudden loud music or instruments not be played, as this may trigger a seizure in the patient. Consequently, flicking lights or reflections off shiny instruments may have the same negative result. The music therapist must intently observe the individual for signs of fatigue. These signs will include a negative shaking of the head or verbalizing "no," turning away from the music therapist, pushing musical instruments away, or physically striking out.

Procedures. The time of day is a factor in the patient's responsiveness. Typically, the morning treatment times are when the patient is more rested and therefore will benefit more from cognitive music therapy interventions. During the afternoon and evening times of the day, the patient usually shows signs of mental and physical fatigue, so providing more passive music therapy interventions will prove to be more effective. The music therapist will need to be aware of the patient's complete therapy schedule. For example, if the patient has just participated in an hour of physical therapy, the music therapist should focus the music therapy interventions on less strenuous physical activity.

Using the patient's name frequently aids in focusing their attention to the presented stimulus. Make sure that the patient is looking at the music therapist and/or music instruments. Gain the individual's visual attention before moving forward with instructions. When asking the patient to follow through on tasks, augment commands by using tactile, auditory, and visual prompts. Keep all verbal directives short and simple and be consistent in the language that is used. Ask the individual to repeat the instructions to make sure that they have heard and understand what is being asked of them. Simply asking "What are you going to do first?" will give the music therapist the confirmation that the individual has not only heard but also comprehends the instructions.

Mental fatigue is an ongoing issue with the individual who has sustained a TBI; therefore, the music therapist must be constantly vigilant in this endeavor. Timing is of the essence, so before the patient exhibits mental fatigue, it is advantageous to alternate cognitive tasks with silence or passive music listening.

Adaptations. There are several adaptations that can ensure that the individual will have a successful experience in music therapy. The amount of cognitive information should be presented from simple to complex. The individual recovering from a TBI should be provided with musical tasks of increasingly longer time frames. The role of music is to cognitively stimulate the patient to want to attend to the presented task in an effort to move toward a more appropriate attention span. This then sets the stage for the relearning of skills, learning new skills, and adaptations of known skills to occur.

Songs for Receptive Language Skills

Overview. With this technique, the therapist presents songs that tell a story and has the patient relay the story back in proper sequence. Often, the individual who has sustained a TBI has difficulty comprehending the spoken language due to damage in the brain's left hemisphere.

The patient may become easily frustrated attempting to understand what is being asked of him/her and may become overwhelmed. When this occurs, the individual is unable to focus on the music intervention and process anything that is being asked of them.

Preparation. The size of written information and the amount of information on a page should be within the patient's ability. It is always better to start with fewer, larger items and progress to smaller print in a larger visual field.

What to observe. The music therapist will have to watch for signs of fatigue and agitation. If the survivor of a TBI exhibits signs of frustration such as motor agitation, vocalizations, sighs, and refusal to attempt the task, the music therapist should change to a more passive music therapy intervention.

Procedures. Songs selected should be based on their ability to tell a story. Folk songs are a good choice for this purpose. The music therapist will provide the song lyrics in written form as well as sing the song live. The patient will be instructed to listen for what happens first, second, and third in the sung story. The individual will then be asked to relay the story back to the music therapist in proper sequence. Initially, only one verse will be presented, and as success is achieved, the length of the song will be increased as well as the complexity of the story. To organize a success-orientated intervention, song lyrics will be presented as one verse per page. This will guard against visual overstimulation and help the individual to maintain focus.

Short, simple instructions should be given and be enhanced by visual prompts or physical demonstrations whenever possible. The music therapist must allow time for the patient to process what has been asked of them, as delayed responses are common with this clinical population. Directions will be given at a slower rate of prosody to aid in comprehension. If commands need to be repeated, they will be repeated using the same language, as changing verbal commands is like asking the patient an entirely new question and is liable to add to their confusion.

Emotional Expression Songs

Overview. With this technique, the lyrics of a popular song are discussed and a meaning or central theme is pinpointed. Next, the patient is encouraged to relate the song to their current emotional state. Feelings typically expressed are those that directly pertain to the accident, physical pain, and family's/friends' reactions to their new appearance, physical and cognitive status, and/or death of loved ones. Fear of future condition and lifestyle are also issues that commonly arise. Using songs as a catalyst for emotional expression may lead to the patient becoming overwhelmed and emotional. The music therapist must make sure that either they or another health care team member is available to provide additional support.

Preparation. Often, popular songs are difficult to comprehend due to the lyrics not being presented in an articulate manner. Typed song lyrics should be presented to the patient to enhance comprehension. The song lyrics should be enlarged and presented on white paper with black letters, as this contrast will aid the individual in their ability to read the words.

What to observe. The music therapist will make sure that the individual who has sustained a TBI is actively looking at the song lyric sheet as the song is being sung or played to ensure focused attention. The music therapist should observe the individual for any changes in facial affect during the experience. For example, the music therapist may observe that the individual fidgets, sighs, or grimaces while a particular lyrical line is being played. These observations may be verbally processed during song lyric discussion.

Procedures. The music therapist will take the individual's music preferences into consideration before selecting a song for lyric discussion. The next consideration is in choosing a theme that is important to the patient's rehabilitation. Common themes include job and/or lifestyle changes; loss of physical capabilities; loss of a loved one; and fear of the future. Whenever possible, the song should be sung and played live for the individual. This will aid in maintaining active attention and will allow the music therapist to slow down the tempo of the song to allow the patient to process all song lyrics. The music therapist will instruct the patient to highlight any lyrics that support their feelings in their current situation or rehabilitation. When the song is completed, the music therapist will ask open-ended verbal processing questions to facilitate a discussion.

Adaptations. The cognitive abilities of the patient who has sustained a TBI should be taken into consideration when choosing songs. Patients with lower cognitive functioning will be given songs that have repetitive lyrics coupled with more simple music instrumentation. Songs with a variety of lyrics and more complex music will be too difficult for the person to comprehend.

Music Relaxation

Overview. With this technique, the therapist designs a relaxation experience with music for the patient with the aim of decreasing physical and mental fatigue. Increasing relaxation through music will give the patient periods of rest so that they are more focused during subsequent treatment. There are different types of music relaxation, including music for relaxation, music-centered relaxation, music with progressive muscle relaxation, and music imagery.

Preparation. Find a quiet area in the hospital or rehabilitation environment. Whenever possible, the lights should also be dimmed, and all environmental distraction held to a minimum.

What to observe. The music therapist should focus on physiological responses of the patient, such as respirations, facial and body tension, and motor restlessness or agitation. This will cue the music therapist to possibly slow down verbal prosody when describing a tranquil process and/or the tempo of the music when instructing the patient in progressive muscle relaxation.

Procedures. The procedure the therapist will follow is dependent on the type of relaxation experience the therapist is providing to the patient.

- *Music for relaxation* introduces the patient to a variety of music that can be used to elicit a relaxation response. The music therapist plays the live or recorded music for a few minutes and has the individual rate which pieces he/she feels are calming. A selection is chosen, and the patient is asked to find a comfortable position and not cross any limbs. They are invited to close their eyes and concentrate on slowing down their breathing while listening to the music.
- In *music-centered relaxation,* the patient is asked to find a comfortable position and not cross any of their limbs. Music is then played, and the music therapist verbally points out instrumentation, tempo, and timbre changes within the music. The length of the relaxation intervention will vary according to the attention span of the individual. Processing after the music relaxation has ended will include which aspects of the music the patient felt were most conducive to a focused relaxed state.
- *Music with imagery and progressive muscle relaxation* is used to help educate the patient on what their body feels like in a tense versus relaxed state. The music therapist will introduce the patient to different styles of instrumental music and/or environmental sounds for feedback from the patient as to their preference. Once the music and/or environmental sounds have been selected, the music will be played and the patient will be asked to get in a comfortable position and not cross any of their limbs. The individual will be invited to close their eyes and initially focus on their breathing to slow it down. The music therapist will begin with a narrative beginning at the patient's head. This may be

done using a more concrete script, such as, "Your forehead is squinting from the sun when a cloud slowly moves in and shields the bright light and your forehead is relaxed." A suggestion for a less concrete script is as follows: "A ball of light is moving from the top of your head, slowly moving to your forehead, and relaxes everything it touches."

- In *music imagery,* the music therapist will create a script using input from the patient about a peaceful environment. The music therapist will ask the person to bring a picture of a peaceful scene to the session. The music therapist will ask the patient to describe what they see, hear, and feel in this environment. When possible, the patient will help in the formation of the relaxation script. The patient, with the aid of the music therapist, may choose music, instruments, and/or environmental sounds to musically create the peaceful environment.

Adaptations. If the individual is at a higher cognitive level, then a more abstract relaxation script can be used. Additionally, music with more depth, such as classical music, can be used during relaxation. The length of the music relaxation session should be within the individual's attention span. Another consideration is if the patient is experiencing any pain in any area of the body. If this is the case, then the individual will be asked to "gently squeeze" the affected area, or it may be determined that music with progressive body tensing and relaxing should not be used.

Music for Gait Training

Overview. This is the use of musical elements to retrain an individual to walk. Often, the inability to walk severely impacts the survivor of a TBI's ability to regain independence. Furthermore, poor balance puts the individual at risk of sustaining another head injury through falls. The anticipation of the rhythmic aspect in music aids the person to move more fluidly through space. Music will be used to enhance gait training, specifically in gait velocity, cadence, stride length, symmetry, and timing.

Physical fatigue is always an issue and can lead to injury. The music therapist must work in conjunction with the physical therapist to ensure that the movement is not contraindicated. Co-treatment in music for gait training is the most beneficial for the patient who has sustained a TBI.

Preparation. The music therapist should ensure that the environment is devoid of visual distractions and physical barriers. The surface that the patient will be walking on should be flat and smooth but not slick. When possible, auditory distractions should be held to a minimum so that the patient can focus on the directions of the music therapist and the music.

What to observe. The music therapist should watch for signs of fatigue and provide periods of rest, when needed. Symptoms of fatigue may include increasingly uneven gait, foot dragging, slowing of physical activity, and/or diaphoresis (excessive sweating).

Procedures. Music preferences will determine the style of music used to facilitate gait training. The music therapist will consult the physical therapist before the session begins to determine if the individual is walking with standby assistance or with a walking device such as a quad-cane or walker. This will determine the number of beats per measure for the music selection. The music will be played live so that the tempo can be regulated to ensure that the individual can successfully execute walking strides. The music is then presented, and the patient is instructed to move their feet and/or supportive walking device to each beat of the music. As the patient with a TBI consistently executes an even gait at a slower pace, the tempo of the music will gradually be increased. The final step is to phase out the music altogether.

Adaptations. Sometimes the survivor of a TBI displays difficulty identifying the beat in the music. The music therapist must first address this by instructing the individual to play the beat of the music to different tempos on rhythm instruments and by using body percussion. Once the individual is successful at determining the beat through these venues, finding the beat to songs in walking cadence will be introduced.

Music for Range of Motion

Overview. This is the use of songs to increase upper- and lower-extremity range of motion and endurance. Music may be instrumental in motivating individuals to engage in physical activity that they find difficult, frustrating, or even painful.

Each individual's treatment should be monitored to ensure that movements they are being asked to perform are not contraindicated. All range-of-motion exercises should be done in conjunction with the treatment team's occupational and physical therapists input.

Preparation. Music to enhance the patient's range of motion and endurance can be done during individual sessions but is most often done in small group settings. This provides an opportunity for peers to support one another and increases a sense of community. The music therapist will need to preplan specific exercises and have knowledge of precautions for each group member.

What to observe. Fatigue is the number one factor and may be manifested by diaphoresis, verbal or physical refusal to continue, and negative change in pallor, such as red for exertion and white for pain.

Procedures. The music therapist will complete music preference surveys of all individuals who will participate in the group and select music based on these preferences. The music therapist will choose music that has a consistent upbeat meter. Whenever possible, provide music choices to the group so that they have input into the selection of the pieces. Move patients into a circle an arm's-length away from each other. The music is played, and the music therapist verbally instructs group members to clap or pat to the beat. Next, previously determined upper-extremity movements are encouraged and alternated with lower-extremity movements to provide needed periods of rest. When the patients are more easily executing the motions, the length of each movement will be increased. When appropriate, group members may suggest and lead in movements. If the group becomes too fatigued, passive music listening will be provided.

Adaptations. Patients may play rhythm instruments while initiating upper- and lower-extremity movements. For example, the music therapist can provide patients mallets to strike drums that are placed above and below midline and to their right and left to increase range of motion. Large, stretchy bands and parachutes can also be used to encourage patients to move in unison to the beat of the music.

Guidelines for Improvisational Music Therapy

Music Instrument Improvisation

Overview. This is music co-created in the moment by therapist and patient for nonverbal means of expression. Often, the individual who has sustained a TBI cannot express their myriad of emotions through just verbal means. Music improvisation is a technique that can provide these individuals with a venue to express these emotions nonverbally. Music therapy may well be the only opportunity a brain-injured patient has to express him/herself emotionally.

Preparation. The music therapist must carefully consider each musical instrument that will be used during therapy. This includes being mindful of the weight of the instrument. If it is too heavy for the patient, they may become easily fatigued, and if it is too light, the music instrument may be difficult to control. The width of the instrument should be considered to determine if a buildup on a mallet will allow the individual to successfully facilitate a grip. Dycem paper under a musical instrument will ensure that the instrument doesn't slide away from the patient.

Wigram (2004) established Guiding Principles for Improvisation as "start with a simple idea; listen carefully to one's music; practice techniques and specific skills; master skills one at a time before attempting to combine and integrate a number of skills" (p. 32). He further states that the music therapist should take into consideration the patient's culture, acquired music skills, music preferences, music education, and personal associations with music.

What to observe. The music therapist should observe the individual for signs of stress and/or fatigue. This may include facial grimaces, verbal protests, or a slowing down or stopping of motor activity.

Seizures are again a consideration, as physical exercise can overtax the individual with a TBI and be an impetus for a seizure to occur. Also, loud, sudden sounds during the improvisation may trigger a seizure in the patient.

Procedures. The music therapist will determine the patient's level of attention and physical abilities and structure the music improvisation accordingly. The individual will be presented with a variety of rhythm instruments, using the considerations mentioned above. In a nonreferential music improvisation, the individual is encouraged to experiment with the instrument's sounds. Next, the patient is asked to begin playing, and the music therapist will support the individual's music by mirroring the same dynamics, timbre, and tempo. The patient is asked to pinpoint a theme at the end of the music improvisation, and verbal processing of the experience will occur.

Adaptations. The individual will be provided with a referential music improvisation with such themes as loss, change, or fear. A variety of music instruments will be provided, and the patient will begin the music-making experience. The music therapist will support the individual by accompanying them on the piano or guitar. The music therapist will engage the survivor of a TBI in verbal processing of the experience.

Story Improvisation

Overview. With this technique, the patient chooses music instruments, vocalizations, and/or body percussion to depict a story based on feelings and emotions related to the rehabilitation process. Story improvisation provides the survivor of a TBI with a creative outlet to express emotions, provides opportunities for decision-making, and increases socialization and cooperation skills with peers. The music therapist must first ascertain that individuals have the cognitive, communication, and attention skills necessary to carry out musical song improvisation to guard against frustration in the patient.

Preparation. Music rhythm instruments will be chosen carefully for the patient's ability to physically manipulate them. A variety of musical instruments with different sounds should be made available to more successfully support their song improvisation.

What to observe. The music therapist should observe the individual for signs of cognitive and/or physical fatigue. The patient being off-task, looking around the room, talking to a peer about another topic, or simply shutting down and looking at the floor are possible signs of cognitive fatigue Physical fatigue may manifest itself through decreased motor movements and verbal complaints.

Procedures. Story improvisation involves four steps. In step one, patients are given several index cards and asked to write feelings and emotions pertaining to their rehabilitation in phrases and sentences, one idea per card. In step two, the patients are asked to arrange each idea in whatever order they choose and are encouraged to add connecting words or phrases to make the story line flow. In step three, the patient chooses music instruments, vocalizations, and/or body percussion to support the song. In step four, the patient(s) perform the song.

Story improvisation can be done in an individual session but is best done as a group project. A group art mural depicting the visual representation of the story can be done to support the theme(s). A melodic line can also be added to the story improvisation.

Adaptations. Survivors of TBI with lower levels of cognition and communication skills can still successfully engage in this music therapy intervention. Short storybooks with poignant themes can be presented to the patient(s). The patient can then choose a story that appeals to them and decide how to support the story line with rhythm instruments.

Guidelines for Re-creative Music Therapy

Song Orientation

Overview. With song orientation, specific songs are used and/or created to prompt and reinforce knowledge of temporal, spatial, and perceptual information. Music acts as a catalyst by which the TBI patient can retrieve important daily information about their immediate environment. The goal with song orientation is to increase orientation to time, place, and person through songs. Two specific techniques are often used. The first technique utilizes interactive song activities whereby the music therapist asks orientation questions to elicit the correct patient response. Responses may be verbal, specific body gestures, or communicated by the use of augmentative devices. The second technique uses informative songs that contain information regarding time of day, day of week, physical location, holidays, or seasons. The role of the music therapist is also to choose songs that take into consideration the patient's age, music preference, culture, and ethnicity.

The individual may become frustrated by the orientation questions asked of him/her. Cognitive tasks require ignoring environmental distractions and the ability to maintain attention long enough to listen to the question fully, process what is being asked, and then formulate a response. This is a lot to require of the patient who has sustained a TBI, and their frustration may lead to verbal or physical aggression.

Preparation. Auditory and visual stimuli should be minimized as much as possible. The extra noise from machines, lights, televisions, radios, and people talking may be a source of distraction. It is best to present only one stimulus at a time and remove it from the patient's visual field before introducing something else. This aids in increasing attention span and the individual's ability to switch from one task to another.

What to observe. Signs of fatigue may manifest themselves in motor restlessness, and/or the patient looking away from the music therapist or totally shutting down and not responding to any questions asked of them.

Procedures. Orientation songs can be used passively to provide information to the patient regarding time of day, place, or season, or for the music therapist to introduce themselves to the patients. Actively, orientation songs can be used to elicit information from the survivor of a TBI. To accomplish a more active approach, the music therapist will choose simple 4 or 5 phrase-known songs. These songs will also have simple melodic lines and steady, nonsyncopated rhythms. The original song lyrics will then be substituted with orientation questions regarding time, place, and person. An example of this would be to use the song "When the Saints Go Marching In." Song lyrics may be the following: Oh, what is today? Today is Wednesday. Today, it's Wednesday April 3rd. Oh, today is Wednesday, April 3rd, 2013.

Adaptations. The passive orientation songs are best used when the patient is at a lower level of cognitive functioning such as coma. Active orientation songs will be used with individuals who have either verbal ability or an augmentative device with which to communicate. The music therapist will begin by requesting simple orientation information such as the patient's name, before moving forward to more complex information.

Activities of Daily Living Songs

Overview. This technique uses simple melodic lines to enhance sequential memory. Sequential memory is often severely impaired, which impacts the patient's ability to perform functional tasks of daily living independently. The goal is to increase sequential memory to achieve activities of daily living (ADL) through song.

Preparation. Environmental distractions will be held to a minimum. The music therapist should also consider the patient's music preference. Once this is known, ADL songs will be presented in that preferred musical style.

What to observe. The music therapist will be vigilant for signs of overstimulation and fatigue. This may manifest itself in motor and/or verbal agitation from the individual.

Procedures. The music therapist should use simple melodic lines from known songs or compose a song with the sequence of an ADL task embedded within the lyrics. Examples of such ADL sequences include eating, clothes dressing, brushing teeth/hair, tying shoes, shaving, or applying makeup. The tempo of the ADL song will be increased to speed up the individual's ability to complete the task in a more appropriate time frame. Gradually, the song is withdrawn and the patient is successful in completing ADLs independently.

Song Communication

Overview. Song communication is the use of vocalization techniques and/or singing to improve verbal communication. There is a strong connection between singing and speech, as both use "pitch and pitch changes, rhythm, dynamics, tempo, tone production, breath control, sentence structure, phrasing, expressive use of tone quality, and cortical control of oral articulators to form words" (Taylor, 1989, p. 174). Therefore, songs and song techniques can be used to increase the patient's expressive communication.

Preparation. The music therapist must ensure an environment that is calm, quiet, and devoid of auditory and visual distractions. Songs chosen are based on patient familiarity, melodic lines with close intervals, and simple rhythmic lines. Completing a music interest survey will provide the music therapist with useful information and ensure appropriate patient preferred music is used.

What to observe. When using songs to enhance communication, the music therapist will observe the individual to determine if the presented song is too complex. The patient may be struggling to keep up with the tempo of the song, become frustrated, and stop attempting to vocalize. Through observation, the music therapist will be able to ascertain when to move to a more advanced level.

The music therapy interventions must not frustrate or overstimulate the patient, as this would impede progress. Removing the patient to a quiet, non-stimulating room or simply providing the patient with silence are effective remedies when a patient does show signs of overstimulation.

Procedures. The brain's left hemisphere is credited with word finding, expressive language, and verbal learning. Rogers and Fleming (1981) developed a five-step progressive technique to improve verbalizations of patients with left hemispheric damage. First, the individual is asked to hum or sing the song using syllables. Second, the music therapist adds phrases that express common individual wants, needs and greetings. Third, the music therapist expands these expressions of needs and greetings to longer phrases. Fourth, vocabulary is increased using a two-note pattern. Finally, the song is gradually faded out and more complicated verbal-only phrases are introduced.

Adaptations. Traditionally, songs used to communicate daily requests and to facilitate greetings are done in individual sessions. Rogers and Fleming (1981) found that this music–speech therapy technique was beneficial in group therapy and also with family involvement.

Songs for Speech Production

Overview. This technique is the use of songs with simple or repetitive melodic lines to increase vocal articulation, volume, and prosody. The end goal is to enhance the communication of everyday wants and needs.

Preparation. The therapy area should be free of visual and auditory distractions. A music interest survey will be completed prior to the first session to determine which songs will be compatible with the individual's preferred musical style. Chosen songs must have simple or repetitive melodic lines and have a consistent, steady beat. As the speech production of a person with TBI improves, more complex melodic and rhythmic lines will be introduced.

What to observe. The music therapist must retain eye contact with the individual at all times to enhance attention and to provide visual cues. Fatigue is also a factor to be considered and may be shown by a decrease in the volume and/or number of vocalizations. Other signs of fatigue include decreased attention and refusing to participate in vocal exercises or singing. When this occurs, the music therapist will change to another music intervention such as passive music listening.

Procedures. The patient will be placed facing the music therapist to ensure that they can receive visual as well as auditory cues. If the person happens to be distracted and looks away, verbal or physical prompts will be provided to bring the patient's attention back to the task. Lucia (1987) developed the Music Therapy Vocal Skills group to aid in speech rehabilitation. The procedure begins with diaphragmatic breathing, vocalizing, singing familiar songs, and rhythmic speech drills. First, songs were sung with rhythmic content and when the patient with a TBI is successful with this step, the melodic component is removed but rhythmic chanting remains. This leads to the individual verbally responding to questions contained within a rhythmic framework.

Adaptations. Baker and Wigram (2005) advocated the use of songs to improve speech intonation in patients who had sustained a TBI. Patients were seen for individual 40- to 50-minute sessions for a total of 15 sessions over a one- to two-month duration. The patients chose three songs that were used repeatedly throughout all music therapy sessions. Each patient was given written lyrics and encouraged to sing. The music therapist sang with the patient and accompanied each song on the guitar.

Melodic Intonation Therapy

Overview. Melodic Intonation Therapy is a structured technique where words, short phrases, and sentences are coupled with melodic and rhythmic components (Albert, Sparks, & Helm, 1973). The individual recovering from a TBI often faces the challenge of regaining expressive language skills. Speech fluency and intonation are important to convey messages. The survivor of a TBI who has expressive language deficits is unable to successfully communicate their wants and needs. The individual and family/friends with whom they are attempting to communicate become frustrated. Soon, the person with a TBI will cease attempting to engage in social situations and will become withdrawn and even depressed (Baker & Wigram, 2005).

Preparation. The music therapist and the individual will sit facing each other, approximately three feet from one another. The environment should be void of environmental distractions and the music therapist should maintain the patient's eye contact. It is best to begin with simple, one-syllable words and progress to multisyllable words, to phrases, and finally to complete sentences given in the framework of melodic and rhythmic lines.

What to observe. The music therapist will be sensitive to signs of frustration from the patient. Signs of frustrations may include facial grimaces, strained vocalizations, heavy sighing, agitated motor movements, and even tears. Positive responses may include smiles, affirmative nodding of the head, and clapping.

Fatigue is again a factor; therefore, verbal tasks should be alternated with nonverbal tasks. The length of the music therapy session should also be a consideration. Initially, the patient may respond more positively to two 15-minute sessions daily instead of one 30-minute session.

Procedures. Once the music therapist has gained the patient's full attention, he/she places their hand over the patient's hand and wrist. The music therapist moves the patient's hand slightly up and down for each syllable of the presented word. This is done while simultaneously singing melodic notes improvised on the spot, one note per syllable. The music therapist presents 10 words in succession by first presenting the word rhythmically and melodically and then signaling the patient to repeat the words with hand gestures. If the patient has difficulty with a presented word, then the music therapist will back up and repeat the word using rhythm and melody at a slower rate to give the patient another opportunity to respond correctly.

Once the individual fluently repeats all the words successfully, the melody is faded out, followed by the rhythmic movement, until the patient is just repeating the presented words. Melodic notes and movement reinforce the word through visual (looking at the music therapist's mouth), tactile (movement and tapping of the syllables), and auditory (melodic notes) stimuli. By using this multimodal approach, the patient is experiencing the sung word through a variety of media in which to relearn language skills.

Adaptations. Baker (2011) suggests using Modified Melodic Intonation Therapy (MMIT) to improve articulation skills and increase motivation of the individual. This researcher has also noted the added benefit to the individual of expressing frustration, anger, and grief about the decreased abilities and the loss of a close family member. In the study, the patient received traditional MIT for three months with a Speech and Language Pathologist (SLP). Together, the music therapist and SLP chose keywords and the music therapist formulated phrases using these words coupled with music. The music therapist took into consideration the patient's vocal and pitch range. First, the music therapist sang the phrase alone; second, the music therapist and the patient sang the phrase in unison; third, the music therapist fades out his/her singing. The final step is to use the phrases in conversational speech. Baker suggests following backup prompts, such as returning to unison singing, if the individual experiences difficulty. The music therapist will cue the patient by jointly singing the first word(s) or target phrase right before the problem area.

Musical Instrument Instruction

Overview. With this technique, the music therapist teaches the patient how to play a selected instrument. Learning to play a music instrument targets many therapeutic goals for the survivor of a TBI. Music instrument playing may increase vital capacity (the amount of gas that is exhaled), eye-hand coordination, and fine and gross motor skills, as well as enhance new learning and memory skills. This in turn will aid the survivor of a TBI to verbally communicate their wants and needs and to perform ADLs. Increasing the patient's vital capacity skills is important not only for their ability to verbally communicate but also for their pulmonary health. The patient's vital capacity endurance is paramount in aiding the patient to perform upper-extremity ADLs and influences motor endurance in the patient, such as walking longer distances. Anyone blowing into an instrument can quickly show signs of fatigue. Therefore, frequent rest periods will be indicated.

Often, the survivor of a TBI has upper-extremity weakness or even paralysis as a result of their injury. The patient may present with hypotonia (muscles are floppy and weak) or ataxia (upper extremities shake when the individual attempts to reach and grasp objects). The individual may experience one or all of these motor deficits at varying degrees.

The individual participating in motor interventions should not strain. This may result in muscle injury and may impede the patient's progress. The music therapist will be observant to carefully monitor the patient for any muscle strain and should frequently ask the individual if they are feeling any ill effects from the movement. The person with ataxia upper-extremity movements may put him/her at risk for hitting themselves in the head with a musical instrument or mallet. The music therapist will take this into consideration before choosing music instruments for engagement in music-making.

Preparation. There are many factors to consider before choosing a music instrument for instruction. The individual's preference for playing an instrument should be considered. If the sound of the instrument is too offensive when played, the individual will not be motivated to continue and put forth their best effort. The person's fine and gross motor skills and range of motion are primary concerns. Hemiparalysis or paralysis may preclude the instruction of many instruments. The left hand is the dominant hand to successfully depress keyholes to produce a tone on wind instruments. Some brass instruments require the opposite, as the left hand is used to stabilize the instrument and the right is used to depress the instrument's keys. The needed upper-extremity extension and weight of the instrument is yet another consideration. Holding an instrument at a 90-degree angle from the body and parallel to the floor, such as is needed to play the flute, is more difficult than holding a recorder or clarinet.

What to observe. The music therapist will closely observe the patient for proper breathing techniques. Physical aspects to observe are the full extension of the abdomen when a deep breath is taken. Shallow breathing may cause the person to become dizzy. The individual's pallor will indicate if he/she is straining (redness) or running out of breath (white or blue).

Physical signs of fatigue are common and it may manifest itself in the form of an unsteady beat or in the patient stopping the movement altogether. It is advantageous to structure the music therapy session with active motor interventions between short periods of passive music listening. These times of rest will help the individual to be more productive during periods of musical engagement.

Procedures. Begin instruction on correct assembly of the music instrument. Encourage the patient to sit erect by squaring his/her shoulders and maintaining head posture. Next, engage the patient in deep breathing exercises by encouraging the individual to place his/her hands on their trunk to watch their hands expand and contract with each breath. Actual playing of the instrument should begin with long tones, with gradual progression to a five-note scale. From there, music notation, music theory, and simple songs can be introduced.

Adaptations. The playing of rhythm instruments can be effective in enhancing motor skills, especially when the patient's memory skills are not advanced enough to retain music instruction. Initially, the music therapist may need to do hand-over-hand prompting so that the person is able to execute an elbow flexion-extension movement to make the instrument sound. Gradually, the music therapist can halt prompting so that the patient builds motor independence. Buildup on mallets to make the handle wider may be necessary to facilitate a more successful grip. Singing is another avenue to pursue to increase the vital capacity skills of a survivor of a TBI. The same procedure should be followed as outlined above in procedural steps.

Guidelines for Compositional Music Therapy

Songwriting

Overview. Songwriting is a therapist-assisted process of creating music and lyrics with the goal of communicating thoughts and feelings. An individual who has sustained a TBI experiences many losses. These losses can be in the form of their inability to walk, physically perform ADLs, remember daily occurrences, make good decisions, communicate their thoughts, and, more tragically, cope with the loss of loved ones who may have died in the trauma associated with the patient's TBI. Songwriting is a good vehicle to emotionally express and work through these losses.

A patient who has sustained a TBI who is unable to communicate short phrases or has an attention span of under 10 minutes may not have the necessary abilities to successfully complete a composed song. Generally, an individual with a TBI at the RLA Level V or greater will be able to successfully engage in songwriting experiences.

Preparation. The music therapist will need to determine how much structure is needed for the patient to successfully complete a song. The lower the cognitive level of a patient, the more structure is needed.

Procedures. The music therapist must consider the individual's cognitive abilities, such as their ability for concrete or abstract thinking and the length of their attention span, to successfully structure the procedure for song composition. Providing more structure for a concrete thinker with a shorter attention span can be accomplished by providing simple carrier phrases, such as "I feel sad when ..." or "I'm proud of ...." The music therapist will provide a variety of rhythmic meters and melodic lines. In the final step, the patient will decide on the music to support their lyrics.

The patient at a higher cognitive level will be encouraged to compose 100% of the music lyrics, melody, and rhythmic components. In the first step, the patient will pinpoint a theme and formulate a poignant statement that will be used as the song's chorus. Next, they will write lyrics to express the chosen theme. The final step is to compose the music. The patient may elect to compose a melody or rap. They may choose to play rhythm or melodic instruments and/or use vocalizations and/or body percussion. Finally, they may instruct the music therapist to play on an accompanying instrument.

Baker, Kennelly, and Tamplin (2005) suggest a nine-stage process to creating lyrics in the song writing process. They are as follows: 1) brainstorm ideas, 2) select topics, 3) expand topics, 4) identify themes and develop chorus, 5) further develop themes, 6) brainstorm ideas, 7) choose one theme, 8) outline and refine themes, and, finally, 9) compose lyrics.

Adaptations. Lyric substitution of familiar songs is a possible adaptation. It is suggested that the music therapist not sing the song in its original format when doing a lyric substitution. Due to cognitive deficits, the patient may not be able to formulate their own song lyrics after they have recently heard the original lyrics. The music therapist can provide carrier phrases from the original song to provide the TBI patient with a starting point to which to add their own lyrics. The melodic line will already be provided but the patient can direct the music therapist to change the music style and meter. The patient can also provide 100% of the song lyrics to a known song, which will be coupled with the original melodic line.

Research Evidence

Receptive Music Therapy

Many studies have reported on the efficacy of music and songs to elicit responses from those individuals in a comatose state. Boyle (1995) reported on the use of improvisational music to arouse an individual with a TBI from a vegetative comatose state. According to Tomaino (1998), when a song is presented, the rhythm first helps to focus the patient's attention. After the patient's attention is maintained, then the melody stimulates an emotional response. Knox and Jutai (1996) concurred with this premise, stating that music motivates the individual to maintain attention, therefore allowing the survivor of a TBI to comprehend what has been presented to them. Seibert, Fee, Basom, and Zimmerman (2000) reported on the use of music listening with a young adult who had sustained a brain injury. His experiences with past oboe performances were used to enhance sensory stimulation and awareness.

Two studies with patients in comatose states were completed by Riganello, Quintieri, Candelieri, Conforti, and Dolce (2008) and later by Riganello, Candelieri, Quintieri, and Dolce (2010). These two research studies examined the use of passive music listening with comatose patients. The researchers concluded that the heartbeat of the patients changed with the music. This suggests that emotional content is still processed even in patients with low alertness levels. Mitchell, Bradley, Welch, Button, and Peter (1990) studied the effects of a vigorous sensory stimulation program administered to comatose patients. The results indicated that the length of coma was shorter and the recovery more rapid when music stimulation was used. This study concluded that coma arousal procedures are effective and therefore should be used with patients who have sustained a severe TBI.

Receptive methods have also been reported to address emotional needs with those who have sustained a TBI. Barker and Brunk (1991) used known songs to facilitate a lyric fill-in to aid survivors of a TBI to express their positive rehabilitation successes. Goldberg, Hoss, and Chesna (1988) investigated the use of traditional psychotherapy with a 41-year-old brain-damaged patient. The patient engaged in Guided Imagery and Music (GIM) to aid her in working through recent life changes as a direct result of her injury. Results indicated that the role of music provided an appropriate container through its inherent form and structure. This in effect provided the patient with a safe environment to express her images and thoughts. Pickett (1996-1997) also used GIM to aid a survivor of a TBI to work through both physical and emotional losses. The conclusion was that psychotherapy is a viable approach to use with this clinical population.

Improvisational Music Therapy

The use of improvisational music therapy methods with the TBI population is very sparse. Gilbertson (2005) completed a review of the literature on music improvisation with individuals with TBI and advocated for music improvisation to be used to provide a venue for emotional expression. Formisano, Vinicola, Penta, Matteis, Brunelli, and Weckel (2001) investigated the use of music instruments and vocal improvisation to increase communication skills of those individuals emerging from a coma. It was found that while music improvisation did not significantly facilitate a "musical dialogue" (p. 627), it did decrease inertia and/or psychomotor agitation. Magee (1999) utilized music improvisation with a cognitively higher-functioning brain-injured client. The researcher stated that the client was able to communicate expressively when improvisatory approaches were used. Magee stressed the importance of music therapy being a flexible intervention with these individuals, as it may well be the only opportunity a brain-injured patient has to express him/herself emotionally.

Re-creative Music Therapy

The most widely used music therapy method to aid in the recovery of survivors of TBI is re-creative. Clayes et al. (1989) examined the role of music and music therapy in the rehabilitation of traumatic brain-injured patients. The researchers concluded that music could be effective in the reintroduction of patients to the environment. This is facilitated through call-and-response activities that can be related to daily living skills, such as clothes selection, random movement, and verbalization. Gervin (1991) has reported the use of songs to provide the structure for the acute traumatic brain-injured client to successfully dress his or herself. The role of the music is paramount in helping the patient correctly recall the sequence of activities of daily living, thus rendering him/her more independent. Hurt, Rice, McIntosh, and Thaut (1998) found that the anticipation of the beat in music and song aided the individual with a TBI to produce a more fluid gait.

The singing of songs has also proven to be the catalyst for survivors of TBI to regain expressive communication and motor skills and enhance mood. Lucia (1987) reported the use of vocal warm-ups, vocalizing, rhythmic speech drills, and singing known songs to increase speech communication skills. A secondary goal was to enhance motor rehabilitation. After the warm-up was completed, songs were coupled with range-of-motion exercises to increase gross motor skills. A total of 14 successive exercises were developed in conjunction with an occupational therapist. Exercises of the shoulder, wrist, and neck were targeted. Cohen (1988, 1992, 1994), Cohen and Masse (1993), and Cohen and Ford (1995) have extensively researched the effects of speech and song to decrease the rate of speech and increase speech production and purposive speech with neurologically impaired persons. Therapeutic goals also focused on the physical tools needed for functional speech, specifically, articulation, vital capacity skills, and oral-motor exercises, to strengthen facial muscles necessary for speech production. This was accomplished through the playing of wind instruments and singing.

Baker and Wigram (2004) also used songs to increase vocal expression and intonation in patients. The researchers noted that singing decreased physical tension and improved posture, which in turn led to vocal freedom and mood enhancement. Baker and Wigram (2004) found singing to reduce muscle tension, thus enhancing vocal range in persons with TBI. Furthermore, the researchers found singing to elevate mood and increase vocalizations. Baker, Wigram, and Gold (2005) concluded that singing positively affected intonation and thus expressive communication in survivors of TBI. Tamplin (2008) used vocal exercises to increase the communication skills of dysarthric patients. Results showed that these techniques were successful in improving speech intelligibility and naturalness and decreased the amount and length of pauses in expressive language.

Compositional Music Therapy

Several researchers have reported on the use of music composition to provide an outlet for emotions for those recovering from a TBI. Thaut (1990) states that by utilizing different aspects of music, the patient is given an outlet for expression and validation of his/her personal thoughts and feelings. He advocates that the process of songwriting be used to facilitate an individual's or group's perception about their personal rehabilitation experience. Glassman (1991) reported on a case study of a woman who survived a TBI. The use of songwriting was successful in providing an outlet to use words to express feelings. Baker, Kennelly, and Tamplin published a series of studies highlighting songwriting themes (2005a) according to age group (2005b), gender differences within songwriting (2005c), and songwriting to provide a venue for identity and self-concept (2005d), written by survivors of TBI. Barker and Brunk (1991) used art and music group projects to treat patients recovering from a TBI. Music composition was one of the techniques employed, where the group created their own lyrics and rhythmic chant. This process was successful in facilitating each TBI survivor's motor, cognitive, communication, and emotional skills.

Summary and Conclusions

Advances in medical treatment have increased the likelihood of people surviving a TBI. Severity scales have been developed to better assess the survivor's alertness level and ability to think, communicate, move, express emotions, and socialize effectively with others. The music therapy literature is heavy on re-creative and receptive methods. The re-creative method targets sequential memory skills needed to perform ADLs and speech and language skills needed for expressive communication. Receptive methods have been reportedly used to arouse the comatose patient to more consistently respond to their environment and for the higher-functioning patient, to provide a venue for emotional expression. There are a few studies that highlight composition, and even fewer that address improvisation methods. Both of these music therapy methods focus on emotional expression, socialization, and providing a sense of community with others who have sustained a TBI.

Although music therapy has proven to be a viable treatment with this clinical population, there needs to be more reported research with the use of composition and improvisation methods with survivors of TBI. The lack of research using composition and improvisation methods may be in part due to the level of individuals with TBI that music therapists traditionally see in treatment. Inpatient treatment usually is for a length of 30 days or less, and the patients are usually more severely impaired. When the patient advances to a more independent stage, such as a RLA level V or greater, they are usually discharged to outpatient rehabilitation for a short period or to their home. Often, music therapists do not have the opportunity to work with individuals who are able to return, even in a limited capacity, to their home and/or work environments.

References

Albert, M., Sparks, R., & Helm, N. (1973). Melodic intonation therapy for aphasics. *Archives of Neurology, 29,* 130–131.

Baker, F. (2011). Facilitating neurological reorganization through music therapy: A case example of modified Melodic Intonation Therapy in the treatment of a person with aphasia. In A. Meadows (Ed), *Developments in music therapy practice: Case study perspectives* (pp. 280–296). Gilsum, NH: Barcelona Publishers.

Baker, F., Kennelly, J., & Tamplin, J. (2005a). Songwriting to explore identity change and sense of self-concept following traumatic brain injury. In F. Baker & T. Wigram (Eds.), *Songwriting: Methods, techniques and clinical applications for music therapy clinicians, educators and students* (pp. 116–133). Philadelphia, PA: Jessica Kingsley.

Baker, F., Kennelly, J., & Tamplin, J. (2005b). Adjusting to change through song: Themes in songs written by clients with traumatic brain injury. *Brain Impairment, 6*(3), 205–211.

Baker, F., Kennelly, J., & Tamplin, J. (2005c). Themes in songs written by people with traumatic brain injury: Differences across the lifespan. *Australian Journal of Music Therapy, 16,* 25–42.

Baker, F., Kennelly, J., & Tamplin, J. (2005d). Themes within songs written by people with traumatic brain injury: Gender differences. *Journal of Music Therapy, 32*(2), 111–112.

Baker, F., & Wigram, T. (2004). The immediate and long-term effects of singing on the mood states of people with traumatic brain injury. *British Journal of Music Therapy, 18*(2), 55–64.

Baker, F., & Wigram, T. (2005). *Songwriting: Methods, techniques and clinical applications for music therapy clinicians, educators and students.* Philadelphia, PA: Jessica Kingsley.

Baker, F., Wigram, T., & Gold, C. (2005). The effects of a song-singing programme on the affective speaking intonation of people with traumatic brain injury. *Brain Injury, 19*(7), 519–528.

Barker, V. L., & Brunk, B. (1991). The role of a creative arts group in the treatment of clients with traumatic brain injury. *Music Therapy Perspectives, 9,* 26–31.

Boyle, M. (1995). On the vegetative state: Music and coma arousal interventions. In C. A. Lee (Ed.), *Lonely Waters* (pp. 163–172). Oxford: Sobell Publications.

Brain Injury Association of America (BIAA). (2011). *About Brain Injury*. Retrieved from http://biausa.fyrian.com/about-brain-injury

Centers for Disease Control and Prevention (CDC). (2012). *Injury Prevention and Control: Traumatic Brain Injury*. Retrieved from http://www.cdc.gov/traumaticbraininjury

Centers for Disease Control and Prevention (CDC), National Center for Injury Prevention and Control. (2003). Report to Congress on *Mild traumatic brain injury in the United States: Steps to Prevent a Serious Public Health Problem*. Atlanta, GA.

Claeys, M. S., Miller, A. C., Dalloul-Rampersad, R., & Kollar, M. (1989). The role of music and music therapy in the rehabilitation of traumatically brain-injured clients. *Music Therapy Perspectives, 6*, 71–77.

Cohen, N. (1988). The use of superimposed rhythm to decrease the rate of speech in a brain-damaged adolescent. *Journal of Music Therapy, 25*, 85–93.

Cohen, N. (1992). The effect of singing instruction on the speech production of neurologically impaired persons. *Journal of Music Therapy, 29*, 87–102.

Cohen, N. (1994). Speech and song: Implications for therapy. *Music Therapy Perspectives, 12*, 8–12.

Cohen, N., & Ford, J. (1995). The effect of musical cues on the nonpurposive speech of persons with aphasia. *Journal of Music Therapy, 32*, 46–57.

Cohen, N., & Masse, R. (1993). The application of singing and rhythmic instruction as a therapeutic intervention for persons with neurogenic communication disorders. *Journal of Music Therapy, 30*, 81–89.

Coronado, V. G., Xu, L., Basavaraju, S. V., McGuire, L. C., Wald, M. M., Faul, M. D., Guzman, B. R., & Hemphill, J. D. (2011). *Surveillance for Traumatic Brain Injury Related Deaths: United States, 1997–2007*. Centers for Disease Control and Prevention, May 6, 2011, *60*(SS05), 1–32.

Daveson, B. A. (2008). A description of a music therapy meta-model in neuro disability and neuro-rehabilitation for use with children, adolescents and adults. *Australian Journal of Music Therapy, 19*, 70–85.

Dawodu, S. T. (2012). *Traumatic Brain Injury—Definition, Epidemiology, Pathophysiology*. Retrieved from http://emedicine.medscape.com/article/326510-overview

Faul, M., Xu, L., Wald, M. M., & Coronado, V. G. (2010). Traumatic brain injury in the United States: Emergency department visits, hospitalizations, and death. Atlanta, GA: Centers for Disease Control and Prevention, National Center for Injury Prevention and Control.

Gervin, A. P. (1991). Music therapy compensatory technique utilizing song lyrics during dressing to promote independence in the patient with a brain injury. *Music Therapy Perspectives, 9*, 87–90.

Gilbertson, S. K. (2005). Music therapy in NeuroRehabilitation with people who have experienced traumatic brain injury: A literature review. In D. Aldridge (Ed.), *Music therapy and neurological rehabilitation: Performing health* (pp. 83–138). Philadelphia, PA: Jessica Kingsley.

Glassman, L. R. (1991). Music therapy and bibliotherapy in the rehabilitation of traumatic brain injury: A case study. *The Arts in Psychotherapy, 18*, 149–156.

Goldberg, F. S., Hoss, T. M., & Chesna, T. (1988). Music and imagery as psychotherapy with a brain damaged patient: A case study. *Music Therapy Perspectives, 5*, 41–45.

Hagen, C., Malkmus, D., Durham, P., & Stenderup, K. (1974, November 15). Assessment Scales: Rancho Los Amigos–Revised. Retrieved November, 29, 2001, from http://www.neuroskills.com/tbi/ranchero.html

Hurt, C. P., Rice, R. R., McIntosh, G. C., & Thaut, M. H. (1998). Rhythmic auditory stimulation in gait training for patients with traumatic brain injury, *Journal of Music Therapy, 35*(4), 228–241.

Knox, R., & Jutai, J. (1996). Music-based rehabilitation of attention following brain injury. *Canadian Journal of Rehabilitation, 9*(3), 169–181.

Lucia, C. (1987). Toward developing a model of music therapy intervention in the rehabilitation of head trauma patients. *Music Therapy Perspectives, 4,* 34–39.

Magee, W. (1999). Music therapy within brain injury rehabilitation: To what extent is our clinical practice influenced by the search for outcomes? *Music Therapy Perspectives, 1,* 20–26.

Medical-Dictionary. (2012). Retrieved from http://medicaldictionary.thefreedictionary.com

Meyer, M. J., Megyesi, J., Meythaler, J., Murie-Fernandez, M., Aubut, J., Foley, N., Salter, K., Bayley, M., Marshall, S., & Teasell, R. (2010). Acute management of acquired brain injury Part III: An evidence-based review of interventions used to promote arousal from coma. *Brain Injury, 24*(5), 722–729.

Mitchell, S, Bradley, V. A., Welch, J. L., Button, & Peter, G. (1990). Coma arousal procedure: A therapeutic intervention in the treatment of head injury. *Brain Injury, 4,* 273–279.

Mosby's Medical Dictionary — Ninth Edition. (2012).

National Brain Injury Foundation (NBIF). (2012). Retrieved from http://nbif.blogspot.com/

National Institute of Neurological Disorders and Stroke (NINDS). (2012). *Traumatic Brain Injury: Hope Through Research.* Retrieved from http://www.ninds.nih.gov/disorders/tbi/tbi.htm.

Pickett, E. (1996–1997). Guided imagery and music in head trauma rehabilitation. *Journal of the Association for Music and Imagery, 5,* 51–60.

Rappaport, M., Hall, K., & Hopkins, K. (1982). Disability rating scale for severe head trauma patients: Coma to community. *Archives of Physical Medicine and Rehabilitation, 63,* 118–123.

Riganello, F., Candelieri, A., Quintieri, M., & Dolce, G. (2010). Heart rate variability, emotions, and music. *Journal of Pschophysiology, 24*(2), 112–119.

Riganello, F., Quintieri, M., Candelieri, A., Conforti, D., & Dolce, G. (2008). Heart rate response to music: An artificial intelligence study on healthy and traumatic brain-injured subjects. *Journal of Psychophysiology, 22*(4), 166–174.

Rogers, G. P., & Fleming, P. (1981). Rhythms and music in speech therapy for the neurologically impaired. *Music Therapy, 1,* 33–38.

Seibert, P. S., Fee, L., Basom, J., & Zimmerman, C. (2000). Music and the brain: The impact of music on an oboist's fight for recovery. *Brain Injury, 14*(3), 295–302.

Tamplin, J. (2008). A pilot study into the effect of vocal exercises and singing on dysarthric speech. *NeuroRehabilitation, 23*(3), 207–216.

Taylor, D. B. (1989). A neuroanatomical model for the use of music in the remediation of aphasic disorders. In M. H. M. Lee (Ed.), *Rehabilitation, music and human well-being* (pp. 168–178). St. Louis, MO: MMB Music.

Taylor, D. B. (1997). *Biomedical foundations of music as therapy.* St. Louis, MO: MMB Music.

Teasdale, G., & Jennett, B. (1974). Assessment of coma and impaired consciousness. A practical scale. *Lancet, Jul 13, 2*(7872), 81–84. PubMed PMID: 4136544.

Thaut, M. H. (1990). Physiological responses to music stimuli, In R. F. Unkefer (Ed.), *Music therapy in the treatment of adults with mental disorders: Theoretical base and clinical interventions* (pp. 33–39). New York: Schirmer Books.

Thompson, A., Arnold, J., & Murray, S. (1990). Music therapy assessment of the cerebrovascular accident patient. *Music Therapy Perspectives, 8,* 23–29.

Tomaino, C. M. (1998). Music and memory: Accessing residual function. In C. Tomaino (Ed.), *Clinical applications of music in neurologic rehabilitation* (pp. 19–27). St. Louis, MO: MMB Music, Inc.

Wigram, T. (2004). *Improvisation: Methods and techniques for music therapy clinicians, educators and students* (pp. 23–37). Philadelphia, PA: Jessica Kingsley

Wilson, B. (1990). Music therapy in hospital and community programs. In R. F. Unkefer (Ed.), *Music therapy in the treatment of adults with mental disorders: Theoretical bases and clinical interventions* (pp. 88–95). New York: Schirmer Books.

Appendix A

Glasgow Coma Scale

EYES	
Open:	
Spontaneously	4
To Verbal Command	3
To Pain	2
No Response	1
BEST MOTOR RESPONSE	
To Verbal Commands:	
Obeys	6
To Painful Stimulus:	
Localizes Pain	5
Flexion-Withdrawal	4
Flexion-abnormal	3
Extension	2
No Response	1
BEST VERBAL RESPONSE	
Oriented and Converses	5
Disoriented and Converses	4
Inappropriate Words	3
Incomprehensible Sounds	2
No Response	1
GCS TOTAL	3–15

In public domain. Taken from: Teasdale, G. & Jennett, B. (1974). Assessment of coma and impaired consciousness. A practical scale. *Lancet.* Jul 13;2(7872) 81-4. PubMed PMID: 4136544.

Appendix B

RANCHO LOS AMIGOS–REVISED

The Rancho Scale is free and available online at the Rancho Los Amigos National Rehabilitation Centers See: http://rancho.org. Taken from: Hagen, Malkmus, Durham & Stenderup (1974)

LEVELS OF COGNITIVE FUNCTIONING

Level I—No Response: Total Assistance

- Complete absence of observable change in behavior when presented visual, auditory, tactile, proprioceptive, vestibular, or painful stimuli.

Level II—Generalized Response: Total Assistance

- Demonstrates generalized reflex response to painful stimuli.
- Responds to repeated auditory stimuli with increased or decreased activity.
- Responds to external stimuli with physiological changes generalized, gross body movement and/or not purposeful vocalization.
- Responses noted above may be the same regardless of type and location of stimulation.
- Responses noted above may be significantly delayed.

Level III—Localized response: Total Assistance

- Demonstrates withdrawal or vocalization to painful stimuli.
- Turns toward or away from auditory stimuli.
- Blinks when strong light crosses visual field.
- Follows moving object passed within visual field.
- Responds to discomfort by pulling tubes or restraints.
- Responds inconsistently to simple commands.
- Responses directly related to type of stimulus.
- May respond to some persons (especially family and friends) but not to others.

Level IV—Confused/Agitated: Maximal Assistance

- Alert and in heightened state of activity.
- Purposeful attempts to remove restraints or tubes or crawl out of bed.
- May perform motor activities such as sitting, reaching and walking but without any apparent purpose or upon another's request.
- Very brief and usually nonpurposeful moments of sustained alternatives and divided attention.
- Absent short-term memory.
- May cry out or scream out of proportion to stimulus even after its removal.
- May exhibit aggressive or flight behavior.

- Mood may swing from euphoric to hostile with no apparent relationship to environmental events.
- Unable to cooperate with treatment efforts.
- Verbalizations are frequently incoherent and/or inappropriate to activity or environment.

Level V—Confused, Inappropriate Nonagitated: Maximal Assistance

- Alert, not agitated but may wander randomly or with a vague intention of going home.
- May become agitated in response to external stimulation, and/or lack of environmental structure.
- Not oriented to person, place, or time.
- Frequent brief periods, nonpurposeful sustained attention.
- Severely impaired recent memory, with confusion of past and present in reaction to ongoing activity.
- Absent goal-directed, problem-solving, self-monitoring behavior.
- Often demonstrates inappropriate use of objects without external direction.
- May be able to perform previously learned tasks when structures and cues provided.
- Unable to learn new information.
- Able to respond appropriately to simple commands fairly consistently with external structures and cues.
- Verbalizations about present events become inappropriate and confabulatory when external structure and cues are not provided.

Level VI—Confused, Appropriate: Moderate Assistance

- Inconsistently oriented to person, time, and place.
- Able to attend to highly familiar tasks in non-distracting environment for 30 minutes with moderate redirection.
- Remote memory has more depth and detail then recent memory.
- Vague recognition of some staff.
- Able to use assistive memory aide with maximum assistance.
- Emerging awareness of appropriate responses to self, family and basic needs.
- Moderate assist to problem-solve barriers to task completion.
- Supervised for old learning (e.g., self-care)
- Shows carry over for new learning with little or no carryover.
- Unaware of impairments, disabilities and safety risks.
- Consistently follows simple directions.
- Verbal expressions are appropriate in highly familiar and structured situations.

Level VII—Automatic, Appropriate: Minimal Assistance for Daily Living Skills

- Consistently oriented to person and place, within highly familiar environments. Moderate assistance for orientation to time.
- Able to attend to highly familiar tasks in a nondistraction environment for at least 30 minutes with minimal assist to complete tasks.

- Minimal supervision for new learning.
- Demonstrates carryover of new learning.
- Initiates and carries out steps to complete familiar personal and household routine but has shallow recall of what he/she has been doing.
- Able to monitor accuracy and completeness of each step in routine personal and household ADLs and modify plan with minimal assistance.
- Superficial awareness of his/her condition but unaware of specific impairments and disabilities and the limits they place on his/her ability to safely, accurately and completely carry out his/her household, community, work, and leisure ADLs.
- Minimal supervision for safety in routine home and community activities.
- Unrealistic planning for the future.
- Unable to think about consequences of a decision or action.
- Overestimates abilities.
- Unaware of others' needs and feelings.
- Oppositional/uncooperative.
- Unable to recognize inappropriate social interaction behavior.

Level VIII—Purposeful, Appropriate: Standby Assistance

- Consistently oriented to person, place, and time.
- Independently attends to and completes familiar tasks for 1 hour in distracting environments.
- Able to recall and integrate past and recent events.
- Uses assistive memory devices to recall daily schedule, "to do" lists and record critical information for later use with standby assistance.
- Initiates and carries out steps to complete familiar personal, household, community, work, and leisure routines with standby assistance and can modify the plan when needed with minimal assistance.
- Requires no assistance once new tasks/activities are learned.
- Aware of and acknowledges impairments and disabilities when they interfere with task completion but requires standby assistance to take appropriate corrective action.
- Thinks about consequences of a decision or action with minimal assistance.
- Overestimates or underestimates abilities.
- Acknowledges others' needs and feelings and responds appropriately with minimal assistance.
- Depressed
- Irritable
- Low frustration tolerance/easily angered
- Argumentative
- Self-centered
- Uncharacteristically dependent/independent
- Able to recognize and acknowledge inappropriate social interaction behavior while it is occurring and takes corrective action with minimal assistance.

Level IX—Purposeful, Appropriate: Standby Assistance on Request

- Independently shifts back and forth between tasks and completes them accurately for at least two consecutive hours.
- Uses assistive memory devices to recall daily schedule, "to do" lists and record critical information for later use with assistance when requested.
- Initiates and carries out steps to complete familiar personal, household, work, and leisure tasks independently and unfamiliar personal, household, work and leisure tasks with assistance when requested.
- Aware of and acknowledges impairments and disabilities when they interfere with task completion and takes appropriate corrective action but requires standby assist to anticipate a problem before it occurs and take action to avoid it.
- Able to think about consequences of decisions or actions with assistance when requested.
- Accurately estimates abilities but requires standby assistance to adjust to task demands.
- Acknowledges others' needs and feelings and responds appropriately with standby assistance.
- Depression may continue.
- May be easily irritable.
- May have low frustration tolerance.
- Able to self-monitor appropriateness of social interaction with standby assistance.

Level X—Purposeful, Appropriate: Modified Independent

- Able to handle multiple tasks simultaneously in all environments but may require periodic breaks.
- Able to independently procure, create, and maintain own assistive memory devices.
- Independently initiates and carries out steps to complete familiar and unfamiliar personal, household, community, work, and leisure tasks but may require more than usual amount of time and/or compensatory strategies to complete them.
- Anticipates impact of impairments and disabilities on ability to complete daily living tasks and takes action to avoid problems before they occur but may require more than usual amount of time and/or compensatory strategies.
- Able to independently think about consequences of decisions or actions but may require more than usual amount of time and/or compensatory strategies to select the appropriate decision or action.
- Accurately estimates abilities and independently adjusts to task demands.
- Able to recognize the needs and feelings of others and automatically respond in appropriate manner.
- Periodic periods of depression may occur.
- Irritability and low frustration tolerance when sick, fatigued, and/or under emotional stress.
- Social interaction behavior is consistently appropriate.

APPENDIX C

Disability Rating Scale (DRS)			
Category	Item	Instructions	Score
Arousability, Awareness and Responsivity	Eye Opening	0 = spontaneous 1= to speech 2 = to pain 3= none	
	Communication Ability	0 = oriented 1= confused 2 = inappropriate 3 = incomprehensible 4 = none	
	Motor Response	0 = obeying 1 = localizing 2= withdrawing 3= flexing 4 = extending 5 = none	
Cognitive Ability for Self Care Activities	Feeding	0 = complete 1= partial 2= minimal 3= none	
	Toileting	0 = complete 1= partial 2 = minimal 3 = none	
	Grooming	0= complete 1= partial 2= minimal 3= none	
Dependence on Others	Levels of Functioning	0 = completely independent 1= independent in special environment 2= mildly dependent 3= moderately dependent 4= markedly dependent 5= totally dependent	
Psychosocial Adaptability	Employability	0= not restricted 1= selected jobs 2= sheltered workshop (non-competitive) 3= not employable	
		Total DR Score	

Total DR Score	Level of Disability
0	
1	
2-3	
4-6	
7-11	
12-16	
17-21	
22-24	
25-29	

Rappaport, M., Hall, K. M., & Hopkins, K. (1982). Disability rating scale for severe head trauma patients: coma to community. *Archives of Physical Medicine and Rehabilitation, 63*, 118-123.

Chapter 8

Adults with Neurogenic Communication Disorders

Nicki S. Cohen

DIAGNOSTIC INFORMATION

A neurogenic communication disorder (NCD) is a speech-language disorder resulting from neurological damage. These disorders usually result from the following: (a) cerebrovascular accident (CVA, i.e., stroke), (b) chronic neurodegenerative condition (e.g., Parkinson's Disease), or (c) traumatic brain injury (TBI). According to the University of Rochester Medical Center (2010), NCDs fall into three categories: articulation, fluency, and vocal disorders. Articulation disorders are characterized by difficulties with the way sounds are formed and assembled, and are often characterized by the omission, addition, substitution, or distortion of sounds. Fluency disorders can be described as an interruption in the flow of speech, resulting in an unusual rate or rhythm, hesitations, repetitions, or prolongations of sounds or words. Vocal disorders are characterized by aberrations in vocal quality, pitch, loudness, resonance, or duration that sound abnormal.

Each category contains a listing of specific communication disorders. Every communication disorder is assigned its own diagnostic code from the World Health Organization's *The International Classification of Diseases, Ninth Revision, Clinical Modification* (ICD-9-CM, 2010). The federally regulated ICD-9-CM represents the official system for assigning codes to diagnoses and procedures associated with hospital management in the United States. The National Center for Health Statistics (NCHS) and the Centers for Medicare and Medicaid Services are the U.S. governmental agencies responsible for overseeing all changes and modifications to the ICD-9-CM. The following represents the aforementioned categories of neurogenic communication disorders along with their corresponding diagnoses and current ICD-9-CM codes.

NEUROGENIC COMMUNICATION DISORDERS

Category	Diagnosis	ICD-9-CM Code
Articulation	Dysarthria	438.13, 784.51
	Apraxia	438.81, 438.12
Fluency		438.14
	Broca's Aphasia	438.11
	Acquired Neurogenic Stuttering	438.14
Vocal	Aphonia, Dysphonia, Hoarseness	438.19, 784.4
	Vocal Cord Weakness/Paralysis	478.30

Articulation Disorders

Articulation disorders, or motor speech disorders, refer to aberrations in the systems and strategies that control the production of speech (Kent, 2000). Simply put, they are disorders of the muscles that regulate speech output. The two most common articulation disorders are dysarthria and apraxia (Cohen, 1994). Speech production involves a series of articulatory movements that convey an intended linguistic message through an acoustic signal that can be interpreted by a listener. The normal rate of speech is six to nine syllables (or 20 to 30 phonetic segments) per second, which is faster than any other discrete human motor performance (Kent, 2000). Speech production also involves more motor fibers than any other human mechanical activity.

Dysarthria results from neurologic impairments associated with weakness, slowness, or coordination of the musculature used to produce speech (Kent, 2000). It is reported to be the most frequently acquired speech disorder (Enderby & Emerson, 1995); at least 20% of CVA patients present with dysarthria (Warlow et al., 2000). Dysarthria occurs when the part of the brain that controls motoric speech production is damaged, causing the muscles that produce certain sounds to become weak or paralyzed. The characteristics of dysarthria reflect abnormalities in the strength, speed, range, timing, or accuracy of speech movements (Mackenzie & Lowit, 2007). People with dysarthria often have trouble coordinating their lips, tongue, palate, jaw, and vocal cords. This can result in speech that is slurred, breathy, jerky, strained, and hard to understand. Most commonly, dysarthria presents with an abnormal rate of speech (Cohen, 1994). It occurs in individuals diagnosed with Parkinson's disease, CVA, amyotrophic lateral sclerosis, multiple sclerosis, cerebral palsy, and traumatic brain injury (Duffy, 1995; McNeil, 1997). General types of dysarthria are ataxic, spastic, flaccid, spastic-flaccid, hypokinetic, and hyperkinetic (Darley, Aronson, & Brown, 1969a, 1969b). Duffy (1995) describes the types of dysarthria as: (a) *ataxic dysarthria,* which affects respiration, phonation, resonance, and articulation, but articulation and prosodic abnormalities are the most pronounced; (b) *spastic dysarthria,* which is characterized by difficulties with fine motor movements due to exaggerated stretch reflexes, resulting in increased muscle tone and incoordination; (c) *flaccid dysarthria,* which results in breathy, hoarse, or harsh vocal qualities; (d) *hypokinetic dysarthria,* which is characterized by difficulties with the initiation of voluntary speech, causing an abnormally slow rate of speech or the freezing of movements during speech; and (e) *hyperkinetic dysarthria*, whose predominant symptoms are involuntary motor movements that result in a harsh, strained, or strangled vocal quality.

Acquired apraxia of speech (AOS) results from cerebral damage that impairs the processes of planning or programming speech movements in the face of essentially normal strength, speed, and coordination of the speech musculature (Duffy, 1995). AOS is a higher-level representational communication disorder that is associated with lesions to the temporal lobe (Tamplin & Grocke, 2008). It occurs most commonly in adults who have already developed language skills. Previously known as verbal apraxia, it is now called acquired apraxia of speech to differentiate it from developmental apraxia in children. It is also referred to, in less severe cases, as *dyspraxia* (Kent, 2000). AOS usually results from a cerebrovascular accident, head injury, tumor, or an illness that causes damage to the parts of the brain that control speech, especially the temporal lobes. AOS impairs existing speech abilities. Simply put, although a person with AOS knows what she/he wants to say, a disconnection exists between the brain and the speech muscles. These symptoms are often accompanied by excessive tension and struggle behaviors when attempting to speak.

Whereas acquired apraxia of speech impairs the programming of speech movements, or the movement plan, dysarthria affects the execution of those movements (Kent, 2000). The movement plan is disturbed in AOS, but the muscular system is essentially intact. Conversely, in dysarthria, the movement plan is intact, but the speech muscles cannot produce the movement plan. Although dysarthria is sometimes confused with AOS, the speech errors that occur with dysarthria are highly consistent from one time to the next, while the speech errors associated with AOS are not (Darley et al., 1975). In addition, while AOS tends to result from localized damage to the speech centers of the left hemisphere, dysarthria results from less localized damage to a number of neurological systems (Darley, Aronson, & Brown, 1975).

Aphasia and Fluency Disorders

Aphasia, the most common form of language disorder, impairs the ability to speak, understand, read (alexia), and write (agraphia) (University of Rochester Medical Center, 2010). According to recent data, at least 19% of those who survive CVAs are diagnosed with long-term aphasia (Wallace, 2010). General types of aphasia are receptive, global, and expressive (ASHA, 2010). Receptive (or Wernicke's) aphasia is caused by damage to the Wernicke area, which is the posterior portion of the superior temporal gyrus of the left hemisphere, and impacts a person's ability to comprehend spoken language and to read written language (Brookshire, 1992). Persons with Wernicke's aphasia may believe they are speaking words because their utterances are fluent and have the same rhythm as normal speech; however, they often produce sounds that are nonsensical. Global aphasia is caused by extensive, nonlocalized damage to the brain and is the most severe form of aphasia. Patients with global aphasia produce few recognizable words and comprehend little to no spoken language. Expressive (or Broca's) aphasia is caused by lesions to the Broca area, which is in the anterior section of the left frontal lobe (Gleason & Goodglass, 1984). People diagnosed with Broca's aphasia tend to lack normal speech prosody and encounter difficulties when attempting to initiate sentences, to combine words into phrases, or to write words (Gleason & Goodglass, 1984). This condition can be identified further by slurred speech or verbal perseveration.

Whereas articulation disorders result from difficulties in constructing speech sounds, fluency disorders result from interruptions to the flow of speech, resulting in dysfluency. Expressive aphasia, as described above, is a major fluency disorder. Another is acquired neurogenic stuttering, which is associated with various conditions such as brain lesions, pharmacologic effects, and psychogenesis. Kent (2000) reported that neuroimaging results indicate atypical patterns of activation in the brains of people who stutter when compared with nonstuttering control participants.

Vocal Disorders

Vocal disorders are described as problems with vocal pitch, intensity, or quality and are often concomitant with other neurogenic speech disorders. Dysphonia and aphonia, the most severe types of voice disorders, are characterized by severe breathiness and lack of phonation of the vocal tone (Baker & Tamplin, 2006; Sapir & Aronson, 1985). Dysprosodia, or disturbances of the prosodic, or melodic, components of speech, often impacts the patient's speaking pitch and speaking frequency range. Other vocal disorders include hypernasality, hoarseness, harshness, or reduced loudness levels.

Needs and Resources

Neurogenic communication disorders occur in patients with brain damage. Tanner identifies the three most common NCDs as aphasia, acquired apraxia of speech, and dysarthria (2009). According to Wallace (2010), in the United States alone, nearly one million people have been diagnosed with aphasia. While many CVA survivors regain functional independence, they are left with permanent disabilities due to the isolated or combined effects of hemiparesis that may impair walking, the use of upper extremities for activities of daily living, and communication. This creates unique challenges for patients with NCDs as they attempt to reenter their home, community, and vocational life. Because of the propensity for concomitant impairments following damage to the brain, effective rehabilitation of people diagnosed with NCD require comprehensive and individualized care that extends beyond traditional, discipline-specific boundaries.

Some experts maintain that all neuropsychological rehabilitation should be completed during the first 6-month period after an accident or illness, while the brain tissue is still healing (Gardner, 1976). Within the context of the U.S. health care system, once a person reaches outpatient status, serious reductions occur in the amount of insurance coverage available for rehabilitation. A good example is found in the Medicare system, which provides medical coverage for individuals 65 and older, the population at greatest risk for CVAs and resultant neurogenic communication disorders. According to recent Medicare guidelines (January, 2010), a $1,860 cap exists on the amount of outpatient rehabilitation an individual can receive for the combined services of physical therapy and speech-language therapy. This presents a dilemma for outpatients who have both physical and speech-language needs. This situation forces some individuals with combined needs to have to choose between therapies. Many private insurance companies also do not provide coverage for long-term outpatient therapy (Wallace, 2010).

Brain injuries pose a threat to a patient's psychological equilibrium, as feelings of self-consciousness and inadequacy, paranoid ideation, diminished interpersonal contact, social withdrawal, alcoholism, depression, and even suicidal tendencies can occur (Baker, Wigram, & Gold, 2005). Persons with NCDs often experience a sense of loss, disadvantage, and increased stress responses when attempting to communicate. They are often misunderstood, and may not be able to successfully hold conversations with others. Furthermore, as contemporary culture values communicative competence, people may demonstrate negative attitudes toward those who lack this. For this reason, a speaker with a neurogenic communication disorder may experience social discrimination or devaluation (Hustad, Kent, & Beukelman, 1998). When the attitudes and reactions of others lead to a fear of failure, there may be reduction in communication attempts not only for the speakers with NCDs, but also for their communication partners (Yorkston, Beukelman, Strand, & Bell, 1999). When communication is compromised, one's quality of life is often impacted (Yorkston, 1996). Unfortunately, due to the effect of NCDs on social communication, patients may inevitably face difficulties participating in traditional verbal therapy sessions. Thus the diagnosis of a neurogenic communication disorder can harm a person's quality of life, especially in the areas of psychological, social, and financial health (Lubinski, 1991).

Rehabilitation

Once the medical status of a patient with brain damage has stabilized, one of the first steps is to determine his/her baseline level of neurofunctioning. Three standard measures routinely used to determine the overall level of functioning are the *Rancho Los Amigos Levels of Cognitive Functioning* (LOC; Hagen, 1982), *The Galveston Orientation and Amnesia Test* (GOAT; Levin et al., 1979), and *The Glasgow Coma Scale* (GCS; Teasdale & Jennett, 1976). After the baseline level is identified, patients with brain damage will receive intensive inpatient therapy that is functional in nature and comprehensive in scope (Wallace, 2000). Due to the limited coverage for outpatient reimbursement, a collaborative treatment approach is critical for patients to achieve the level of functional independence necessary to return home in a timely manner. At no other time are specialists as cogent in their efforts to muster combined resources and enhance performance across disciplines. The typical rehabilitation team is composed of a number of professionals, including medical staff, social workers, physical therapists, occupational therapists, counselors, music therapists, and speech-language pathologists. Medicare pays for the hospitalization and inpatient rehabilitative care for 90 days following neurological impairment for individuals 65 and over in the U.S., which is the stage when people are more likely to experience CVAs.

Speech-Language Pathology

A speech-language pathologist (SLP) is a professional who works with the full range of human communication and its disorders. The SLP's roles include evaluating, diagnosing, and treating persons with speech, language, cognitive-communication, and swallowing disorders (ASHA, 2010). Speech-language pathologists aim to improve the patient's ability to communicate by focusing on remaining language abilities, the restoration of language function as much as possible, compensation for language problems, and the acquisition of other methods of communicating (National Institute for Neurological Disorders and Stroke, 2010). Individual therapy focuses on the specific needs of the patient, while group therapy offers the opportunity to use new communication skills in a small-group setting. Stroke clubs, which are regional support groups for persons with CVAs, are available in most major cities. These clubs offer the opportunity for persons with neurogenic speech disorders to try out new communication techniques. In addition, stroke clubs can help outpatients and their families adjust to the resultant life challenges. Family involvement is often a crucial component of treatment so that family members can learn the best way to communicate with their communication-impaired loved one.

Melodic Intonation Therapy. A well-known SLP treatment approach for persons with expressive aphasia is *Melodic Intonation Therapy* (MIT), which is a hierarchically structured method that trains verbal production by repeating melodically intoned phrases while rhythmically tapping the patient's hand (Van der Meulen, Van de Sandt-Koenderman, & Ribbers, 2012). The treatment occurs in three stages: (a) unison speech with melodic patterns, (b) imitative speech with melodic patterns, and (c) imitative speech without melody. Developed in the 1970s, MIT was one of the first systematic aphasia treatment approaches (Albert, Sparks, & Helm, 1973; Laughlin, Naeser, & Gordon 1979; Sparks, Helm, & Albert, 1974; Sparks & Holland, 1976). It is still employed in its original (Van der Meulen, Van de Sandt-Koenderman, & Ribbers, 2012) as well as modified forms (Hurkmans et al., 2012). Although MIT has been successful for persons with expressive aphasia, it has not been effective for patients with dysarthria (Sparks & Holland, 1976). In addition, MIT was designed as individual therapy and is not deemed suitable for groups or for global aphasia patients (Jungblut et al., 2009). Brookshire (1992) also questions the credibility of the research conducted on MIT, which has primarily been based on small sample designs.

Dysarthria often results from chronic conditions that cannot be treated successfully with surgery, medications (Kent, 2000), or MIT (Sparks, Helm, & Albert, 1974). The *Lee Silverman Voice Treatment* (Ramig, 1998) is one of the most systematically investigated SLP treatments for dysarthria. This approach teaches patients to focus their efforts on increasing voice volume. As patients progress in therapy, the length and complexity of their speech increases, as does their volume. Practice and feedback begin with a single sound to train the patient about the desired volume and the breath support required to produce increased sound. The training moves on to simple and frequently used phrases so that increasing loudness eventually becomes habitual. Speaking full sentences, reading aloud, and engaging in conversation are also part of the therapy (Rainbow Rehabilitation Centers, 2011).

Like dysarthria, acquired apraxia of speech does not respond well to most SLP treatments due to its inconsistencies in speech production and accompanying tension and struggle behaviors. AOS is often a concomitant diagnosis to expressive aphasia (Brookshire, 1992). Four recommended SLP treatments for AOS are articulatory kinematic approaches, rate and/or rhythm treatments, alternative and augmentative communication systems, and intersystemic reorganization (van der Merwe, 2011). Efficacy data for these treatments are rare or nonexistent, however (Kent, 2000).

SLP Assessments. SLP training meticulously teaches clinicians to administer tests designed to evaluate communication tasks and diagnose communication disorders. The following are tests typically used by SLPs to diagnose aphasia, which is the most common neurogenic communication disorder

(ASHA, 2012; Brookshire, 1992): *Aphasia Language Performance Scales* (ALPS; Keenan & Brassel, 1975), *The Boston Diagnostic Aphasia Examination, Third Edition* (BDAE-3; Goodglass, Kaplan, & Barresi, 2000), *Examining for Aphasia* (Eisenson, 1994), *The Porch Index of Communicative Ability—Revised* (PICA-R; Porch, 2001), and *The Western Aphasia Battery-Revised* (WAB-R; Kertesz, 2006). Functional communication is assessed via *The Functional Communication Profile—Revised* (FCP-R; Kleiman, 2003) and *Communicative Abilities in Daily Living, Second Edition* (CADL-2; Holland, Frattali, & Fromm, 1999). For patients with dysarthria, SLPs commonly use the *Assessment of Intelligibility of Dysarthric Speech* (AIDS; Yorkston, Beukelman, & Traynor, 1984). Additional published assessments are available to evaluate auditory comprehension, auditory discrimination, vocabulary, reading, word retrieval, and verbal/nonverbal intelligence (Brookshire, 1992). All of these aforementioned speech and language assessments must be administered by a certified speech-language pathologist (CCC-SLP).

Music and Resiliency

Following damage to the brain, patients receive immediate medical services followed by a period of intense rehabilitation. Once the initial brain swelling has subsided, and depending on the extent and severity of the damage, some patients are fortunate enough to resume their *premorbid* lifestyles. The postswelling period is also when the healthy areas of the brain can be *retrained* to compensate for those that are damaged (Luria, 1963). In the presence of an injury to the left hemisphere of the brain, the right hemisphere, which is more commonly associated with the affective and prosodic elements of speech, may be used to assist the damaged left hemisphere (Hartley, 2010). In fact, the development of Melodic Intonation Therapy was based on the premise that the unimpaired right hemisphere would assist the damaged portions of Broca's area in the left hemisphere (Hébert, Peretz, & Racette, 2008; Sparks, Helm, & Albert, 1973).

For those individuals with neurogenic communication deficits, music can facilitate recovery. The premise behind this thinking is that music and speech share many common elements, such as pitch, rhythm, tempo, and dynamics. In addition, according to Hartley (2010), mutual neural substrates exist for the processing of music and speech. As both hemispheres of the brain share in the regulation of human musical behaviors, musical processes can help compensate for damaged speech areas (Besson, Faïta, Peretz, Bonnel, & Requin, 1998; Hébert, Peretz, & Racette, 2008; Liégeois-Chauvel, Peretz, Babaï, Laguitton, & Chauvel, 1998; Patel, Peretz, Tramo, & Labrecque, 1998; Peretz, 1990).

Researchers have indicated that the ability to sing is preserved in persons with Broca's aphasia (Racette, Bard, & Peretz, 2006; Yamadori et al., 1977). For that reason, singing may provide an alternative way to rediscover verbal fluency and breath flow, akin to that in the Melodic Intonation Therapy approach. Even prior to the MIT studies, Gerstman (1964) described one aphasic patient who was unable to articulate her words through speech, but could sing words. This patient's ability to mimic and sustain singing was remarkably more developed than her language skills. In this example, Gerstman used singing successfully for articulation training. Similarly, Rogers and Fleming (1981) developed a music-speech protocol akin to MIT. Their protocol used a carrier melody in which the melody, rhythm, and intervals were as close as possible to conversational speech. Not only can singing facilitate speech fluency in persons with NCDs, but its emphasis on deep breathing, controlled exhalation, and audible phonation can improve dysphonic and dysprosodic speech. Along with singing, pacing techniques have been recommended by speech-language pathologists for the treatment of abnormal speech rates (Beukelman & Yorkston, 1984). In one related example, Kim and Tomaino (2008) observed that the rhythmic flow of CVA patients' singing remained relatively intact despite their severely impaired speech rhythms (p. 559).

MIND Model

Because of music's similarities to speech plus its inherent structure, flexibility, and creative potential, music therapy is an invaluable resource in the treatment of persons with NCDs. Daveson's *Meta-Model of Music Therapy in Neuro-disability* (MIND) defines music therapy neuropsychological practice according to three concurrent goal areas: (a) to restore function, (b) to attend to areas of psycho-social-emotional need, and/or (c) to compensate for loss (Daveson, 2008, p. 70). The rationale behind Daveson's multifocused approach is that patients with neurological impairments often present with multiple needs (p. 72).

The first goal is based on the premise that music facilitates a movement toward wholeness. This music therapy function is *restorative,* which alludes in this chapter to the restoration of speech function to a level similar or close to the premorbid level through the engagement of healthy brain mechanisms. An example of a restorative approach would be Cohen's (1988) application of singing, chanting of functional sentences, and clapping rhythms to assist an adolescent with dysarthria and Kluver-Bucy syndrome to speak at a more normalized rate. Many music therapists working in rehabilitation settings have modified the MIT approach to make it less time-intensive and more music-oriented (Magee, Brumfitt, Freeman, & Davidson, 2006). When using strategies that originate from SLP techniques (e.g., melodically intoned or rhythmically assisted speech), the music therapist is encouraged to collaborate with a speech-language pathologist to find appropriate speech materials and to avoid possible contraindications or professional misunderstandings (Hobson, 2006b; Magee, Brumfitt, Freeman, & Davidson, 2006).

The second goal is based on the premise that music helps patients cope with the frustrations, social alienation, and depression that often accompany a neurological impairment. In this case, the music therapy function is psycho-social-emotional. For patients who are nonverbal, music may serve as a preverbal, tonal language that can arouse fundamental emotional responses (Jochim, 1994, as cited in Purdie, 1997). In this chapter, an example of this would be Hitchen, Magee, and Soeterik's case study of a man with aphasia (2009), in which they introduced a therapist-composed song that focused on patient-centered themes to help him express his needs and emotions.

Finally, music helps patients develop strategies to compensate for losses, while enabling them to retain their social roles; thus, music therapy also functions in a compensatory capacity. In the context of this chapter, this occurs when a patient's communicative functioning continues to deteriorate or the patient has lost certain skills, with little chance of regaining them (Daveson, 2008, p. 73). Consequently, compensatory strategies may help patients either retain their present levels of functioning or learn new strategies to compensate for the lost skills. One example of this approach would be Tamplin's (2006b) song-collage technique, which enables functionally nonverbal patients with NCDs to express how they are coping with their injuries.

Referral and Assessment

The MIND model is a relatively new protocol for music therapy assessment and practice in the field of neurological rehabilitation. Published music therapy assessments are difficult to find, especially for patients with NCDs. A few general assessments have been published for use in rehabilitation settings, but they tend to be either focused on patients with very low awareness states (Magee, 2005) or used as a general tool for all patients in rehabilitation settings. The one exception is Lucia (1987), who developed a music therapy assessment protocol for the treatment of patients with NCD. She specifically evaluated patients' preserved music skills and certain other deficits for potential placement in a Vocal Skills Group. Lucia used the following selection criteria for the group members: (a) ability to match pitch, (b) singing range, (c) breath capacity while singing/chanting, (d) attention to musical task, (e) automatic recall of melody and words of premorbidly learned songs/proverb chants, (f) respiration-phonation patterns while singing/chanting, (g) syllabic production rate and rhythm during singing/ chanting, and (h) oral apraxic interferences while singing/chanting. In addition, she assessed visual field deficits and alexic elements to determine the value of visual cues such as large-print song charts, regular size–print song sheets, or directions to follow the mouthing cues of the therapist (p. 36). Lucia stated that those patients with damage to the left frontal lobe (Broca's area) or with bilateral damage leaving the right temporal lobe relatively intact tended to respond the best to the Vocal Skills treatment.

Overview of Methods and Procedures

The following sections contain clinical music therapy examples for the treatment of persons with neurogenic communication disorders; each example references one of the MIND goal areas (Daveson, 2008). Although all three MIND goals may be equally relevant, the present author has selected one goal for each of the examples to demonstrate how a specific goal area can be identified and emphasized in music therapy practice. Although all examples can apply to individual or group formats, for the sake of uniformity, the following examples will be based on a group format unless otherwise stated. These interventions have not been sequenced to reflect relative significance, effectiveness, or complexity. For all of these examples, the therapist will need to have experience with neurological rehabilitation and communication strategies or work under the supervision of a music therapist with this experience.

Re-creative Music Therapy

- Functional Sentences with Tapping: rhythm-based pacing techniques to accompany the recitation of functional speech
- Therapist-Composed Song: singing of song composed by therapist based on specific emotional needs of the patient group
- Singing Skills Group: using vocal instruction to facilitate expressive speech production

Compositional Music Therapy

- Song Collage: lyric phrases from preferred songs set to 16-bar precomposed melodies

Improvisational Music Therapy

- Musical Mirroring: Therapist musically supports emotional playing of client

Receptive Music Therapy

- Song as Language: Music forms a bridge to bring emotional support to a person's deeper self
- Music and Imagery: client-centered inductions and music to stimulate imagery

Guidelines for Re-creative Music Therapy

Functional Sentences with Tapping

Overview. Patients diagnosed with expressive aphasia or dysarthria may benefit from rhythm-based pacing techniques to accompany the recitation of functional speech. A pacing technique is a form of rhythmic self-cuing (e.g., walking, clapping, tapping, or counting one syllable on each finger) that creates a self-monitored rate of speech. The level of this intervention is restorative, according to Daveson's levels of therapy (2008), and the intervention model is based on Cohen's case study of a girl with Kluver-Bucy syndrome (1988). This technique is contraindicated for patients with acquired apraxia of speech, as attempting to tap while speaking may prove to be too difficult. This may lead to exacerbated motoric dysfunction and increased frustration levels (Cohen, 1995, p. 54).

Preparations. Materials needed include a frame drum and single mallet, a metronome or similar pacing device, a list of functional sentences created jointly by the patient and music therapist that reflect the patient's needs and speech abilities, and a preselected speaking pace, as determined by the patient and music therapist, with collaboration from the speech-language pathologist. It is better to use preselected sentences for this intervention, as it may prove confusing for the patient if the therapist uses conversational speech paired with musical phrasing (Kim & Tomaino, 2008). Additionally, the repetition of the musical and speech material is essential in this type of rehabilitation.

What to observe. The intended outcome for this intervention is for the patient to speak the functional sentences at an appropriate pace while tapping as the therapist plays speech rhythms on a frame drum. If the patient shows signs of cognitive or motor fatigue (e.g., latency, confusion, grimacing, motor tremors), the therapist will stop the intervention and allow the patient to rest.

Procedures. The therapist will place his/her chair directly facing the patient's to make facial cues clear (Tomaino, 2012) and to keep auditory and visual distractions to a minimum. Step-by-step procedures are as follows:

1) Begin with the first functional sentence on the list.
2) Say the sentence while tapping the speech rhythm on the frame drum as a model.
3) Repeat the sentence while tapping the speech rhythms on the frame drum and ask the patients to speak the sentence while tapping (e.g., on leg, chair, wheelchair tray).
4) Repeat procedure for the other functional sentences.

Variations. This intervention may be adapted in a variety of ways. If working with apraxic patients, the therapist may not be able to pair the sound of the drum with speaking or ask the patients to tap and speak, as that may prove to be too frustrating for them. The list of functional sentences may have to be simplified based on the patient's reading needs (e.g., the therapist may need to show patient only one sentence at a time; the therapist may need to use pictures instead of written language). If the patient has difficulty tapping and speaking at the same time, it may be necessary to break these skills down into simpler steps. The music therapist could teach the patient rhythmic values (e.g., *Solfège rhythmique*) via chanted rhythmic syllables, transfer the chanted rhythmic syllables to single words, and then combine the words into short phrases or sentences. A second variation could involve using a question-and-answer format, where the music therapist speaks the first half of a functional sentence while playing the drum and the patient speaks the second half of the sentence while tapping.

Therapist-Composed Song to Address Patient Issues

Overview. Patients with expressive neurogenic communication disorders may benefit from opportunities for self-expression within a group of peers who share similar issues. The level of therapy is psycho-social-emotional, according to Daveson's levels of therapy (2008), and the intervention is based on Hitchen, Magee, and Soeterik's clinical work (2009). This intervention is meant to address the patients' specific emotional needs by (a) engaging them in singing songs composed specifically for them by the music therapist, (b) allowing the patients to express themselves musically via the voice and breath, and (c) validating the patients' concerns and issues. This intervention is contraindicated for persons diagnosed with concomitant receptive language disorders who may not be able to comprehend lyrics, learn new words to songs, or read lyrics. In addition, the music may trigger agitated behaviors in patients with brain injuries if it is too loud or stimulating, or if competing auditory stimuli are present in the environment, such as voices or television (Hitchen, Magee, & Soeterik, 2009). The singing act may fatigue patients both cognitively and physically, so music therapists may need to plan to sing for short periods of time and to provide physical rests between songs.

Preparations. Materials needed include song sheets or sheet music and an accompanying instrument (e.g., guitar, keyboard, electric bass). It is best to choose a setting with minimal distractions or traffic. The music therapist will rehearse accompaniment patterns from popular musical genres in order to successfully facilitate a songwriting intervention that matches the musical preferences of the patients. For this group, the music therapist will choose patients with expressive neurogenic communication disorders who have the capacity to communicate either verbally, in writing, by pointing, or via an alternative communication system.

What to observe. The intended outcome for this intervention is for the patients to respond either verbally, by gesturing (e.g., pointing to a word or picture), or in writing, while participating in the creation of a song that is being composed specifically for them by the music therapist. If patient fatigue or frustration responses occur, the therapist can either break the task into smaller steps or provide rest breaks so that the songwriting remains a positive experience for the patient.

Procedures. Step-by-step procedures are as follows:

1) Invite patients to share their concerns/issues/feelings regarding their accidents, brain injuries, speech disorders, relationships, etc.
2) Compose a song in the patients' preferred musical style that addresses these issues while using lyrics that are brief and repetitive, at a slower tempo, and within the vocal range of the patients.
3) At the next group session, distribute song sheets or sheet music of the song. The words need to be presented in large black print on white or yellow paper due to possible visual perception problems.
4) Discuss the song with the patients, reminding them that the lyrics came from the group's feedback.
5) Perform the song, inviting patients to sing along if they wish.

Variations. This intervention may be modified in a variety of ways. If the patients are unable to answer questions verbally, the music therapist may need to have blank paper and a pencil handy, with necessary prosthetic modifications (e.g., clipboard, pencil cuff) so that the patient can write the first few letters of the word or draw a picture representing the intended word. If those attempts are not successful, the music therapist may need to have a list available so that the patient can point to a word or picture on the list. The therapist can record the song on digital media for the patients to share with others outside of the music therapy session. If the patients seem reluctant to sing (e.g., adolescents, patients with TBI), the music therapist can sing the song to the patients and/or ask them to accompany the song with percussion instruments. Another adaptation would be for the therapist to introduce a popular, patient-preferred song, with the recorded version of the song provided as the accompaniment. Once the patients seem to be comfortable singing along with the recorded accompaniments, the music therapist can substitute live guitar or keyboard accompaniment for these familiar songs. Once the patients will sing along with the live accompaniment, the music therapist can introduce the song composed specifically for them and invite them to sing along (Hitchen, Magee, & Soeterik, 2009).

Singing Skills Group

Overview. The singing skills group intervention is designed to benefit patients with neurogenic communication disorders by using vocal instruction to facilitate expressive speech production. The level of this intervention is restorative, according to Daveson's levels of therapy (2008), and the intervention models include the Music Therapy Treatment Protocol (Baker & Tamplin, 2006), the Singing Instruction Group (Cohen, 1992), and the Vocal Skills Group (Lucia, 1987). The goals of this intervention are to (a) apply singing skills to improve the fluency, prosody, and audible power of speech; (b) use breathing exercises to help build consistency and strength in speech; and (c) use vocal exercises as models for speech fluency, duration, and production. This intervention is contraindicated for patients with vocal dysprosodia or dysphonia caused by organic, chronic conditions, such as vocal cord paralysis, as it may be prove frustrating for these patients to attempt to change these particular speech characteristics. In this case, the music therapist may want to focus on other aspects of speech that can be changed, like speech pace or rhythm, or to offer an alternative music therapy experience. The singing may also trigger agitated behaviors in patients with brain injuries, especially if competing auditory stimuli are present in the environment, such as live voices or television (Hitchen et al., 2009).

Preparation. Materials needed for this intervention include a keyboard or piano, seats arranged in a semicircle for the vocal skills group members, and visual aids situated in front of the group. The music therapists leading this intervention will need to be comfortable with their own singing voices and have sufficient vocal skills to demonstrate correct breathing, phonation, vowel production, and consonant articulation. Because the therapists will be explaining and demonstrating exactly how the vowels and consonants are formed, they either will need to be trained vocalists or will need to co-treat this group with a speech-language pathologist.

The music therapist will choose a group of patients with neurogenic communication disorders who have the capacity to benefit from restorative singing instruction. The therapist will consult with a speech-language pathologist when forming this group to determine if the patients selected are suitable. The group will be scheduled to meet very regularly (e.g., four times a week for 8 weeks), since ongoing repetition of a motor task is mandatory for the restoration of motor function (Tomaino, 2010).

Prior to the first meeting of the Singing Skills Group, the music therapist will meet separately with each group member to discuss the purpose of the group, to answer any questions, to explain the procedures, and to receive each patient's consent. The music therapist will consult with a speech-language pathologist to determine which monosyllabic words, polysyllabic words, and song lyrics are appropriate and within the patient's capacity to produce and in what progression to present them. The vocal skills treatment plan will include (a) stretching of head, neck, shoulders; (b) breathing exercises (supported vowel sound for one to two seconds); (c) vowel exercises (on mi-re-do pattern); (d) functional words and short phrases intoned into melodies (on mi-re-do and sol-fa-mi-re-do melodic patterns); and (e) singing familiar songs that are appropriate for the patients' musical preferences, age level, and culture. The music therapist will select songs that are simple, slow, repetitive, and syllabic, with target words in case the patients cannot sing all the words (e.g., "and help me make it through the ______").

The music therapist will next create visual aids of the vowels, words, vocal exercises, and song lyrics. A white board, flip chart, song sheets, projected slides, or poster board can be used for this purpose. Prior to the session, the music therapist will place two chairs facing the group. One chair will be situated behind the keyboard but facing the group so that the therapist can lead while playing the musical examples (Tomaino, 2012). A second chair will be located in front of the keyboard so that the therapist can model and the patients can more clearly observe the exact motor skills needed to produce a desire sound. The group will also need to meet in a setting where auditory and visual distractions are kept to a minimum.

What to observe. The intended outcome for this intervention is for the patient to sing isolated vowels (e.g., [i], [e], [a], [o], [u]) within a mi-re-do pattern for two seconds per vowel. If the patients' expressive skills are more advanced, the projected outcome could include singing monosyllabic words or short phrases within a simple descending diatonic pattern. If the music therapist notices frustration responses, especially from patients with apraxia, dysprosodia, or dysphonia, it may be more suitable to switch these patients to a group that focuses on different outcomes, such as compensatory or psycho-social-emotional (Daveson, 2008).

Procedures. Once the preparatory steps are concluded and the group has been assembled, the music therapist will conduct the following:

1) Lead the group members in gentle stretching exercises.
2) Instruct patients about the importance of good breathing for health and demonstrate correct breathing techniques. For example, cue patients to inhale while seated in a chair with their hands placed on their abdomen. Encourage them to feel their backs expand against the backs of their chairs and feel their abdomens expand against their hands. Rehearse the stretches and basic breathing exercises at the beginning of every group meeting.
3) Cue patients to exhale using a [ts] sound for at least one second.
    a. Using the pitches of B-flat ascending to G, ask patients to inhale and to vocalize on a single vowel ([a]) for one second while continuing the feeling of the [ts] exhalation.
4) Repeat for other vowels ([i], [e], [o], [u]).
5) Introduce and demonstrate mi-re-do melodic pattern (approximately one and a half to two seconds) for each vowel sound (see Exercise One).
6) Lead the patients in the singing of the mi-re-do melodic patterns for each vowel sound in the keys of B-flat major to F major.
7) Introduce and demonstrate the singing of monosyllabic words using the mi-re-do melodic pattern.
8) Lead the patients in the singing of monosyllabic words using the mi-re-do melodic pattern in the keys of B-flat major to F major.
9) Demonstrate and lead patients in the singing of polysyllabic words and short phrases using a sol-fa-mi-re-do melodic pattern in the keys of B-flat major to D major (see Exercise Two).
10) Lead patients in the singing of familiar, preferred songs.

Exercise One for Vocal Group

(Men sing one octave lower.)

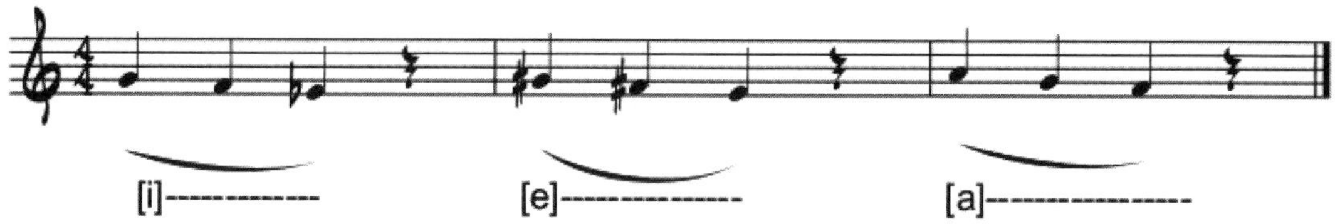

Exercise Two for Voice Group

(Men Sing One Octave Lower)

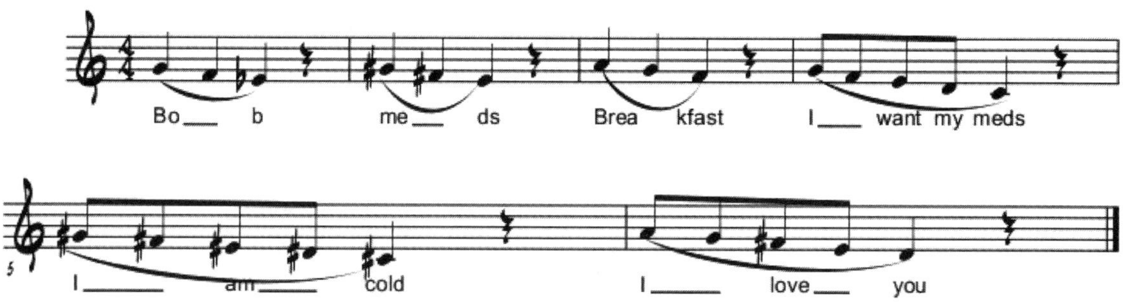

Variations. A number of variations are possible with this intervention. If the patients experience difficulties with the breathing, phonation, vowel production, or consonant articulation tasks, they may need additional singing demonstrations, physical cues, video recording examples, or props (stretch bands, mirrors) to produce the desired speech sounds. Along with the procedural steps outlined above, the therapist may ask for individual volunteers to sing for the group, or the therapist may use a question-and-answer format in which the therapist sings a question and the group members sing the answer (e.g., Question: "The stars at night are big and bright"; Answer: "Deep in the heart of Texas").

GUIDELINES FOR COMPOSITIONAL MUSIC THERAPY

Song Collage

Overview. The song-collage intervention is designed for patients with neurogenic communication disorders who may need an avenue for self-expression of feelings about their impairments or who may demonstrate poor initiation/ memory/idea generation, or for those short-term patients whose allotted time does not allow for a full songwriting process (Tamplin, 2006). The level of treatment is compensatory, as based on the MIND model (Daveson, 2008). The intervention is based on a clinical model described by Tamplin (2006). The goals of this intervention are as follows: (a) to allow patients to process their thoughts and emotions, (b) to teach patients coping strategies, (c) to offer patients opportunities for self-expression, (d) to provide choice-making opportunities for patients, and (e) to give patients ownership in a creative process. One potential contraindication is that the patient's heritage traditions may not condone self-expression via secular song lyrics. If that is the case, allow the patients to choose lyrics from appropriate literary sources (e.g., sacred texts, traditional poetry) or use a different intervention altogether.

Preparation. Prior to the song-collage session, the music therapist will prepare lists of lyric phrases from familiar songs that are organized under common themes (e.g., love, anger, helplessness, fun). These phrases need to be printed with large, black print and on white or yellow paper, with plenty of spacing between the lines of text to accommodate visual perception deficits. Plan in advance to have assistants or higher-functioning patients as partners to assist with the choice of the song theme and lyrics. Set up tables and chairs in the room and distribute a printed list of lyric phrases for each seat. Provide one clipboard and writing implement per patient, with a generous amount of blank paper available.

Next, compose an assortment of 16-measure melodies with accompaniment patterns representing different popular musical genres (e.g., blues, rock and roll, bluegrass, country) to provide musical structure for the song collages. Be sure to research the cultural and religious backgrounds of the patients regarding secular vocal music prior to offering the intervention so that the song-collage intervention does not unintentionally offend a patient or patient's family.

What to observe. The intended outcome from this intervention is for each patient to select three different lyric phrases for the song collage. If patient seems confused with the directions and needs additional assistance, have assistants or higher-functioning patients there to assist.

Procedures. Once the room is readied for the song collage intervention, the music therapist will follow these steps:

1) Group the patients in dyads with an assistant or a higher-functioning patient as partner.
2) Explain that the patients can choose as many lyric phrases as they wish from the provided sheets.
3) Once the dyad members have chosen their lyric phrases, perform the precomposed 16-measure melodies for the group. Each dyad will then choose a melody/genre for their song collage.
4) Encourage dyad members to organize their phrases thematically, revise their lyrics to fit into a poetic or musical structure, or add new lyrics as needed to match the selected melody/genre.
5) Allow the song collage process to take place over multiple sessions, if possible.

Variations. The therapist can provide as little or as much structure as needed to allow the song-collage process to work for patients with differing levels of cognitive and communication deficits. For example, rather than composing original melodies, the music therapist might use a piggy-back technique with already familiar melodies, as long as the addition of new words doesn't confuse the patients. To encourage socialization, the dyads could be made up of the patients and their family members or friends. Following the creation of the song collages, the dyad members and music therapist can perform the songs for the group, staff, or family members/friends. The music therapist can also commemorate the occasion by making an audio or video recording of the song collages and sharing a copy with the patients and their loved ones.

Guidelines for Improvisational Music Therapy

Musical Mirroring

Overview. The music therapist's intention for musical mirroring is to offer emotional support, to validate, and to allow the patients the opportunity to express themselves via music. The musical mirroring intervention is intended for patients with neurogenic communication disorders who are at risk for emotional deprivation due to their inability to communicate verbally. The level of this intervention is psycho-social-emotional, according to the MIND model (Daveson, 2008). It is based upon treatment techniques established by Hartley, Turry, and Raghavan (2010) and by Jungblut (2009). At this level, it is not meant to be a cognitive exercise where the patients listen and imitate each other's music, nor is the music meant to represent a metaphor for an abstract concept.

The goals of this intervention are as follows: (a) to decrease levels of frustration associated with communication disorders (Daveson, 2008), (b) to provide patients with a greater sense of control (Magee, 2007), (c) to provide patients with feelings of accomplishment, ability, skill, and success (Magee, 2007), (d) to allow patients a highly physical experience through music-making (Magee, 2007), and (e) to give creative articulation to human feelings (Hartley, Turry, & Raghavan, 2010).

Contraindications are possible with this intervention. Neurologically impaired patients may not be capable of playing instruments or vocally improvising due to their physical and cognitive impairments. Also, the lack of structure in the improvised music may be too threatening for the patients, especially if they are already experiencing confusion.

Preparation. To prepare for this intervention, the music therapist will collect drums with large striking areas (e.g., turbanos, djembes) or Orff fixed-pitch percussion instruments with large striking areas (e.g., bass bars, bass metallophone, bass xylophone). The therapist will then set up chairs or wheelchairs in a circle around the instruments. The music therapist should try to make the space as open, comfortable, and free from intrusion as possible so that patients feel free to express themselves without being self-conscious.

What to observe. The intended therapeutic outcome for this intervention is for each patient to play an instrument for a total of three minutes while the music therapist mirrors the patient musically. Patients with confusion may not be comfortable participating in an unstructured musical interaction and may need increased structure or assistance from the music therapist to continue playing.

Procedures. Once the patients are seated in a circle around the instruments, the music therapist will proceed with the following:

1) Address one patient at a time. Ask that patient to choose an instrument from the center and offer assistance if needed.
2) Explain to the group that they will proceed around the circle one at a time. One designated patient will start playing, and the music therapist will play along with him/her. The rest of the patients will listen. The therapist will assure the patients that anything they play is fine, and that there is no wrong or right way to play.
3) As each patient plays, the music therapist will musically mirror the patient's emotional tone and nonverbal gestures to create a sense of empathy and understanding between the therapist and each patient.
4) The music therapist will musically mirror the patient for as long as the patient is playing.

Variations. The therapist can either play a separate instrument or share an instrument with each patient. If a patient perseverates musically, the music therapist may need to introduce increased musical structure (e.g., slow down tempo, get softer, emphasize downbeat) to bring the musical mirroring to a close. The therapist may also need to introduce musical structure to engage the patient initially.

GUIDELINES FOR RECEPTIVE MUSIC THERAPY

Song as Language

Overview. With this technique, music forms a bridge to bring emotional support to a person's deeper self. Not all patients are capable of using singing as a means to rediscover speech production, as with the Singing Skills Group intervention described above. In fact, for patients in very low awareness states (e.g., those who have been diagnosed on the lower levels of the *Rancho Los Amigos Levels of Cognitive Functioning*), a desired goal may simply be to help them connect to their inner resources, especially during the acute stages of recovery. Jochims and Aldridge (1994, as cited in Purdie, 1997) wrote about their case studies with patients who had experienced extreme brain trauma resulting from automobile accidents. The authors described how they had "established contact in the early stage of craniocerebral trauma" by using "sound as a bridge to mute patients" (as cited in Purdie, 1997, p. 217). The authors claimed that music aroused fundamental cognitive and emotional responses in persons with no speech, and that music communicated with a patient's "inner self," therefore functioning as a source of emotional support (as cited in Purdie, 1997, p. 212).

The song-as-language intervention is based on Jochim and Aldridge's premise that music forms a bridge to bring emotional support to a person's deeper self. This will be described as an individual intervention and is not recommended for a group. The level of this intervention is psycho-social-emotional, according to Daveson's levels of therapy (2008). The goals of this intervention are to (a) arouse fundamental cognitive and emotional processes, (b) to connect with the patient at a preverbal level, and (c) to provide emotional support to the patient. For patients in these stages, even soft, a cappella singing may result in overstimulation and auditory fatigue responses. This intervention needs to be coordinated with other therapeutic modalities so that the patient is not overly subjected to stimulation in a short period of time (Wong, 2004).

Preparation. Prior to the first session, the music therapist will ask the patient's family and friends about his/her musical preferences and inquire about any taboos or indigenous customs regarding music in the patient's culture. Based on the feedback received, the music therapist will prepare songs that are familiar and hopefully meaningful to the patient. Prior to the session, the therapist will visit the patient's room and identify any auditory distractions. The music therapist will turn off any television, radio, phones, or other sound-producing objects that are not medically necessary, and will limit the number of people in the room to reduce the potential for auditory fatigue.

What to observe. The intended outcome for this intervention is for the patient to demonstrate localization responses (e.g., turns head, vocalizes, opens eyes, smiles, moves fingers) during or following the therapist's singing. The therapist needs to watch the patient carefully for agitation or fatigue responses, as music can easily overstimulate persons who are in low awareness states. If the patient demonstrates any agitated, perseverative, or fatigue responses (e.g., motor tremors, facial grimacing), the music therapist will stop the intervention and let the patient rest.

Procedures. Once the preparation is completed and the patient's room is quiet and comfortable, the music therapist will proceed with the following steps:

1) Set up a chair close to patient's head, facing the patient.

2) Introduce self briefly to patient so that the patient is not startled by the initial sound of the music.
3) Softly begin humming, vocalizing on a vowel, or singing familiar melodies that were recommended by the family or friends and that may be personally meaningful to the patient.
4) Sing in a simple, unobtrusive, and soothing manner that will support and connect with the patient.
5) Sing no longer than one to two minutes at first, followed by 1-2 minutes of silence (Wong, 2004). These intervals can be repeated.

Variations. The amount of singing time may increase as the patient's awareness responses become consistent. Continue to provide resting intervals between singing phases. At first, repeat the patient's preferred melodies across the sessions, rather than introduce new ones, so as not to overwhelm or fatigue the patient. Although the therapist will start out with soft a cappella singing, it may be possible later to add or substitute an accompanying instrument (e.g., guitar, lyre, harp) once the patient's cognitive and emotional responses stabilize. In fact, the patient may respond more positively to the sound of a familiar instrument than to the sound of a singing voice. If the family members and friends also seem to crave engagement with the music, the therapist can provide a separate session for them so as not to overstimulate the patient.

Music and Imagery

Overview. Music and imagery uses client centered inductions and music to stimulate imagery. It is a technique that can only be studied after a music therapist passes the board certification exam administered by the Certification Board for Music Therapists. The Music and Imagery training model was created by Dr. Lisa Summer, Director of the Anna Maria College (AMC) Institute for Music and Consciousness, to allow board-certified music therapists to learn supportive-level music and imagery concepts and techniques so as to apply them immediately into their clinical music therapy practices. According to the Institute's website, the first level of the training "provides the expertise to design and implement individualized, single-session music and imagery techniques. The curriculum focuses on quick assessment and the development of effective spontaneous, client-centered inductions and music to stimulate imagery. There is an emphasis on treatment for stress, anxiety, or pain with individual clients" (AMC, 2011, Level I).

Music and Imagery grew out of the core concepts of the Bonny Method of Guided Imagery and Music; however, the Bonny Method training is considerably more time-intensive and psychodynamic in nature. To become a Fellow of the Association for Music and Imagery (i.e., Bonny Method practitioner), a trainee must complete three levels of comprehensive training, which requires a period of years. In contrast, music therapists can implement supportive Music and Imagery techniques in their clinical environments after successfully completing AMC's first level of study and corresponding field experience.

This final clinical intervention example represents the Music and Imagery paradigm. It is based on a case study with a musician diagnosed with brain damage and expressive aphasia (Cohen, 2003). The patient could converse only for brief periods of time without becoming physically fatigued. She had been a professional musician for many years before the onset of the brain damage, and was struggling with issues such as self-identification, loss, struggle, and faith. The patient requested Bonny Method sessions from the therapist, who was both board-certified and a Fellow of the Association for Music and Imagery.

Due to the psychodynamic nature of the Bonny Method and the potential vulnerability of a patient with brain damage, the music therapist was ethically responsible to establish beforehand that the patient was physically and psychologically healthy and emotionally grounded enough to benefit from this approach. With the patient's written consent, the therapist acquired background information and reports from other professionals who were treating this patient. After reviewing the reports and conducting an initial intake session with the patient, the music therapist decided to use the Music and Imagery approach due to her concerns that the Bonny Method might be contraindicative due to this unique patient's inability to speak fluently or to process imagery in a traditional manner. The patient agreed with this decision. The therapist was also aware that the evocative nature of the typical music used in Bonny Method sessions might prove to be too powerful or last too long for the patient. The therapist's intention was to provide a supportive and holding container for the patient during this difficult transition.

What was unique about this case study was that the therapist and patient used electronic communication (e.g., scanning pictures, electronic mail) for communicating and processing between sessions so as not to overstimulate the patient on the day of her session. The level of treatment was compensatory, as based on the MIND model (Daveson, 2008). The overall goals for the intervention were as follows: (a) to provide a supportive, holding musical space; (b) to create avenues to compensate for the patient's lack of verbal skills; (c) to allow the patient access to a healthy, creative space to explore her faith; (d) to provide the patient with opportunities for self-growth and self-awareness; and (e) to provide a means for this patient to connect with music at a deeper level. This final goal was especially essential, as the patient was no longer able to perform music and was grieving over the loss of that relationship.

During the intake session and via email, the therapist was able to discern the patient's musical preferences and also musical selections that might be contraindicative for the patient due to past associations. For example, the patient was from a Lutheran background and had performed Bach's instrumental music regularly in ensembles, so that music was intensely referential for her due to her familiarity with the genre. The goal (e.g., support, healing) for each session was established between the therapist/patient dyad via email before the session.

Preparation. Once the goal had been identified, the music therapist completed the following preparations:

1) Preselect a minimum of three recorded digital music selections, each one approximately two to three minutes in length, with the following musical characteristics: structured, repetitive, dependable, supportive, with few abrupt changes. The music therapist in this case study initially used homophonic string chamber pieces featuring lower-pitched instruments and lighter textures for this client. The therapist listened to potential selections on the day of the session before leaving to drive to the patient's home.
2) Bring sheets of blank paper on a clipboard and a writing implement so that the patient has the choice to narrate (while the therapist writes) or to write during or following the music session.
3) Create a therapeutic environment that is free from intrusion, visitors, and distractions. For example, the patient had a very sweet dog that liked to bark at people walking by, so the patient put the dog outside in a fenced yard before the session to help prevent that distraction.
4) Position the patient in a supine position on a bed with the head propped on a pillow, and check that the patient is comfortable in that position. The patient chose using a bed over using a lounge chair.
5) Bring in a portable digital music device with a remote control and place the speaker near or behind where the patient's head will be.
6) Test the remote control to make sure it works.

7) Check with the patient to ascertain that the music is audible but at a comfortable level. Music that is at a preferred volume for the therapist may be too strong for a patient with brain damage.

What to observe. The intended outcome was for the patient to share one imagery experience related to the predetermined goal, either verbally, in writing, or via drawing, that had occurred during the session.

Procedures. After the preparation, the therapist followed these steps:

1) Meet briefly with the patient to reconfirm the goal of the session.
2) Allow the patient a short rest period (e.g., five minutes) prior to the beginning of the induction and music listening.
3) Sit close to the bed, facing the patient, and keep a clipboard with blank sheets of paper, a writing implement, and the remote control for the music device within reach.
4) Lead a verbal relaxation induction. Speak slowly and calmly and include long pauses between the instructions to allow for necessary processing time. Repeat instructions more than once.
5) Once the patient is in a relaxed state (e.g., respiratory rate slows, facial muscles relax), restate the goal of the session and inform the patient that the music will be starting.
6) After the recording music has ended, tell the patient that the music has stopped and guide the patient back to an alert state. Speak simply, slowly, and calmly. Allow a long period of time for the patient to reach alertness.
7) When the patient appears alert, ask him/her to share the imagery experience and offer choices for communication (e.g., verbally, in writing, by drawing).

Variations. During the music portion of the session, the therapist observed the patient's responses. If the patient displayed any signs of fatigue or agitation (tremors, twitching, grimacing), the therapist stopped the music, informed the patient why the music has stopped, and stayed seated while allowing the patient to rest. The amount of recorded music time and number of selections increased across sessions, but never extended past six minutes, total. The therapist often provided resting intervals or time for processing, as needed, between the individual recorded pieces. It was sometimes too difficult for the patient to verbalize after listening to a piece of music. When that was the case, the therapist and patient created a system to communicate whether the patient wanted a different piece of music, the same music repeated, or no more music. This system varied across sessions, and the patient used physical gestures, single-word cues, and pointed to the compact disk case to communicate her preferences.

After the music, the patient was sometimes too fatigued to talk or write. When this occurred, the therapist left quietly, and they processed the imagery experience later via email or Skype. Although Music and Imagery sessions usually involve drawing during or following the music session, it was too difficult for this patient to draw during or following the music. The patient often drew a few hours following the session, scanned the drawing, and then sent the drawing and a written synopsis/interpretation of the session's imagery to the music therapist a few days later. The therapist then responded via email, and the process continued.

References

Albert, M. L., Sparks, R. W., & Helm, N. A. (1973). Melodic intonation therapy for aphasia. *Archives of Neurology, 29,* 130–131.

American Speech-Language-Hearing Association. (2010). Therapy cap advocacy center. Retrieved May 26, 2012, from http://www.asha.org/advocacy/federal/cap

American Speech-Language-Hearing Association. (2012). Directory of speech-language assessment instruments. Retrieved May 26, 2012, from http://www.asha.org/assessments.aspx?type=&lang=English

Anna Maria College Institute for Music and Consciousness. (2011). *Music and imagery training: Level one.* Retrieved December 27, 2012, from http://www.annamaria.edu/academics/instituteformusic

Baker, F., & Roth, E. A. (2004). Neuroplasticity and functional recovery: Training models and compensatory strategies in music therapy. *Nordic Journal of Music Therapy, 73*(1), 20–32.

Baker, F., & Tamplin, J. (2006). *Music therapy methods in neurorehabilitation: A clinician's manual.* Philadelphia, PA: Jessica Kingsley.

Baker, F., Wigram, T., & Gold, C. (2005). The effects of a song-singing programme on the affective speaking intonation of people with traumatic brain injury. *Brain Injury, 19*(7), 519–528.

Besson, M., Faïta, F., Peretz, I., Bonnel, A-M., & Requin, J. (1998) Singing in the brain: Independence of lyrics and tunes. *Psychological Science, 9*(6), 494–499.

Beukelman, D., & Yorkston, K. (1981). Ataxic dysarthria. Treatment sequence based on intelligibility and prosodic considerations. *Journal of Speech and Hearing Disorders, 46,* 398–404.

Brookshire, R. H. (1992). *An introduction to neurogenic communication disorders* (4th ed.). St. Louis, MO: Mosby Year-Book, Inc.

Centers for Disease Control and Management (2010). *ICD-9-CM diagnostic codes.* Atlanta, GA: Author.

Classification of diseases, latest developments, functioning, and disability. (Sept. 23, 2011). Centers for Disease Control and Prevention. Retrieved May 26, 2012, from http://www.cdc.gov/nchs/icd/icd9.htm

Cohen, N. (1988). The use of superimposed rhythm to decrease the rate of speech in a brain-damaged adolescent. *Journal of Music Therapy, 25*(2), 85–93.

Cohen, N. (1992). The effect of singing instruction on the speech production of neurologically impaired persons. *Journal of Music Therapy, 29*(2), 87–102.

Cohen, N. (1994). Speech and song: Implications for therapy. *Music Therapy Perspectives, 12*(1), 10–16.

Cohen, N. (2003). *The floating leaf: A case study of the Bonny Method for a musician with brain damage.* Unpublished report.

Cohen, N., & Ford, J. (1995). The effect of musical cues on the nonpurposive speech of persons with aphasia. *Journal of Music Therapy, 32*(1), 46–57.

Cohen, N., & Masse, R. (1993). The application of singing and rhythmic instruction as a therapeutic intervention for persons with neurogenic communication disorders. *Journal of Music Therapy, 3*(2), 81–89.

Darley, F. L., Aronson, A. E., & Brown, J. R. (1969a). Differential diagnostic patterns of dysarthria. *Journal of Speech and Hearing Research, 12,* 249–269.

Darley, F. L., Aronson, A. E., & Brown, J. R. (1969b). Cluster of deviant speech dimensions in the dysarthrias. *Journal of Speech and Hearing Research, 12,* 462–496.

Darley, F. L., Aronson, A. E., & Brown, J. R. (1975). *Motor speech disorders.* Philadelphia, PA: Saunders.

Daveson, B. (2008). A description of a music therapy meta-model in neuro-disability and neuro-rehabilitation for use with children, adolescents, and adults. *Australian Journal of Music*

Therapy, 19, 70–85.

de l'Etoile, S. (2010). Neurologic music therapy: A scientific paradigm for clinical practice. *Music and Medicine, 2*(2), 78–84.

Dronkers, N. G. (1996). A new brain region for coordinating speech articulation. *Nature, 384,* 159–161.

Duffy, J. R. (1995). *Motor speech disorders: Substrates, differential diagnosis, and management.* St. Louis, MO: Mosby-Year Book.

Eisenson, J. (1994). *Examining for aphasia: Assessment of aphasia and related impairments* (3rd ed.). Austin, TX: PRO-ED.

Gardner, H. (1976). The shattered mind. New York: Alfred A. Knopf.

Gerstman, M. (1964). A case of aphasia. *Journal of Speech and Hearing Disorders, 29,* 89–91.

Gilbertson, S. (2008). Evidence missing, or missing evidence? The role of the literature in defining neuro-disability and neurorehabilitation: Commentary on Daveson's 2008 article. *The Australian Journal of Music Therapy, 19,* 86–88.

Gleason, J. B., & Goodglass, H. (1984). Some neurological and linguistic accompaniments of the fluent and nonfluent aphasics. *Topics in Language Disorders, 4,* 71–81.

Goodglass, H., Kaplan, E., & Barresi, B. (2000). *Boston diagnostic aphasia examination* (3rd ed.). Austin, TX: PRO-ED.

Haneishi, E. (2001). Effects of a music therapy voice protocol on speech intelligibility, vocal acoustic measures, and mood of individuals with Parkinson's disease. *Journal of Music Therapy, 38*(4), 273–290.

Hartley, M. L., Turry, A., & Raghavan, P. (2010). The role of music and music therapy in aphasia rehabilitation. *Music and Medicine, 2*(4), 235–242.

Hébert, S., Peretz, I., & Racette, A. (2008). Should we make aphasic patients sing? *Neuropsychological Research: A Review, 1,* 185–200.

Hitchen, H., Magee, W. L., & Soeterik, S. (2009). Music therapy in the treatment of patients with neuro-behavioural disorders stemming from acquired brain injury. *Nordic Journal of Music Therapy, 19*(1), 63–78.

Hobson, M. (2006a). The collaboration of music therapy and speech-language pathology in the treatment of neurogenic communication disorders, Part I. *Music Therapy Perspectives, 24*(2), 58–65.

Hobson, M. (2006b). The collaboration of music therapy and speech-language pathology in the treatment of neurogenic communication disorders, Part II. *Music Therapy Perspectives, 24*(2), 66–72.

Holland, A. L., Frattali, C., & Fromm, D. (1999). *Communication abilities of daily living* (2nd ed.). Austin, TX: PRO-ED.

Hurkmans, J., de Bruijn, M., Boonstra, A. M., Jonkers, R., Bastiaanse, R., Arendzen, H., & Reinders-Messelink, H. A. (2012). Music in the treatment of neurological language and speech disorders: A systematic review. *Aphasiology, 26*(1), 1–19.

Hustad, K. C., Kent, R. D., & Beukelman, D. R. (1998). DEC talk and MacinTalk speech synthesizers: Intelligibility differences for three listener groups. *Journal of Speech, Language, & Hearing Research, 41,* 744–752.

Enderby, P., & Emerson, J. (1995). *Does speech and language therapy work? A review of the literature.* London: Whurr.

Jungblut, M. (2009). SIPARI: A music therapy intervention for patients suffering with chronic, nonfluent aphasia. *Music and Medicine, 1*(2), 102–105.

Jungblut, M., Suchanek, M., & Gerhard, H. (2009). Long-term recovery from chronic global aphasia: A case report. *Music and Medicine, 1,* 61–69.

Kent, R. D. (2000). Research on speech motor control and its disorders: A review and prospective. *Journal of Communication Disorders, 33,* 391–428.

Keenan, J. S., & Brassell, E. G. (1975). *Aphasia-language performance scales.* St. Louis, MO: Pinnacle Press.

Kertesz, A. (2006). *Western aphasia battery-revised.* San Antonio, TX: Harcourt Assessment, Inc.

Kim, M., & Tomaino, C. M. (2008). Protocol evaluation for effective music therapy for persons with nonfluent aphasia. *Top Stroke Rehabilitation, 15*(6), 555–569.

Kleiman, L. I. (2003). *Functional communication profile-revised.* LinguiSystems.

Krauss, T., & Galloway, H. (1982). Melodic intonation therapy with language delayed, apraxic children. *Journal of Music Therapy, 19*(2), 102–113.

Laughlin, S. A., Naeser, M. A., & Gordon, W. P. (1979). Effects of three syllable durations using the melodic intonation therapy technique. *Journal of Speech and Hearing Research, 22,* 295–310.

Liégeois-Chauvel, C., Peretz, I., Babaï, M., Laguitton, V., & Chauvel, P. (1998). Contribution of different cortical areas in the temporal lobes to music processing. *Brain, 121,* 1853–1867.

Lubinski, R. (1991). *Dementia and communication.* Hamilton, Ontario: B. C. Decker.

Lucia, C. M. (1987). Toward developing a model of music therapy intervention in the rehabilitation of head trauma patients. *Music Therapy Perspectives, 4,* 34–39.

Luria, A. R. (1963). *Restoration of function after brain injury.* Pergamon Press.

Magee, W. (2005). Music therapy with patients in low awareness states: Approaches to assessment and treatment in multidisciplinary care. *Neuropsychological Rehabilitation, 15,* 522–536.

Magee, W. (2007). A comparison between the use of songs and improvisation in music therapy with adults living with acquired and chronic illness. *Australian Journal of Music Therapy, 18,* 19–38.

Magee, W. L., Brumfitt, S. M., Freeman, M., & Davidson, J. W. (2006). The role of music therapy in an interdisciplinary approach to address functional communication in complex neuro-communication disorders: A case report. *Disability and Rehabilitation, 28*(19), 1221–1229.

Mackenzie, C., & Lowit, A. (2007). Behavioural intervention effects in dysarthria following stroke: Communication effectiveness, intelligibility and dysarthria impact. *International Journal of Language and Communication Disorders, 42*(2),131–153.

McNeil, M. R. (1997). *Clinical management of sensorimotor speech disorders.* New York: Thieme.

McNeil, M. R., Robin, D. A., & Schmidt, R. A. (2009). Apraxia of speech. In M. R. McNeil (Ed.), *Clinical management of sensorimotor speech disorders* (2nd ed.). New York: Thieme.

National Institutes of Health: National Institute for Neurological Disorders and Stroke. (May 6, 2010). Aphasia. Retrieved from http://www.ninds.nih.gov/disorders/aphasia/aphasia.htm

Patel, A. D., Peretz, I., Tramo, M., & Labrecque, R. (1998). Processing prosodic and musical patterns: A neuropsychological investigation. *Brain and Language, 61*(2), 123–144.

Peretz, I. (1990) Processing of local and global musical information in unilateral brain-damaged patients. *Brain, 113,* 1185–1205.

Porch, B. (2001). *Porch index of communicative ability-revised.* Albuquerque, NM: PICA Programs.

Purdie, H. (1997). Music therapy in neurorehabilitation: Recent developments and new challenges. *Critical Reviews in Physical and Rehabilitation Medicine, 9*(3–4), 205–217.

Racette, A., Bard, C., & Peretz, I. (2006). Making nonfluent aphasics speak: Sing along! *Brain, 129,* 2571.

Rainbow Rehabilitation Centers. (2011). *Lee Silverman voice treatment.* Retrieved May 28, 2012, from http://www.rainbowrehab.com

Ramig, L. O. (1998). Treatment of speech and voice problems associated with Parkinson's disease. *Topics in Geriatric Rehabilitation, 14,* 28–43.

Robey, R. R., & Schultz, M. C. (1998). A model for conducting clinical-outcome research: An adaptation of the standard protocol for use in aphasiology. *Aphasiology, 12*(9), 787–810.

Rogers, A., & Fleming, P. L. (1981). Rhythm and melody in speech therapy for the neurologically impaired. *Music Therapy, 1*(1), 33–38.

Rosenbek, J. C., Lemme, M. L., Ahern, M. B., Harris, E. H., & Wertz, R. T. (1973). A treatment for apraxia of speech in adults. *Journal of Speech and Hearing Disorders, 38*(4), 462–470.

Rousseaux, M., Daveluy, W., & Kozlowski, O. (2010). Communication in conversation in stroke patients. *Journal of Neurology, 257,* 1099–1107. DOI: 10.1007/s00415-010-5469-08.

Sapir, S., & Aronson, A. E. (1985). Aphonia after closed head injury: Aetologic considerations. *British Journal of Disorders of Communication, 20,* 289–296.

Sparks, R. W., Helm, N., & Albert, M. (1974). Aphasia rehabilitation resulting from melodic intonation therapy. *Cortex, 10,* 313–316.

Sparks, R. W., & Holland, A. L. (1976). Method: Melodic intonation therapy for aphasia. *Journal of Speech and Hearing Disorders, 41,* 287–297.

Tanner, D. C. (2009). *The psychology of neurogenic communication disorders.* iUniverse, Inc.

Tomaino, C. (2010). Recovery of fluent speech through a musician's use of prelearned song repertoire: A case study. *Music and Medicine, 2*(2), 85–88.

Tomaino, C. (2012). Effective music therapy techniques in the treatment of nonfluent aphasia. *Annals of the NY Academy of Sciences, 1252,* 312–317.

Tamplin, J. (2006). Song collage technique: A new approach to songwriting. *Nordic Journal of Music Therapy, 15*(2), 177–190.

Tamplin, J. (2008). A pilot study into the effect of vocal exercises and singing on dysarthric speech. *NeuroRehabilitation, 23,* 207–216.

Tamplin, J., & Grocke, D. (2008). A music therapy treatment protocol for acquired dysarthria rehabilitation. *Music Therapy Perspectives, 26*(1), 23–29.

Thaut, M. H. (2005). Neurologic music therapy in speech and language rehabilitation. In M. H. Thaut (Ed.), *Rhythm, music, and the brain: Scientific foundations and clinical applications* (pp. 165–178). New York: Routledge.

U.S. Department of Health and Human Services: Centers for Medicare and Medical Services. *Medicare coverage: General information.* Retrieved January 26, 2010, from http:// www.hhs.gov

Van der Meulen, I., Van de Sandt-Koenderman, M. E., & Ribbers, G. M. (2012). Melodic intonation therapy: Present controversies and future opportunities. *Archives of Physical Medicine and Rehabilitation, 93*(1), 46–52.

Van der Merwe, A. (2011). A speech motor learning approach to treating apraxia of speech: Rationale and effects of intervention with an adult with acquired apraxia of speech. *Aphasiology, 25*(10), 1174–1206.

Wallace, G. L. (2010). Profile of life participation after stroke and aphasia. *Top Stroke Rehabilitation, 17*(6), 432–450. DOI: 10.1310/tsr1706-432.

Warlow, C. P., Dennis, M. S., Van Gijn, J., Hankey, G. J., Sandercock, P. A. G., Bamford, J. G., & Wardlaw, J. (Eds.). (2000). *Stroke: A practical guide to management.* Oxford: Blackwell Scientific.

Weller, C. M., & Baker, F. A. (2011). The role of music therapy in physical rehabilitation: A systematic literature review. *Nordic Journal of Music Therapy, 20*(1), 43–61.

Wong, E. H. (2004). *Clinical guide to music therapy in adult physical rehabilitation settings.* Silver Spring, MD: American Music Therapy Association.

Yamadori, A., Osumi, Y., Masuhari, S., & Okubo, M. (1977). Preservation of singing in Broca's aphasia. *Journal of Neurology, Neurosurgery, and Psychiatry, 40,* 221–224.

Yorkston, K. M. (1996). Treatment efficacy: Dysarthria. *Journal of Speech & Hearing Research, 39,* 46–57.

Yorkston, K. M., Beukelman, D., Strand, E. & Bell, K. R. (1999). *Management of motor speech disorders in children and adults.* Austin, TX: Pro-Ed.

Yorkston, K. M., Beukelman, D., & Traynor, C. (1984). *Assessment of intelligibility of dysarthric speech.* Austin, TX: Pro-Ed.

Chapter 9

Adults with Neurodegenerative Diseases

Wendy L. Magee

Diagnostic Information

Long-term neurological conditions (LTNC) are chronic and degenerative diseases, with no cure at the present time. Individuals diagnosed with LTNC can live for many years, with intermittent yet gradually increasing symptoms resulting from their disease. In the early stages, the person will be living independently alone or with family; the person will continue to do so for as long as possible until their needs change to a level where 24-hour nursing care is required. Unlike people living with other diseases who will require palliative care (e.g., cancer), the disease trajectories of people living with LTNC have longer and more variable time courses, with more diverse symptoms, and complex disabilities which may include cognitive, behavioral, and communication problems in addition to physical impairments (Turner-Stokes et al., 2007). Care for individuals with LTNC encompasses disability management and symptom control, with the aim to maintain a person's independence and quality of life. Often, long-term care and support is required over many years, particularly in the more slowly progressive or stable conditions.

The illness trajectories and duration of the disease processes for each of the LTNC covered differ. However, motor and communication disorders are central to all LTNC, as well as cognitive disorders to a differing degree between diseases and, sometimes, within the same condition. Living with an LTNC results in profound changes to most aspects of daily living for the individual and their loved ones, and therefore the social and emotional consequences are highly significant. For people with slowly changing conditions, there may be many years of rehabilitative treatment aiming to maintain a person's functioning and optimize their independence and autonomy (Turner-Stokes et al., 2007). Palliative models are most appropriate for the final stages and have been termed "neuropalliative rehabilitation," because as the patient's neurological condition becomes more advanced, rehabilitation and palliative care approaches often overlap (Turner-Stokes et al., 2007). This model is a useful one for music therapists to understand in order to consider the most appropriate goals of intervention and shape the intervention they offer accordingly.

Huntington's Disease (HD)

Huntington's disease is a hereditary, progressive neurodegenerative disorder characterized by increasingly severe motor impairment, cognitive decline, and behavioral manifestations leading to functional disability and complete dependency (Bonelli, Wenning, & Kapfhammer, 2004). It is characterized by involuntary movements and abnormality of voluntary movements, which, in combination with the gradual cognitive deterioration and neuropsychiatric disorders, cause complex social consequences for the individual and their support network (Magee, 1995). Although occurring across all racial groups, it is most common in people of northern European origin, with conservative estimates of prevalence in the Western Hemisphere at 7–10/100 000 (Novak & Tabrizi, 2010).

Because HD is an autosomal dominant disorder, every child born to a parent carrying the HD gene has a 50% chance of developing the disease. Thus, this disease devastates entire extended families. It is not uncommon for a spouse to nurse their husband/wife through many years of debilitating disability to death, only to then have to nurse one, two, or more of their offspring in a similar way. The disease progresses over 15–20 years (Novak & Tarbrizi, 2010), with death caused most commonly by secondary complications such as pneumonia or cardiorespiratory illness (Folstein, 1989; Harper, 1992). Although the average age of onset is 36–45 years of age, symptoms may begin at any time of the affected person's life, from childhood to old age (Folstein, 1989). The disease course is relentless, with symptomatic rather than curative treatment, and rates of depression are reported to be as high as 40%, although pharmaceutical treatment of this is pathetically lacking and as low as 2% (Bonelli et al., 2004).

People with HD develop subcortical dementia characterized by the dyexecutive syndrome, forgetfulness, slowness of thought processes, altered personality with apathy or depression, and impaired ability to manipulate acquired knowledge (Bonelli et al., 2004). Damage to the frontocortical circuitry is evident when working with a person with HD through their difficulties with cognitive flexibility and abstraction, manual dexterity, attention/concentration, performance skills, and verbal skills, among a multitude of other cognitive deficits (Bonelli et al., 2004), including a marked loss of spontaneity and a reduced ability to participate in novel situations (Magee, 1995). However, knowing and insight may be relatively well preserved even into the most advanced stages of the illness (Shoulson, 1990). Similarly, it seems that memory may not deteriorate until the advanced stages of the illness (Bamford, Caine, Kido, Cox, & Shoulson 1995). Treatment should aim to reduce symptoms and improve quality of life, with both drug-based and non–drug-based approaches to treat the movement disorder, and an emphasis of specialist multidisciplinary care to provide holistic care (Novak & Tabrizi, 2010).

Motor Neurone Disease/Amyotrophic Lateral Sclerosis

Motor Neurone Disease (MND) is a rapidly progressive adult-onset neurodegenerative disorder (Sathasivam, 2010) involving the progressive degeneration of upper and lower motor neurons (McLeod & Clarke, 2007). Amyotrophic Lateral Sclerosis (ALS) is the most common variant of the illness and is often used interchangeably with the term MND. Two other variants include primary lateral sclerosis and progressive muscular atrophy (Sathasivam, 2010). Epidemiological studies have been conducted with Hispanic, black African, African-American, and Asian populations; however, its highest incidence is reported in Caucasian populations (Sathasivam, 2010). The age of onset ranges from 40 to over 70, peaking in the late 60s. The majority of cases start with symptoms in the limbs progressing to contiguous areas of the body (Sathasivam, 2010). Disease progression is highly variable and rapid, usually being fatal within 2–4 years (Chaudri et al., 2003). MND can result in as little as 14 months between diagnosis and death (Department of Health, 2005), singling it out from the other LTNC discussed in this chapter. Death is most likely caused due to respiratory failure, and studies suggest that care settings at time of death are most likely to be home, hospice, or nursing home settings.

Reports of cognitive impairment in MND range widely, varying from 10%–75%; overlap with frontotemporal dementia is suggested (Lillo & Hodges, 2009). Where present, cognitive impairment in MND progresses mildly over the course of the disease process and only in some MND patients. Cognitive impairment may be related to a faster disease process and a shorter survival (Lillo & Hodges, 2010). Frontal executive abilities have been found to be most common in people with MND, including problem-solving, cognitive flexibility, multitasking, planning, and working memory, with a number of language problems including verbal fluency and recall (Lillo & Hodges, 2009, 2010). People with MND can sometimes present with behavioral symptoms similar to frontotemporal dementia, including apathy that is independent of mood, blunting of emotions, reduced concern for feelings of others, irritability, and emotional lability (Lillo & Hodges, 2009).

For a person living with MND, suffering, social support, and hopelessness correlate more highly than the physical state of the patient (McLeod & Clarke, 2007). Emotional distress is not necessarily associated with the illness severity, with rates of depression reported as high as 50% (McLeod & Clarke, 2007), although distress is strongly correlated with quality of life. Social support, hope, and hopelessness are all important issues, with hopelessness contributing significantly to suffering and a desire for hastened death (McLeod & Clarke, 2007), although a significant number cope well and find positive meaning in life.

Although Locked-In Syndrome (LIS) has not been included in this chapter, the physical presentation of LIS can be similar in many ways to that of someone living with advanced MND. Thus, many of the methods outlined in this chapter for MND may be appropriate (with minor adaptations) for people living with LIS as well.

Multiple Sclerosis

Multiple Sclerosis (MS) is a complex neurodegenerative autoimmune disease, characterized by inflammatory lesions known as "plaques" (scarlike tissue) that spread throughout the central nervous system (CNS), including the brain (de Sa et al., 2011). It is incurable, with an unknown prognosis, although several disease courses have been identified and broadly categorized into four types. Relapsing-remitting MS (RRMS) is the most common form of MS, affecting around 85% of those diagnosed. It follows a course of symptoms that relapse and then disappear or remit. Secondary progressive MS (SPMS) typically follows on from RRMS, and is diagnosed in approximately 65% of those with RRMS. SPMS results in a sustained increase of disability independent of any relapses, with a widely variable disease course. Primary progressive MS (PPMS) affects around 10%–15% of those diagnosed with MS. Symptoms gradually worsen over time rather than appearing in sudden relapses. Benign MS involves a small number of relapses with complete recovery. From 250,000 to 350,000 patients in the US have MS, with twice as many women affected as men affected, and people of northern European descent are at highest risk (Goldenberg, 2012). Negative prognostic factors for disease trajectory include having progressive disease symptoms and a faster initial disability rate, along with a higher initial relapse rate and a shorter interval between initial and second relapse (Degenhardt, Robnagopalan, Scalfari, & Ebers., 2009).

The course of MS is highly varied and unpredictable, with symptoms following the location and severity of the MS plaques within the brain and spinal cord. Thus, any number of physical, cognitive, and sensory symptoms affect regular functioning, impacting negatively on quality of life (de Sa et al., 2011). Physical symptoms result in motor disorders such as spasticity, tremor, ataxia, dysarthria, dysphagia, occulomotor disorders, and a number of other symptoms including incontinence, sleep and sexual disorders, and pain (de Sa et al., 2011). Depending on the location of plaques, people with MS can experience significant cognitive problems, especially in the domains of learning/memory, processing speed, and working memory, with estimates as high as 65% (Genova, Sumowski, Chiaravalloti, Voelbel, & DeLuca., 2009).

Multiple Sclerosis taxes the individual on a number of fronts that can be grouped under psychosomatic symptoms. Mood disorders are prevalent, with depression being the most common disorder, ranging between 27% and 54% (Bol, Dutis, Hupperts, Vlaeyen, & Verhey, 2009). Fatigue is a frequent and disabling symptom in people with MS. The underlying pathophysiological causes of fatigue in MS are not well understood, but it is acknowledged that a complex interaction of factors comes into play between fatigue and a number of other psychological aspects such as anxiety, cognitive-behavioral factors, and personality (Bol et al., 2009).

Styles of coping are important in MS, as perceived stress and uncertainty are associated with worse adjustment (Dennison, Moss-Moriss, & Chalder, 2009). In particular, wishful thinking, such a hoping a miracle might happen, and escape-avoidance coping, such as trying to "forget the whole thing," have been found to be predictors of worse adjustment. On the other hand, having satisfactory social support and positive interactions with significant others is associated with better adjustment (Dennison, Moss-Morris, & Chalder, 2009). Having a parent with MS has a negative impact on children's social and family relationships and their psychological well-being, with adolescent children seeming to be more at risk for psychosocial problems than school-age children (Bogosian, Moss-Morris, & Hadwin, 2010). Factors associated with poor adjustment included parental negative emotions, increased illness severity, family dysfunction, children's lack of knowledge about the illness, and lack of social support.

Parkinson's Disease

Parkinson's Disease is a degenerative disorder of the central nervous system. It results from gradual degeneration of nerve cells in the portion of the midbrain that controls body movements (Jankovic, 2008). The first signs are likely to be barely noticeable—a feeling of weakness or stiffness in one limb or a fine trembling of one hand when it is at rest (activity causes the tremor to disappear). Eventually, the shaking worsens and spreads, muscles tend to stiffen, and balance and coordination deteriorate (Davie, 2008). Parkinson's Disease is often defined as a Parkinsonian syndrome that is idiopathic (having no cause), although some atypical cases have a genetic origin (Jankovic, 2008). Parkinson's Disease usually begins between the ages of 50 and 65, striking about 1% of the population in that age group; it is slightly more common in men than in women. While Parkinson's disease itself is not fatal, the Centers for Disease Control rated complications from the disease as the 14th top cause of death in the United States and as the second most common neurodegenerative disorder after Alzheimer's Disease (de Lau & Breteler, 2006). There is currently no cure for Parkinson's; however, medication can help control symptoms (Davie, 2008).

Normally, there are brain cells (neurons) in the human brain that produce dopamine. These neurons concentrate in a particular area of the brain, called the substantia nigra. Dopamine is a chemical that relays messages between the substantia nigra and other parts of the brain to control movements of the human body. Dopamine allows for smooth, coordinated muscle movements. When approximately 60% to 80% of the dopamine-producing cells are damaged and do not produce enough dopamine, the motor symptoms of Parkinson's Disease appear (Samii, Nutt, & Ransom, 2004). Scientists are also exploring the idea that loss of cells in other areas of the brain and body contributes to Parkinson's. Researchers have discovered that the hallmark sign of Parkinson's Disease—clumps of the protein alpha-synuclein, which are also called Lewy bodies—are found not only in the midbrain but also in the brain stem and the olfactory bulb. The presence of Lewy bodies in these areas could explain the nonmotor symptoms experienced by some people with PD. The intestines also have dopamine cells that degenerate in Parkinson's, and this may be important in the gastrointestinal symptoms that are part of the disease (Aarsland, Londos, & Ballard, 2009).

Tremor is usually the first symptom of Parkinson's Disease, appearing in just one limb (arm or leg) or on only one side of the body. Tremor may also occur in the lips, tongue, jaw, and eyelids. As the disease progresses, the tremor usually spreads to both sides of the body, although in some cases the tremor remains on just one side. Joint pain, weakness, and fatigue may occur. In addition to tremor, slow movement, stiff muscles, and poor coordination may occur early on in the disease (Poewe, 2006). A person in the early stages of Parkinson's disease may move slowly and may not make normal, frequent posture adjustments. As the disease progresses, problems with posture and balance develop. A person with Parkinson's disease tends to walk in a stooped manner with quick, shuffling steps. After several years, as muscle stiffness and tremor increase, the person may become unable to care for himself or herself. Weak, stiff muscles eventually may confine the person to a wheelchair or bed. Ten years after diagnosis, most people with PD have autonomic disturbances, sleep problems, mood alterations, and cognitive decline (Poewe, 2006).

Medication, mainly levodopa and dopamine agonists, are effective at managing the early symptoms of Parkinson's. As the disease progresses and dopaminergic neurons continue to be lost, medications become less effective. Disability is more related to motor symptoms that do not respond well to medication, such as swallowing/speech difficulties, gait/balance problems, and motor complications. These appear in up to 50% of individuals after five years of levodopa usage (Poewe, 2006). In severe cases, where medications are ineffective, surgery and deep brain stimulation have been used. Medications to treat non–movement-related symptoms, such as mood and behavioral issues, are also used in the treatment of Parkinson's.

Needs and Resources

Working with people who have acquired neurodegenerative conditions is full of joy and sorrow. On the one hand, you have the privilege of working with people who have lived full lives and have a life story full of the usual highs and lows, including education, work, family, and building a life full of hope. On the other hand, you share the experience of the client, facing strange physical or cognitive symptoms, annoying at first, then bewildering, then frightening, until the final devastation of a diagnosis giving a name to the symptoms. The person may have been bounced around from specialist to specialist until a clear diagnosis was gained. Sometimes, they may have been given an incorrect diagnosis and faced the trauma of coming to terms with one diagnosis, only to find out at a later date that this was incorrect, creating devastation all over again. Some people are never given a clear diagnosis, as their symptoms are too complex and don't seem to fit any clear disease trajectory. This may happen less as medical advances and diagnostic procedures improve. However, the experience of clients is likely to be influenced by a complex combination of factors including differences in national health care systems, the wealth of a nation, and the decade in which the client was diagnosed. Thus, the journey traveled by the person living with a neurodegenerative condition will be individual and affected by factors outside their control. All of this occurs as they attempt to live day by day, getting on with the business of life that is familiar to all of us: working, loving, building a family, managing the home, tending to children, worrying about money, coping with extended family matters, and building and maintaining friendships.

The experience of living with an acquired and degenerative condition requires continual adaptation to change, increasing isolation, and coping with an uncertain future. This may result in genuine resilience, but it can also mean that the person presents with a resilient coping front that helps them to cope with intolerable situations by using strategies to mask feelings which are too difficult to acknowledge (Magee & Davidson, 2004a). This can situate music therapy as a place to explore more vulnerable feeling states that may not be of priority in the person's mind.

Physical

The consequences for people living with Huntington's disease are most usually the large, uncontrolled choreic movements involving the arms, legs, fingers, trunk, neck, head, and face. Sometimes, the disease results in movements that are slow and rigid. Both types of movement disorders make it difficult for the person to control their movements and engage in activities. People living with conditions such as Motor Neurone Disease and Multiple Sclerosis experience problems such as weakness and extreme fatigue that can affect their physical participation. Muscle spasms causing pain are common for people with Multiple Sclerosis, as is ataxia, a movement disorder resulting in a lack of coordination while performing voluntary movements. Tremors, difficulties in fine-motor control, and weakness in the upper-limb motor responses cause problems for people with PD, in combination with generalized fatigue.

There are a number of other medical considerations of which you should be aware when working with people who are living with the diseases discussed in this chapter.

Continence: For all conditions, continence is likely to be an issue. This will usually be managed by nursing staff with continence aids such as catheters. However, it is important to be aware of what the continence needs are of the person and remember that incontinence is humiliating and horrible to live with for anyone who is not a young child, causing self-consciousness.

Skin Integrity: Once mobility is affected, seating in a wheelchair becomes a reality of daily life. Sitting for long periods can result in the buildup of pressure on particular points of the body which come into contact with hard surfaces of the wheelchair, or even soft-cushioned areas such as seating pads. Combined with other factors such as difficulties with nutrition due to swallowing problems, limited mobility, and incontinence, the person can become at risk of pressure wounds. These are a serious matter as if such wounds are not properly managed, infection can set in and cause risk to life.

Swallowing: Swallowing becomes a problem as a consequence of motor disorders involving a complex coordination of lips, tongue, jaw, and throat muscles. Poor lip seal results in drooling; poor coordination of lip, tongue, and throat muscles results in difficulty swallowing, including swallowing saliva. Coughing as a result of gag reflex can be sudden and violent. Choking becomes a daily struggle for people who continue to take food and liquids orally, rather than choosing to have a feeding tube installed. The decision to have a feeding tube inserted is fraught with ethical dilemmas, and some people choose not to have a feeding tube inserted. This can be seen as a conscious decision not to prolong life unnecessarily. It is difficult for family, friends, and carers when a person makes this decision. It can also affect the person's nutritional and fluid intake, in turn impacting upon general health matters and overall well-being, including all cognitive capacities, weight, and management of skin integrity and emotional well-being.

Conditions of Normal Aging: It is important to remember when working with people living with disabilities who are "middle-age" (40–65 years) or aging (65 years and above) that they face the usual health problems associated with age. So, for example, women ages 45–55 will be facing the onset of the menopause, with its own set of physical, cognitive, and emotional symptoms. However, a diagnosis of MS means that they may also be dealing with temperature dysregulation, with 60%–80% experiencing worsening of clinical symptoms (Davis, Wilson, White, & Frohman, 2010). Temperature dysregulation results from impaired neural control of autonomic and endocrine functions stemming from plaques in the sympathetic nervous system regions caused by MS. Symptoms of normal aging will interact with those of the acquired disease.

Communication

Motor disorders also affect verbal communication due to impairments to the speech mechanisms. When speech starts to fail, speech and language therapists will begin to assess for augmentative and alternative communication aids to best suit the person's changing and longer-term needs. Such devices may be low- or high-technology, ranging from "listener scanning" through to communication aids involving electronic aids and computer software. Listener scanning depends on a communication partner to speak the alphabet out loud while the client selects letters through eye blinks, spelling out the words of their intended message letter by letter. High-technology solutions are expensive and depend on others to set the person up to enable access for the client. All systems require the client's cooperation and engagement and, most important, insight that an alternative communication system is required.

Air pressure system problems are typical for people who are seated in wheelchairs and have limited capability for whole-body mobility. Additionally, poor trunk control from neurological illness results in the person having difficulty maintaining their trunk in an optimal position for taking deep breaths and pushing the air out adequately to support phonation. Dysarthria is caused by muscle disturbances in the mechanisms involved with speech production, resulting in weakness, lowered coordination, and altered muscle tone (Tamplin & Grocke, 2008). It is typically characterized by limited verbal intelligibility, vocal intensity, range, abnormal rate of speech, poor prosody, and impaired naturalness of speech (Tamplin & Grocke, 2008). Dysarthria is no small matter, as it can lead to major difficulties in speaking in social situations and coping with everyday life, with depression being a commonly reported outcome as a person becomes increasingly isolated (Hustad, Beukelman, & Yorkston, 1998).

Articulation is a problem across all conditions. However, each of the conditions discussed in this chapter has particular patterns of dysarthric speech that might be typical of that condition. For example, PD dysarthric speech patterns include difficulties with volume (hypophonia), with pitch variability that can result in speaking in a monotone, and with the speed of speech, which is typically rapid. All of these problems combine to reduce speech intelligibility. People with MS and MND/ALS, on the other hand, can have difficulties with speaking too slowly, vocal resonance, pitch control, and speech volume. Hypernasality can be typical of all PD, MDN/ALS, and MS. For people with HD, the rate of speech is a problem, but speech is typically broken in its flow, with "bursts" of speech, rather than being uniformly slow as in MS and MND/ALS or rapid as in PD. Vocal quality is also impaired in HD, becoming hoarse and strained, with "bursts" of loudness. Vocal output is combined with the continual choreic movements that also confound the listener's experience. In summary, all the LTNC result in dysarthria that limits the person in communicating the things they want a listener to understand.

Cognitive

Alongside the visible and stigmatizing physical and communication difficulties already outlined, people living with LTNC can experience cognitive impairments. The impairments differ across and within conditions, that is, there is no one similar pattern for a person with MS or one with HD. There are trends that are outlined in the literature pertaining to each condition and as already briefly reviewed in this chapter. Cognitive decline is related entirely to the disease process. Some conditions have patterns of decline that can be anticipated due to homogeneity of the disease process. For example, in HD, there is a progressive atrophying (or shrinking) of the brain (Shoulson, 1990), leading to progressive dementia, whereas in MS, cognitive decline is related entirely to the location of plaques in the brain, which differs in every individual. This means that someone with MS may present with no cognitive impairment at all throughout their disease trajectory or may present with significant global cognitive decline—and everything in between. As new insights continually emerge about patterns of cognitive decline in LTNC, music therapists are guided to read the most up-to-date sources on a specific condition. Similarly, working closely with other members of the multidisciplinary team, and in particular neuropsychologists, will assist with learning more about the disease progression as it relates to cognition, as well as to the specific problems that may be encountered by the individual with whom the therapist works.

Language problems encountered in LTNC are separate from speech difficulties; whereas speech problems are a motor impairment, language disorders result from cognitive impairments. Language disorders specific to each condition have been outlined earlier but typically involve general difficulties with word-finding, initiation, perseveration, verbal fluency, and spontaneity.

Of relevance to music therapists is how cognitive impairments will affect the person's ability to respond in sessions. Adjustment to the ways in which activities are presented in a session can make the difference between a client not being able to respond and being able to participate to their optimum ability.

Mood

Lability is an affective dysregulation syndrome that reduces the capacity for emotional regulation (Arciniegas & Topkoff, 2000). Lability presents as "exaggerated or inappropriate episodes of laughter, crying, or both without an apparent motivating stimulus or in response to stimuli that would not have elicited such an emotional response before the onset of the underlying disease" (Parvizi et al., 2006, p. 1482). During an episode of lability, the person will present with emotional expression (e.g., laughing, crying) that seems particularly exaggerated to the stimulus (e.g., a song) and endures for a prolonged period. It is important to understand that the person may feel the emotion being expressed, but not to the degree which their behavior suggests. Furthermore, it is difficult for the individual to regulate or stop the behavior. This can be distressing for the client and bewildering or even offensive for others present, such as family or peers in a group setting. For example, something that might seem mildly funny to other group members can cause the person with lability to start laughing uncontrollably and to continue laughing long after the stimulus has passed. There is no agreed-upon behavioral management of lability—only recommended drug treatments. There are some ways of managing the environment that can help the person during an episode of lability.

When it is suspected that the client is responding to a musical (or other) stimulus in an emotionally exaggerated way, first, the therapist should feed back to the person that they seem to have found something particularly funny or particularly sad (according to their emotional behavior). Second, the therapist should ask the client directly how he would like her to manage things. Offer a forced option or two slowly and clearly: The therapist should ask whether he would like to stop and talk about what he finds so sad/funny or whether he would like to keep going with the music/activity. This gives the person the chance to have the focus taken off their behavior. It also offers him the opportunity for distraction away from the stimulus that caused the behavior in the first place. Once the person is distracted, the labile behavior will generally cease. Once it has ceased, the therapist has the opportunity to explore with the person their emotional experience of the stimulus without the problem of the emotional behavior (e.g., laughing, sobbing) that can get in the way of communication. The therapist can acknowledge what the person found so sad/funny and explore this more fully and can ask if it is sometimes difficult for him to "turn the tears/laughter off." This also opens the door for exploring some of the symptoms that the client may be experiencing as a consequence of his disease.

Social

Diagnosis of an LTNC is different from diagnoses of a more acute nature. The person will have already been dealing with strange symptoms for a period of time, suspecting that something is wrong, but not knowing what.

In the case of HD, the situation is slightly different. If the person is knowingly born into a family with HD (i.e., has not been adopted or separated from genetic family for some other reason), they will live their life knowing that there is a 50% chance of acquiring the disease and will have witnessed one parent, at least one grandparent, possibly aunts and uncles, possibly siblings, and possibly nephews, nieces, and their own offspring acquire the disease and live with its disabling impact. This disease devastates entire family systems.

Increasing physical symptoms lead to a shift from independence to increased dependence on others. It can be difficult for friends and family to respond to a loved one's changing situation, and it is common for intimate, social, and even family relationships to dissolve (Tyerman, 1996). Prolonged immersion in illness takes its toll upon social relationships and self, with social isolation translating directly into emotional isolation and loneliness (Charmaz, 1991). Complex medical and care needs stemming from the disease as it progresses often cannot be met within the home environment, resulting in frequent respite or continuing residential care. Leaving one's home, losing one's support network, and moving into care can (although not always will) result in a world that is shrunken and isolated. Opportunities for accessing the external world are reduced, and there may be little potential for developing new relationships. Personality and cognitive changes experienced as a result of acquired brain injury can affect the quality of relationships with significant others (Oddy, 1984).

Spiritual

It is interesting to note that little has been written about using music therapy to address spiritual needs with people with neuropalliative conditions. This might be considered surprising given that we are working with people living with long-term chronic illness for which there is no cure and death is the ultimate outcome. In this sense, the work is palliative. However, the author believes that the people with whom we work living with these conditions are focusing on *living*. Thus, time spent in therapy is often spent looking back and coping with the present. Using the music therapy space for reflection upon spiritual needs can be invaluable. It is, however, a very personal and intimate way of working, and one that might develop if the client's needs in this area are prominent and if the therapeutic relationship can support this. This being said, this chapter is not offering methods for working on spiritual comfort. The very experience of music is likely to be spiritually comforting, so the therapist should always remain alert and open to this need in the client.

Musical

Regardless of the nature of the physical problems caused by an LTNC, it will be frustrating for the client and greatly challenging for the music therapist to find instruments which are appropriate, safe, aesthetically pleasing, and also responsive to the client's movements. In addition to traditional acoustic instruments, therapists working with clients with such severe movement problems adopt electronic music technologies to enable clients to play instruments (Lindeck, 2005; Millman & Jefferson, 2000; Nagler, 1998).

Referral and Assessment

The setting in which the therapist is working with someone with HD, PD, MND, or MS will depend on a number of factors. Most prominently, health care provision differs markedly between countries; this will affect the environment in which therapy services are offered and whether individual or group care is offered. For instance, in the United Kingdom, people are provided with health care in their own homes for as long as possible. However, the conditions written about in this chapter result in a complex combination of symptoms. Typically, complexity requires specialist care, so people often move to specialist facilities providing around-the-clock care.

Typically, music therapists will work with people once they are in continuing care settings (e.g., nursing homes) or in day centers. Unless otherwise specified in the following sections, assumptions will be made that people are seen in continuing care settings, living with other people who require continuing care. Many of the guidelines provided should also be applicable within people's homes or day centers.

Overview of Methods and Procedures

The following methods and procedures are used most commonly implemented to address the physical, communication, emotional, cognitive, social, and/or spiritual needs of LTNC patients. These have not been sequenced to reflect relative significance, effectiveness, or complexity.

Receptive Music Therapy

- Song Discussion/Lyric Analysis: The patient selects precomposed songs of a personal meaning to express and acknowledge emotions.
- Biographical Work with Songs: Music of personal meaning associated with events, memories, relationships, and people from across the life span.
- Song Communication: Employing songs of personal meaning with associations for the client and his family.
- Sensorimotor Methods: Music-based methods to address sensorimotor disorders.

Improvisational Music Therapy

- Therapeutic Instrumental Music Performance*:* Musical instrument–playing to exercise and stimulate functional movement patterns.
- Clinical Improvisation: An experience in which the therapist and client generate musical dialogues and forms in mutual partnership.

Re-creative Music Therapy

- Therapeutic Singing: Singing and musical activities to facilitate initiation within, development of, and articulation in a person's speech and language, as well as to increase functions of the respiratory system.
- Vocal Exercises: Various techniques focused on breath support, phonation, and pitch range.
- Motor and Respiratory Exercises: Musical exercises using sound vocalization and wind instrument–playing.
- Musical Speech Stimulation: Use of musical materials such as songs, rhymes, chants, or musical phrases simulating prosodic speech gestures.

Compositional Music Therapy

- Songwriting: The therapist helps the client to write songs, lyrics, or instrumental pieces or to create any kind of musical product, such as music videos.

Guidelines for Receptive Music Therapy

Song Discussion/Lyric Analysis

Overview. Beginning therapy with precomposed songs of personal meaning to the client is a very helpful way to start to build a relationship with someone living with a long-term degenerative illness. First, someone new to the idea of therapy and used to presenting a "cheerful" face to the world is less likely to be threatened by the suggestion of listening to some of their favorite songs than they might be by the idea of "therapy." Songs are familiar and thus reassuring. As a therapeutic tool, they are "containers" for mood states and emotional expression. Songs of personal meaning are friends who have accompanied the person living with LTNC throughout his life, often in the face of loss of friendships and relationships (Magee, 2007; Magee & Davidson, 2004a).

Songs of personal meaning can assist people to express and acknowledge emotions that are unbearable and otherwise remain unacknowledged. Songs enable expression through a sequence of steps which progress only as the client chooses, and therefore allow him to remain in control (Magee, 2007). This process can remain subconscious or become conscious as the client allows. First, a client's request for a song sounds out the mood of that song into the session. This enables the client to explore and experience a range of emotional states musically without explicitly acknowledging the emotion or identifying that emotion. Through this musical experience, the client has brought the therapist into his emotional world. Second, the client and/or therapist can identify verbally the emotions elicited by a song, giving a name to the unmentionable, but related only to the song (as container) and not yet to the client. Last, when the client feels safe enough, he may be able to relate the mood or emotions elicited by a song to his own experience and feelings and acknowledge the unbearable feelings as his own.

Using songs in this way is useful for people with HD, MND, MS, and PD at any stage of their disease process. In particular, using songs in the latter stages of any of these diseases is indicated when the physical effects of the disease process leave the person completely physically dependent, unable to communicate verbally and with limited means for social interaction. This can be a time when physical difficulties render the playing of instruments impossible or unsuccessful. Furthermore, the person may have little means for verbally expressing or exploring their mood states at this time due to speech and/or language impairments. Even when verbal expression is still possible through the use of AAC, devices and the strategies to use them (e.g., listener scanning) can be laborious and time-consuming, thus diminishing the spontaneity of any expression.

There are particular indicators for using precomposed familiar songs for mood exploration. When the disease process has rendered all active movement impossible, eye blinks are often used by carers as a means for the person to communicate yes and no, particularly in late stages of MND and MS. Even when this is the person's only active involvement, it is possible for them to choose songs for listening, and thus enables them to explore a range of mood states of their choice.

The goals that might direct the decision to use this method vary according to the client's emotional state and the level of resistance or acceptance they are currently using to manage their emotional response to their illness. However, goals will typically center on building trust between therapist and client, promoting reassurance, encouraging self-reflection, stimulating memories of life events, and discussion of these where the client's communication skills allow. All of these goals will work toward the ultimate goals of helping a client to explore a wider range of mood states within the music selected for listening.

While not a contraindication, there are some things of which the therapist should remain aware. Emotional responses such as smiling, laughing, and tearfulness are expected when using songs. However, people with what are classed as "neuropsychiatric disorders" typical of HD, MND, MS, and PD may commonly present with emotional behaviors which are not fully representative of how they are feeling when they have difficulties with lability. As a particularly emotional stimulus, songs can often prompt emotional responses and labile responses, and the therapist should keep this in mind.

Preparation. As with many therapy sessions, an ideal environment is one that is quiet, private and free from distractions. This is not always possible in a busy day center or in a residential care setting, where space is likely to be at a premium. It may also be difficult in the home setting, where relatives may be milling around. However, for the purposes of enabling full emotional expression, it is important that the person feels safe to express their immediate feeling state. This can be compromised if there is a risk of disruption from carers or even from loved ones. Difficulties with attention (most important, divided attention) can be common for people with MS and HD, highlighting another reason for working in an environment free from distractions and interruptions. Sometimes, when working with people in the later stages of some of these conditions, it may be more typical to work by the bedside if the person is bed-bound. In such cases, try and optimize privacy by pulling a curtain around the bed.

It is important to encourage an intimate environment when using songs to explore emotion and mood states. For this reason, the use of live rather than recorded music is encouraged. Sometimes, it may be without the therapist's skill to produce credible renditions of the client's preferred music, or the most meaningful versions of the music may be performed by specific artists. In such cases, recorded music may be the most sensible solution.

In early sessions it is important to have adequate resources on hand from which the client's significant music can be sourced. Adequate resources means enough "sheet music" (or digital equivalents) from genres that are known to be within the client's preferred music. If no information can be gained about the client's preferred music, the therapist should be prepared with music that is typical of someone of the client's generation, gender, and sociocultural background.

What to observe. A client's song choices can offer some insights into their mood states, thus it is useful to note the mood of the songs selected by the client from open (i.e., unlimited) or forced (i.e., limited) choices. Naïve categorization of songs as "sad" and "happy" should be avoided. A client's emotional experience of a song will be influenced by extra musical associations that cannot be guessed by the therapist. Gaining an understanding of the song's meaning to the client will help the therapist to categorize songs into more subtle and diverse mood state categories.

During the music, careful observation should be made of the changes in the client's breathing, facial gestures, whether his eyes open or close, and whether there are any attempts to mouth or vocalize the lyrics.

Procedures. It is essential to gauge client's capacity for making choices and tailor the session accordingly. For example, is the client able to choose from an unlimited choice (e.g., "What would you like to listen to today?") or does he need assistance through offering forced choices? It is important to consider the client's cognitive capacity. Is the client able to remember and recall the songs from their past? How quickly can the client communicate a choice? Will their attention sustain making and communicating a choice? How can flow best be maintained in a session? Offering forced choices of two options can assist the client in getting to their meaningful song. Choices can start broad: "Would you like something up-tempo or mellow?" Using categories related to mood rather than to musical genre can assist the client in understanding the activity as an opportunity for emotional reflection.

As the therapist develops a better understanding of the client and his personally meaningful repertoire, she can offer a narrower choice of songs that include the most significant songs for the client. This not only helps to maintain a flow to the session, but it can communicate to the client that she understands him and understands his emotional needs well. It can enable an intimate feeling to the session quickly once she has established a strong enough relationship. For someone who has to wait for everything in the smallest detail of their daily routine, this rapid progression to core issues can be a relief. The therapist should not be afraid to offer the same songs repeatedly, both across sessions and within sessions. Sometimes a client may wish to hear a particularly significant song repeatedly within a session, closing his eyes and allowing himself to experience the mood inherent in the song. However, always try to offer a range of mood states if forced choices are given. That is, in every choice of two, try to offer one upbeat, brighter, more lively song, along with one that is more mellow and reflective.

If the therapist notices a client has moved to a place of personal reflection during a song, allow a long pause at the end of the song, with no verbal intervention. She should allow the client to break the silence and speak (or gesture in cases of nonverbal clients) first. If the client does not speak/gesture after a long pause, the therapist can ask simply and quietly whether he would like to hear the song again and repeat the song if he wishes to listen again. This can foster an intimate environment where the entire focus is on the enabling the client to experience the emotions stimulated by his significant song. Sometimes, a song might be repeated several times in this way. The client can experience the song in its full emotional force, being supported through the nonverbal expression of their chosen mood state by the therapist acting as companion, guide and witness. Repeated singing or presentations of the same song is believed to increase the emotional response elicited (Baker & Wigram, 2004; Sloboda, 1991).

Skills in verbal intervention are useful when utilizing songs in this way. Sensitive exploration can assist a client in exploring dreams, memories, hopes and fears. Sometimes it can be enough for the therapist to simply acknowledge the mood she has witnessed the song express. This, in itself, is recognizing the client as an emotional being. Most music therapists, who are trained in musical skills, make the mistake of using too many words. The therapist should keep her words to a minimum, using a gentle and quiet tone of voice, allowing as much silence as she can.

Adaptations. When using repeated presentations of the same song, from the second listening onward it can be useful to include some extemporization of the original song. This is achieved by including instrumental verses or bridge sections with elaborations of the melody; including a verse with a wordless melody line sung; or by repeating significant verses or the chorus.

Biographical Work with Songs

Overview. Music of personal meaning associated with events, memories, relationships, and people from across the life span can assist with biographical work. Health sociology research highlights that it is important for people living with chronic illness to carry out "biographical work," namely the review, maintenance, repair and alteration of one's life (Charmaz, 1987, 1991; Corbin and Strauss, 1987).

Clients who can benefit from this method are those who initiate reminiscence when songs are played to them. This method is also a natural extension of mood exploration and expression using songs, particularly for clients who have difficulty moving beyond the idea of music therapy being a private personalized performance of their favorite tunes. Goals associated with this method include for the client to identify memories associated with songs; to reflect on the changed meaning of the song; to share reflections about their current situation.

Music for biographical work requires the client to be able to engage through verbal reflections. Thus this method cannot be fully followed with people who have lost the capacity for verbal communication. As this method requires considerable verbal reflection, careful thought should be given before introducing this as a method with people who use communication strategies that are time consuming. The session duration needs to allow enough time for the client to fully explore a memory, communicate and understand the meaning of the memory to him in order to rework the memory into his current biography.

Preparation. Preparation of the session and environment should follow all those recommendations made previously for mood exploration and expression using precomposed songs of personal meaning.

What to observe. A client's reminiscences to songs of personal meaning will be varied, spanning the good times and the difficult times from his life. The therapist should enable the client to reminisce upon the same memory as many times as he needs to: sometimes, repeated reminisces can lead to reconfigured biographical workings and new insights. Similar to the previous section, gaining an understanding of the song's association for the client will aid the therapeutic relationship and assist with the flow of a session. As the therapy progresses, the therapist can make shortcuts by querying gently after a song if the specific memory … intaining the session's flow if the person has communic… focused on the person's therapeutic material rather t… it. Thus, keep note of the memories associated with a s… ificance of this association to him; what is the essence of … ient?

Procedures. The pro… his method as well. As this method works at a more consc… likely to be more cognizant of the songs he wishes to ch… mmended in the previous method are useful here too. … e client to embody their associations with it, but verbal … ferentiates the use of songs for exploration of mood from t…

Once more, verbal i… songs in this way. The therapist needs to use skills … lient's reminiscences, and reflecting these back to the cl… The therapist should avoid using too many words.

Adaptations. Tangib… hical work with songs. For example, photographs, letters … magazine clippings, can be placed together in an album of memorabilia. A CD of the client's significant music can be added if he wishes. Developing such an album can be an activity with which family (spouse, children, grandchildren or siblings) and friends can get involved, or can engage volunteers helping at the facility. Such objects can also provide a useful medium for all members of the treatment team to use in their treatment sessions with the client, and communicate vast amounts of information more easily than the person with communication problems. Last, albums developed in this way can become a legacy for the family once the person has passed away.

Songs for Communication to Loved Ones

Overview. This method relies on employing songs of personal meaning with associations for the client and his family. It is a variation of the methods already outlined in this section.

Most commonly, this method will be indicated as a matter of convenience as family members may be visiting at the times when a music therapy session is scheduled or is offered. It can be quite usual for a client to want their family member to experience the pleasure of a music therapy session. There may also be awareness on a subconscious level as well that this can be a time to share emotions and feelings which are difficult to say in words.

The goals of the session will be for the client and his family members to select songs of personal meaning and to share reminiscences. Messages do not necessarily need to be discussed verbally; it can be enough for them to be sounded out through the music.

As already mentioned, lability can be one side effect of neurological damage with certain conditions. Labile behavior can be distressing for relatives to witness, as they experience the behavior as an indicator of the level of emotion experienced by their loved one. It can also be difficult for the person living with the LTNC to be seen in this state. Thus, before using songs for communication to loved ones, care should be taken to explore with the person whether they feel that they want to take this risk given that music is an emotional stimulus which can often prompt an emotional reaction.

Preparation. Preparation of the session and environment should follow all those recommendations made previously for the song-based methods. Ensuring that the client and his relative are within reaching distance of each other can enable touching during the session such as hand holding.

What to observe. The therapist should observe the flow of the session and ensure that there is continuity, particularly if difficult emotions arise. For example, if a silence between the client and his relative appears to become prolonged or awkward, more music can be offered.

Procedures. Using songs in this way can be conducted on a number of levels. It is the first time you see a person with their loved one, the client and their relative/friend may experience this method as a performance, even applauding after each song. As with the methods already outlined in this section, encourage the participants to choose songs of personal meaning. Offering choices of musical genres (rather than mood as previously outlined) can assist in participants finding songs that stimulate memories or are meaningful. The therapist's role in this type of session becomes one of facilitator, allowing the client and his relative to explore memories between themselves.

Adaptations. If music is a familiar activity for the family, it can be helpful to make resources such as musical instruments available to them outside of usual work hours (e.g., on weekends) so that they can use music themselves in this way.

Sensorimotor Methods to Maintain or Improve Movement

Overview. Movement disorders are possibly the most disabling factor of LTNC. There is a considerable body of research on the effects of music-based methods to address motor disorders for LTNC (http://www.colostate.edu/dept/cbrm/). While not the only method to address sensorimotor disorders in LTNC, Neurologic Music Therapy provides defined methods and systematized protocols for treatment, ensuring that it is delivered consistently an precisely. It requires specialist training in order to implement the methods, however, a description of the most important elements are provided here.

The auditory system is a fast and precise processor of temporal information that is projected directly into motor pathways within the brain, creating entrainment between the rhythmic signal and the motor response (Thaut & Abiru, 2010). There are several theoretical principles for the effect of auditory rhythm on brain functions associated with the motor system (Thaut, 2005a). The most relevant for understanding the effects of rhythm on the brain are: that auditory rhythm entrains immediate and stable motor responses; that rhythm primes the auditory-motor pathways; and that it will work only with movements that are intrinsically rhythmic. Two methods are relevant for neuropalliative rehabilitation programs for people with LTNC.

Rhythmic Auditory Stimulation (RAS) is a method in which rhythmic motor cuing is provided in the form of external metronomic pulse to train movements that are intrinsically and biologically rhythmic, e.g., gait; repetitive functional arm movements (Thaut, 2005a). RAS works to cue gait parameters such as step cadence, stride length, velocity, symmetry of stride length and stride duration. Rhythmic cues are presented in 2/4 or 4/4 meter either using a metronome or as accented beats embedded in music. The evidence for the effects of RAS on gait is impressive for people with PD, including immediate improvements (McIntosh, Brown, Rice, & Thaut, 1997; Richards, Maloving, Bedard, & Cioni, 1992) and long-term carryover effects (McIntosh et al., 1997). Improvements in gait are also reported for people with HD (Thaut et al., 1999).

Patterned Sensory Enhancement (PSE) uses the elements and patterns within music (e.g., melodic, harmonic, dynamic) to provide temporal, spatial and force cues to structure and regulate functional movements. Through breaking the targeted movement down into its component parts, musical elements can be manipulated and shaped to musically structure, in time, space and force, any functional movement regardless of whether it is intrinsically rhythmic. PSE is useful for rehearsing and repetitive training of movements such as reaching, grasping or even sit-to-stand transfers. It is often used as a precursor to RAS, in order to rehearse isolated movements that are part of the larger motor pattern required for gait. For example, a heel to toe foot strike involves a rocking movement of the foot. Thus a rocking rhythm such as 6/8 might be useful, with a downward melodic direction to follow the movement of the foot, with the accent falling on the final part of the movement when the ball of the foot touches the floor.

These are complex and detailed methods requiring advanced skill training. The reader is thus directed to authoritative sources to gain a more thorough description and training should be sought before attempting these methods.

These methods should be used in interventions planned, and possibly delivered, jointly with physical and/or occupational therapists. Liaise closely with these professionals to identify people who need to work on specific functional movements, or people who may not be responding well to conventional physical therapy. Goals should be quite specific to a client's particular movement needs. Pregait training will focus on improving postural elements whereas goals during gait training, planned with the physical therapist, will target increasing or decreasing the rate of walking.

Rhythmic responses in people with HD differ from those with other LTNC. Although the tempo of external rhythmic cues improves gait performance, the temporal control of choreic gate is irregular (Thaut, 2005a). Thus, RAS should be used with care with this population.

Preparation. RAS requires a long space for gait training in a long straight line, free from obstacles, distractions or moving objects such as other people. Quiet corridors might be appropriate, but otherwise the physical therapy gym might offer an appropriate space for both RAS and PSE.

What to observe. The therapist should monitor all changes to physical functioning particularly those which are being targeted by the method.

Procedures. Advanced training is required to implement PSE and RAS, however, the basic elements are described here. Working with the occupational or physical therapist, the music therapist needs to identify the specific movements to be worked on, including both making the movement and returning to the start point as both will be practiced in repetitive cycles during PSE. Elements of the movement to be identified include the direction of the movement; the start and end point of the movement; the speed of the movement; the point of the movement where the accent falls; and other individual components of the movement that can be translated into musical expression. Then, the music therapist needs to translate the movements into musical expression, considering how the musical elements may be manipulated such as melodic contour to express the movement direction; the musical structure to incorporate accent by means of, for example, anacrusis; harmonic progression to expression tension and resolution; and the tempo to reflect the speed at which the movement will be rehearsed. The exercises should involve maximum repetition in order for training to take place.

For RAS, the person is firstly assessed for walking specific distance without musical accompaniment, e.g., 10 meters. Gait parameters are measured such as: the number of heel strikes per second; the number of meters walked in sixty seconds; or the length of strides achieved (Thaut, 2005). Music is then played with a metronomic pulse and at a tempo which matches the rate of the client's heel strike. The tempo of the music is then either increased or decreased, depending on the clinical goal. Measures of the gait parameters are monitored during the musical condition, and then afterward with no musical condition to measure improvements.

Adaptations. Once a patient is responding to RAS and demonstrating change in their gait, treatment can continue at intermittent periods post discharge through the use of home programs using recorded music.

Guidelines for Improvisational Music Therapy

Two methods of improvisation are outlined here, one that is functionally focused and one in which the expressive and emotional experience is central. Therapists are advised to keep in mind that although a client may wish initially to try improvisation as a functional activity, emotional responses may emerge rendering improvisation as an opportunity for emotional expression and exploration of feelings relating to identity.

Therapeutic Instrumental Music Performance (TIMP)

Overview. TIMP is a method from Neurologic Music Therapy that uses musical instruments playing to exercise and simulate functional movement patterns in therapy to address movement disorders (Thaut, 2005a). It differs from other improvisational methods in that the primary goal centers on improving movement and rehearsing functional movement patterns which can be translated to nonmusical conditions and functional tasks. Once the physical goal is identified, the placement of instruments is specially configured to meet the physical goals. It should be noted that TIMP can be used equally as an improvisational method, with music composed specifically for its purpose or as a re-creative method with familiar, well-learned songs. The choice of which music to use should be directed by the client, i.e., which music is more motivating for them to play?

Using TIMP is indicated for individuals who express repeated concern about their loss of motor ability or demonstrate behaviors indicative of illness monitoring (Magee & Davidson, 2004a). It is important that the individual is motivated to engage in this method and that it is not therapist-led. The goals in TIMP center on motor performance, not on emotional expression as with other improvisational methods. Thus, instrumental activities provide opportunities for monitoring physical performance and, as LTNC involve loss of physical functioning, the client may have a negative experience of instrument-playing. Consultation with multidisciplinary colleagues is essential in planning appropriate treatment.

When working with people with LTNC, the goals will be to maintain motor performance for as long as possible, rather than to improve performance as might be typical in rehabilitation models. Motor goals can include increasing or maintaining range of motion, endurance, strength, limb coordination, and fine-motor movements such as finger dexterity. Goals should be set in conjunction with the client, using their personal goals as a lead.

Using TIMP is contraindicated for people whose movement is so severely limited that they cannot achieve functional movements or for those where fatigue is a limiting factor. It is also contraindicated for people who are not motivated to work toward functional goals.

Preparation. Once physical goals have been identified, there are two important steps in preparing the environment. First, instruments should be selected that match the movement the client is trying to achieve. Second, adaptations in relation to playing the instrument should be considered.

LTNC cause varying movement disorders both across conditions and within conditions. Thus, one person with MS will not necessarily have the same motor problems as another with MS. Some of the movement disorders encountered include large, uncontrolled choreic movements (HD); shaky tremors during intentional movement which become larger as the arm moves away from midline (MS, PD); small, slow, weak movements requiring support at the elbow, wrist, or hand (MS, MND); and small, rigid movements (HD, PD). For uncontrolled movements, the instrument needs to be large enough to provide a strong visual target, e.g., a large-headed drum. Small, weak movements would benefit from the range of electronic music technologies currently available, particularly apps that provide touch-sensitive interfaces and produce sounds of excellent quality (see Magee, 2013, for suggestions) and can allow the client to focus on controlling fine-motor movements without the frustration of producing a sound that is inaudible.

A decision should be made as to whether the person has enough wrist flexion to manipulate a beater, or whether using a hand is more effective. This will then influence which instrument is most appropriate, e.g., a drum or a xylophone. Instruments should have a very stable base to counter disordered movements.

Adaptation of instruments and to the traditional ways of playing the instruments might be necessary. For example, placing a tambourine at knee height to be played by raising the leg, and striking the tambourine with the knee; placing an instrument behind the client to be played with the elbow, using a backward arm movement; or using angled boom stands, microphone stands, or another person from which/whom to suspend instruments. Second, in TIMP, the positioning of instruments needs to be carefully planned so that the person has to maximize their physical potential to reach the target and achieve a sound.

What to observe. Observations should be made as to the number of times a client can make contact with an instrument and achieve a sound; the duration that the client is able to sustain activity; and the range of movement and whether this changes across sessions.

Procedures. TIMP lends itself well to group work and also to interdisciplinary working. In group work, clients can be paired together to share instruments or support each other playing by acting as "instrument stands" where this meets an individual's specific motor goals. The music used (improvised, newly composed, familiar precomposed) should employ musical structures that support the client in following the music (Thaut, 2005a). The musical elements should be directed by the movements being targeted. Meter and tempo should be matched to the movements, while also taking into account the client's compromised ability to perform the movement. Harmonic changes can cue changes in direction; melodic lines can illustrate the spatial direction of a movement; and accents should be strong, easily distinguishable, and fall on the beats on which the motor response is expected (Thaut, 2005a).

Clinical Improvisation

Overview. The definition of clinical improvisation included under this method is a very broad one, being an experience in which the therapist and client generate musical dialogues and forms in mutual partnership (Magee, 2002). Within clinical improvisation, the therapist listens to the client's musical utterances, whether these be sounds made on instruments or vocally, or attends to the musical aspects of a client's physical expressions, such as noting the rate and volume of breathing or the velocity and tempo of physical movements. The musical elements of the client's expression are heard as emotional expression. The therapist uses these as the cue for the music that she improvises.

Clinical improvisation is indicated for individuals who still have enough physical capacity to engage with instruments. That is, they have active movement and adequate stamina to engage in improvisation. Also, they might be expressing a need or desire for creative expression or demonstrate an interest in instruments. It is also indicated for individuals who are having increasing difficulty with spoken communication and are experiencing frustration with this. Improvisation may assist with catharsis of feelings, so it may be a useful medium for people experiencing emotions such as anger, fear, and frustration. For people with weak or limited movements, e.g., in cases of advanced MND or MS, the use of electronic music technologies using adaptive devices may be useful if the client is motivated to continue playing music actively (see Nagler, 1998, for an illustration). These tools can enable people to create sounds of good quality that may not be possible to achieve with acoustic instruments.

Goals within clinical improvisation will center on encouraging the client to explore a full range of instruments, establishing preferred instruments, adapting instruments as necessary for the client to achieve a sound, and encouraging the client to achieve a full, expressive range of the instrument. The ultimate goal is for the client to achieve full emotional expression through and feel supported through the therapist's music.

Although recommendations are made in the last subsection, improvisation may be contraindicated when the person no longer has enough functional movement to elicit sounds from an instrument, as can happen in the late stages of MND and MS. In particular, a person in the late stage of HD may have constant, unintentional choreic movements. This means that sounds elicited may not be intentional. At this time, alternative methods will be more appropriate, such as receptive or possibly re-creative methods. Changes in cognitive abilities may also render the use of unfamiliar improvised music as a less meaningful medium than familiar overly learned music from the person's past (Magee & Davidson, 2004a).

Preparation. The therapist should follow the recommendations made under improvisation for appropriate instrument selection. Adaptation of instruments is also appropriate for clinical improvisation. However, as there is less of a functional focus in clinical improvisation and a greater emotional focus, it may be useful to include instruments which have not been adapted. This can encourage exploration of difficult feelings as the individual negotiates the instrument and explores their physical boundaries. A range of instruments should be provided, including pitched and nonpitched; ensure that the instruments provided require different types of movements to play.

For people with tremors and ataxia, it will be easier for them to play instruments that can be placed central to midline and close to the body. Securing a surface onto which the person can stabilize their arm will help them to achieve some physical control in their playing. A table or tray placed over the person's lap, with the instrument placed upon it, can enable this. Instruments should be secured or heavy enough to counteract the person's tremors; otherwise, the instrument will not remain in place. For people with fatigue problems, instruments should also be placed relatively close to the body so that energy levels can be optimized. Having to reach out to the side using a repeated movement, e.g., to play a drum, is tiring.

Time can be spent at the start of the session, establishing with the person how they feel their energy levels are and exploring which instruments they feel they can best manage.

What to observe. The therapist should listen carefully not just to the musical aspects of the sounds produced by the individual, but also to the emotional quality of these as well. When the therapist reflects the emotional expression of the person's sounds, they act as a "performance validator" and thus reinforce the person's emotional expression and the shifts in self-concepts that can occur during playing (Magee & Davidson, 2004a).

Procedures. Instruments first need to be selected by both the client and the therapist. The therapist may play on an instrument on which they are fully skilled (e.g., piano, guitar) or on a range of percussion instruments selected with the client. Using an instrument that enables harmonic accompaniment can provide particular support for the client's musical utterances.

The therapist should follow the client's lead closely as to the musical ebb and flow of the improvisation, but also regarding indications for the ending of the improvisation. The therapist needs to keep in mind the fatigue and energy levels of clients with LTNC; the client may only be able to sustain playing for short periods, resulting in short improvisations. At the end of the improvisation, the therapist should leave a silent pause rather than speaking too quickly. By doing this, the therapist encourages the client to understand the emotional nature of the shared activity; that improvisation in music therapy is a time for reflection and exploration. Allow the client to speak first. In cases of very long pauses, nonverbal gestures can be offered for encouragement before the client speaks, such as gentle smiling and head nodding. The therapist should be prepared for verbal exploration of issues to do with both loss and success. The client may introduce discussion of feelings around disability and how they can no longer achieve physical tasks that were once easily achievable.

Adaptations. Although this section has focused on instrumental improvisation, vocal improvisation may also be used. This may be more challenging for many clients, who already express anxiety about improvisation; the idea of making something up and singing may prove too much for many individuals. However, many use singing as another activity in which to monitor their illness, specifically through comparing the quality of their vocalization (Magee & Davidson, 2004b).

Other adaptations include using a programmatic structure rather than "free" clinical improvisation. Programs can be helpful when working with people with cognitive impairments, who may require greater structure due to memory impairments, or people who just feel too much anxiety to improvise freely without any structure or too heavily defended to make the best use out of improvisation. Using programmatic improvisation enables the person to engage in a creative experience and an experience that encourages relaxation, without risking breaking down psychological defenses. Programs can be stories, images, or themes proposed by the client. If this is too difficult for the client, the therapist might choose a theme or story and align this with the client's material.

Guidelines for Re-creative Music Therapy

Functional singing encompasses a wide range of techniques and methods from a number of models and music therapy approaches. These include song-singing programs (Baker & Wigram, 2004), neurologic music therapy (NMT) methods (Thaut, 2005a, 2005b), and a number of other research protocols devised to address neurocommunication disorders (Elefant et al., in press; Haneishi, 2001; Magee et al., 2006), including one devised specifically to address dysarthria following neurological damage (Tamplin & Grocke, 2008). The neurocommunication disorders associated with HD, MND, MS, and PD can differ, although they have many common presentations. Communication problems which can be helped by functional singing include both speech and language problems. Typically, music therapy to address neurocommunication disorders focuses on factors such as speech intelligibility, speech rate, vocal intensity, vocal range, duration of phonation, voice fundamental frequency and its variability, and language production within musical activities.

When presenting these activities to clients, it can be best to emphasize the motivational and enjoyment factor, with lesser emphasis on the benefits for communication outcomes so as not to promise false hope. It can be helpful to stress that functional singing can also help to keep the voice and speech mechanisms in as "best shape as possible" by giving the voice mechanism "a thorough workout."

Some general recommendations for leading a session with functional singing methods should be made here. A number of authors recommend thorough warm-up and exercises prior to vocal exercises (Elefant et al., in press; Haneishi, 2001; Magee et al., 2006; Tamplin & Grocke, 2008), including relaxation and stretching of the face, neck, throat, jaw, and tongue. Fatigue is a side effect of many LTNC, and the therapist should monitor the client's fatigue levels carefully (Baker, 2001; Magee et al., 2006; Tamplin & Grocke, 2008a). It is recommended that sessions be kept relatively short until the client's energy levels are well understood, aiming for a maximum of 30 minutes initially.

The need to identify the client's specific problems cannot be stressed enough, and consultation with the client's speech therapist will be invaluable. It is too easy to assume that singing can be helpful for any voice and respiratory problem. However, Tamplin and Grocke (2008) illustrate how this is not the case, by stating "Without enough breath support to sustain phonation for short phrases, it is not possible to address articulation, resonance, or prosody" (p. 26).

Therapeutic Singing

Overview. Therapeutic singing involves singing and musical activities to facilitate initiation within, development of, and articulation in a person's speech and language, as well as to increase functions of the respiratory system (Thaut, 2005a). Thus, this method serves both speech and language problems. To the observer, therapeutic singing can appear to be "having a sing-song," so it is important to determine the purpose of the activity and what you hope to achieve. It is a particularly useful technique within the assessment period as it allows the therapist to hear and observe the person's speech and language problems within music.

Therapeutic singing is useful for people living with any of the conditions discussed in this chapter, whenever a person presents with dysarthria or language disorders associated with brain damage (e.g., word-finding difficulties). The goal of therapeutic singing is to address broader speech and language functions demanding coordination of all the components involved, e.g., respiratory function, phonation, resonance, articulation, and prosody. Broader goals are often more appropriate when working in neuropalliative settings. Thus, although the following goals are very broad, these might reflect treatment appropriate to the care setting's program:

- Patient will produce sung language within a well-learned familiar song.
- Patient will achieve approximate pitch of melody within a well-learned familiar song.
- Patient will produce sung verbal output within a well-learned familiar song, demonstrating control in tempo, phrasing, melodic contour, and volume appropriate to overall musical structure.

There are no contraindications for using this method in assessment, i.e., when the therapist is trying to determine what the patient can achieve and identify problem areas. Even if the person has no residual language and unknown voice production capabilities, they may enjoy mouthing the words voicelessly to songs or humming to songs. However, once it has been ascertained that the person is not able to engage actively in therapeutic singing by singing words, other methods outlined in this section might be more appropriate, or the use of receptive methods only.

Preparation. Ensure that the therapist is seated opposite the patient. This will offer a visual model for the patient to enhance prompts for articulatory speech movements and words, as well as musical aspects such as when to come in, phrase lengths, and tempo. If the therapist is using a piano, try to use an electric keyboard that can be placed directly between the therapist and client so that full eye contact can be made above the instrument and there is no barrier between client and therapist. Where only an upright piano is available, the therapist should ensure that her trunk is rotated adequately to present as front-on to the patient as possible. Bring the patient right up to the keyboard and ensure that he faces the therapist as much as possible, rather than faces the piano.

What to observe. During assessment, observe any attempts (successful or otherwise) to mouth or sing the words. This will determine the use of music to prompt or enable language production. Identify whether the person is able to sing the entire lyrics of each line in full, or whether he sings only the last part of each line, or only the last word or syllable. Usually, emotionally laden choruses are easier to recall than verses. Determine whether the chorus optimizes the patient's ability to respond, or whether verses prompt an equal response. Note which verses are most helpful, and maximize the use of these.

In addition to observing language production, listen carefully to the speech sounds produced. Can the client achieve accurate speech sounds? If not, which ones seem the most difficult to achieve? Observe, too, the musical elements of the client's singing. For example, are they able to achieve the full range of the melody? If not, how limited is the client's melodic range, e.g., can they sing only in a monotone, or are they able to achieve a range of a major 2nd /perfect fourth?

Procedures. Therapeutic singing needs to employ songs that are as familiar as possible to the patient so as to prompt an automatic response. Using music that is known to hold personal meaning for the patient will help. If possible, the therapist should determine the patient's preferred or favourite music prior to the session. The therapist should explain the purpose of the activity to the client, emphasising both the enjoyment and functional benefits. During songs at the start of therapy, the therapist should sing with the client at the start of each line in order to prompt the client with words, although the therapist should maintain a supportive role, e.g., singing slightly quieter than the client, rather than in the role of an equal partner such as in a duet. Within each line, the therapist should fade out their own singing in order to ascertain whether the client is able to produce the lyrics independently. This should be done only within choruses or well-known verses of the song, and only toward the ends of lines. In this way, the musical structure is acting as a prompt for the client to produce the words.

Repetition is an important part of rehabilitation, as it can help to change brain structures and make new learning automatic. However, when working with people with LTNC, a fine balance should be sought between rehabilitation and palliative approaches. That is, enjoyment and pleasure should not be compromised for the sake of functional benefits. Thus, although repetition of songs can be helpful from a functional point of view, the therapist should ensure that the range of songs is wide enough to keep the client motivated and engaged, in addition to optimizing the enjoyment of the session. In a similar way, the frequency of sessions is important in optimising the functional benefits of a therapeutic singing program. Preferably, individuals should be encouraged to practice singing daily. While this is usually not possible within music therapy service provision, the use of a practice CD with exercises for the patient to use between sessions has been recommended (Grocke & Tamplin, 2008).

It is recommended that clients be encouraged to tap their hands rhythmically on their knees or to tap percussion instruments rhythmically during singing activities. Although there is no "hard" evidence for this suggestion, brain-imaging research with people with brain lesions following stroke found that tapping during intoned speech (like Sprechstimme) primes the sensorimotor and premotor cortices for articulation (Schlaug, Marchina, & Norton, 2008). That is, tapping rhythmically while singing may assist with the motor movements involved in speech (and singing) articulations. We can make some assumptions that this finding may hold for other adults with acquired neurological damage as well.

Methods to Address Voice Disorders

Overview. Vocal exercises used with clients with LTNC tend to focus on breath support, phonation, and pitch range (Elefant et al., in press; Haneishi, 2001; Magee et al., 2006), using varying exercises such as glissandi, arpeggio, and syllables produced on a single pitch in ascending and descending pitch patterns. Vocal Intonation Therapy (VIT) is a more widely used method from NMT speech and language methods (Thaut, 2005b). It involves musical vocalization through controlled singing and vocal exercises to train all aspects of voice control regarding inflection, pitch, breath control, timbre, and loudness in voice disorder rehabilitation (Thaut, 2005b). When using VIT, the therapist devises exercises that employ intoned phrases simulating the prosody, inflection, and pacing of normal speech. Tamplin and Grocke (2008a) describe a protocol employing VIT for neurocommunication disorders where sentences that gradually increased in length were set to music in which the melody, rhythm, meter, and accents of the musical phrase reflected the inflection, rhythm, and stress of natural speech prosody.

Voice methods are useful in cases of abnormal voice, such as difficulties with phonation, high voice, hypernasality, and difficulties with pitch, which are all typical of dysarthria in LTNC. Typical goals might be for the client to:

- Achieve phonation;
- Achieve a wider pitch range during singing than within speech;
- Increase his dynamic range over the course of a session;
- Achieve inflections within sung vocalizations that are not achieved in speech conditions alone;
- Increase the duration of his vocal sounds on a single exhalation.

Within assessment, the therapist should determine which vocal parameters are responsive to musical intervention. Only those vocal parameters that show potential for change should be targeted within interventions. For example, if the client with PD vocalizes only a monotone in response to musical stimuli, then he may not be able to achieve a wider pitch range. In this case, focusing on an unrealistic goal will only reinforce negative outcomes.

Preparation. Preparation of the session should follow the recommendations made for functional singing methods.

What to observe. Within voice disorder methods, the therapist should observe any of the vocal parameters of interest and document these carefully each week. For example, if working with a client with limited pitch range, observations should focus upon maximum pitch ranges achieved in each session. Parameters of interest should be monitored through exercises specifically tailored to that parameter, e.g., the pitch range achieved within voice glissandi; duration of single phonations; and the quality of the vocal sound, particularly when working with clients with difficulty with hypernasality. The client's fatigue levels should be monitored carefully, and the length of vocal exercises as one part of the session tailored accordingly, possibly to no more than 5–10 minutes.

When working toward improvement in vocal parameters, it is important to record the session in order to evaluate the client's progress accurately. Also, computer software such as Audacity (http://audacity.sourceforge.net/) can provide a useful tool for evaluating the client's response objectively through its Spectrogram view modes for visualizing frequencies. This can enable the therapist to evaluate pitch and volume objectively.

Procedures. Vocal methods are typically one part of a music therapy session, and often function as part of the warm-up to therapeutic singing. Usually, preparatory exercises in the session can involve melodic and rhythmic components and can produce measurable outcomes so that the client is able to compare his progress across sessions as a way of monitoring his voice production.

Therapists can use their musical creativity to develop exercises tailored to the client's needs. A number of protocols suggest specific vocal exercises (Haneishi, 2001; Magee et al., 2006; Tamplin & Grocke, 2008) that are often structured as singing exercises, with an emphasis on simplicity and repetition. The key of each exercise should center on the pitch range that is most achievable for individual patients, working toward a greater pitch range if the patient is able.

Methods to Address Speech Disorders

Overview. Given the prevalence of dysarthria in LTNC, music therapy methods are strongly recommended to improve or maintain function of the articulatory system, involving the tongue, teeth, lips, jaw, and facial muscles. A number of procedures have been outlined in clinical and research protocols. Oral Motor and Respiratory Exercises (OMREX) (Thaut, 2005b) involve musical exercises using sound vocalization and wind instrument–playing. These exercises aim to enhance articulatory control and respiratory strength and function of the speech apparatus. Typically, they involve a range of activities to exercise the lips, tongue, and facial muscles in combination with voice and in coordination with respiratory strength. Lightweight blowing instruments offer alternative feedback to the voice in these activities, which is helpful if vocalizing is difficult and tiring for the client. Blowing instruments demands respiratory strength and oromotor coordination, thus is functionally challenging. The instruments used should be graded for difficulty so that the client can gauge their changing abilities. Games using instruments can be particularly fun in group work. OMREX is helpful not only with dysarthria, but also for dyspraxia, which can be a problem in LTNC.

Music-based speech methods are indicated in all cases of dysarthria. The therapist should ensure that the client's specific problems are clearly identified, e.g., poor lip seal; specific sounds which cannot be achieved, and the articulatory movements involved; and difficulties with alternating between bilabials and vowel sounds. Collaboration with the client's speech therapist is essential in order to accurately identify the client's problems and plan realistic goals.

Goals can then be planned to target the client's specific problems. Where coordination of respiratory and articulatory strength is a problem, activities should aim to build strength through repetitive, short bursts of sound (vocal or instrumental), while working on the problematic aspect of articulation, e.g., lip seal (through blowing instruments), alternating open vowel sounds with contrasting mouth shapes (e.g., ee/oo, ah/ee), alternating open vowel sounds with bilabials (e.g., mm/ah, bah/pah), or alternation of sounds created through alternative placements of the tongue (e.g., see/me, fa/la, da/ta).

People with LTNC may produce speech that is too rapid (typical in PD) or very slow and labored (typical in MND and MS). Typical goals will be to improve the regularity, pace, or rhythmicity of the patient's speech. Tamplin and Grocke (2008) make some useful suggestions about music that is not helpful in song-singing for dysarthria, including complex lyrics or rhythmic patterns, wide pitch range, difficult melodic lines, fast tempo, and negative lyrical content. Current research suggests that people with HD have a compromised perception of rhythmic cues, even when with mild or no overt disease signs (Thaut, 2005a). Temporal control of motor functions is irregular, so rhythmic speech cuing should be used with caution with people with HD.

Preparation. Preparation of the session should follow the recommendations made for functional singing methods.

What to observe. The specific function being targeted should be carefully monitored within each task to address that function. For example, if the goal is to achieve lip seal within an activity, observe whether the client is able to achieve this within the activity, how many times, and the quality of the lip seal (fully, partially, not at all). If the goal is to reduce the rate of speech, monitor whether the client is able to achieve the improved rate of speech and, if so, whether this is for the complete task, part of the task, or not at all. It can be helpful to monitor the client's performance on each goal and exactly those elements he achieves or does not fully achieve for each separate activity. Also, monitor the client's motivation for working on their functional speech. It goes without saying that if the activities become too hard, particularly as the client's speech function deteriorates, it is time to work toward different goals.

Procedures. Methods to address speech disorders are typically one part of a music therapy session and often function prior to therapeutic singing. Activities should be short and repetitive in order to maximize the functional benefit. Set the goals with the client and offer feedback after each activity.

Useful equipment employed should include lightweight wind instruments such as recorders and plastic harmonicas and whistles. Blowing instruments which require greater respiratory strength or tighter lip seal can be introduced once the client has achieved sounds on the instruments that require less effort. A metronome with a clear audible beat is essential when doing rhythmic speech methods. This can be used on its own or within activities where the therapist plays another instrument. However, the auditory cue is essential. The therapist should use visual cues as much as she can, including modeling targeted lip shapes and facial gestures in an exaggerated manner. This is essential if the client also has dyspraxia. When working with people with reduced respiratory capacity, it is recommended to initially use songs with short phrase lengths (Tamplin & Grocke, 2008).

Methods to Address Language Disorders

Overview. It is commonly noted that well-known overly learned music is able to prompt automatic language output in people with neurological damage, even in the absence of functional language output due to conditions such as aphasia (Cohen & Ford, 1995; Magee, 1999). This is a technique that has been used for decades in clinical work, but more recently given the title of Musical Speech Stimulation (MUSTIM) (Thaut, 2005a). This is the use of musical materials such as songs, rhymes, chants, or musical phrases simulating prosodic speech gestures (e.g., inflection patterns for questions, answers, exclamations, etc.) to stimulate nonpropositional speech in aphasia therapy or with apraxic patients. MUSTIM is useful for rehearsing words that are used in functional communication, such as the completion or initiation of overly learned familiar song lyrics, or association of words with familiar tunes. It is also useful for enabling patients who can no longer produce functional language for communication to experience success in producing language. In addition to language goals, this is a wonderful method to use with individuals who have severe memory deficits, particularly with recall. The overly learned nature of the stimulus can elicit responses in the even the most impaired client.

Language-based methods such as MUSTIM are indicated when the person is presenting with language problems such as word-finding, perseveration, or initiation difficulties. Goals will typically focus on the client producing the final words of phrases to songs and rhythmic chants which are familiar and well-known to the client. Novel music might be used in sessions as well, such as hello songs in which the goal will be for the client to sing their own and therapist's names within the song.

Melodic intonation therapy is a different method used in aphasia therapy with a very specific patient population. It should not be confused with the methods discussed in this chapter and is contraindicated in all cases of LTNC unless the person has experienced a stroke.

Preparation. Preparation of the session should follow the recommendations made for functional singing methods.

What to observe. All attempts to verbalize at the target point of a song should be closely monitored, e.g., mouth movements and attempts to vocalize. If the client does achieve a sound, the accuracy of the sound from linguistic, speech, and musical factors should be noted. That is, did they achieve the approximate pitch of the note? Did they achieve the full word or just the last syllable? Did they achieve the articulation required to speak the word?

Procedures. Prior to the session, the therapist must have established that the music is well-known and emotionally meaningful to the client. The best results with this method will be achieved using only those parts of the song that are overly learned, prompting an automatic response, i.e., choruses or emotionally laden verses or bridge sections. These songs can be played to the client, leaving a pause for the final word in a phrase. The musical accompaniment should be slowed as the target word is approached, and a pause should be left for as long as comfortably possible to enable the client to respond. Sometimes, the client can be helped by a given prompt of the first sound or syllable of the target word. Exaggerated presentations of the song (e.g., with facial gestures) can aid the client. It is perfectly acceptable to use just the section of the song that prompts a response in the client and to repeat this. Sections from different songs that elicit optimal responses can be run together as a medley.

Guidelines for Compositional Music Therapy

Songwriting

Overview. The therapist helps the client to write songs, lyrics, or instrumental pieces, or to create any kind of musical product, such as music videos or audiotape programs. Usually, the therapist simplifies the process by engaging the client in the easier aspects of composing (e.g., generating a melody or writing the lyrics of a song) and by taking responsibility for more technical aspects (e.g., harmonization, notation).

Song collage is a method wherein the words and phrases of existing songs are selected by clients and collaged together as part of the lyric creation process (Tamplin, 2006). This has been identified as a helpful method of song composition for people with cognitive impairments and thus might be indicated for people with LTNC in whom cognitive decline has been experienced. However, this method might also be considered less applicable where individuals are dealing with highly personal themes such as those already highlighted to be relevant for people with life-threatening conditions (Dileo & Magill, 2005; O'Callaghan, 1996). Therapists should use their judgment as to whether this method can aid someone who has difficulty generating personal expression, or whether it prevents the individual from expressing more individualized material.

Preparation. Preparation of the session and environment should follow all those recommendations made previously for mood exploration and expression using precomposed songs of personal meaning. An ideal environment, whether working with individuals or dyads or in small groups, is one that is quiet, private, and free from distractions so that a feeling of intimacy can be achieved. Clients need to feel safe to explore their stories and feelings, both of which might contain difficult material.

What to observe. The therapist should listen attentively to all the words, verbal utterances and sounds a person makes when relaying their story, as all of the person's sounds can contribute to creating an authentic personal expression through song. It can help to document, either through written means or recording, all of the client's thoughts and suggestions that they offer; ideas or words that may not seem important during the session might gain greater prominence over the course of therapy. Using people's nonverbal sounds can also be built into the song if appropriate.

Procedures. Comprehensive procedures for a range of songwriting experiences have been outlined elsewhere (Baker & Wigram, 2005), and the reader is guided to that authoritative source for more detailed information about the range of protocols for lyric creation and music creation and the varying levels of support and models of cocreation that therapists have used. However, the therapist should keep in mind the themes that tend to be prevalent for people living with life-threatening illnesses that have already been outlined. Encouraging the client to reflect and talk about the characters and stories that are important to them is often the first step. Identifying a key theme can provide the motif for the refrain, the part of the song that will repeat and thus be emphasized.

Some important considerations include the degree to which an existing song structure is used or whether the song is freely composed. Song parody, a method wherein an existing song melody and harmony is used but with the lyrics fully or partially replaced by the client's own words, provides a higher level of structure and support. This can be useful when the client is disorientated or fatigued, or when there are reasons for creating a song relatively quickly over one or very few sessions. Freely composed songs can take longer to create and provide more opportunities for the client to influence the musical structures. This may be important for some clients, although they can also place more pressures on the client.

When working with clients who rely on "low-technology" methods of AAC devices, for example, eye gaze boards or listener scanning, the therapist might consider proposing song parody methods. This method supports those who have difficulty generating lyrics quickly, but enables some original novel lyric generation that can partially substitute existing lyrics and provide the client with a musical reward relatively quickly.

Adaptations. Fill-in-the-blank methods of song composition enable participation even when cognitive decline causes the person difficulty in initiating new ideas or expressing his ideas. In this method, key words in an existing song are replaced with single words generated by the client relevant to their thematic material. As with song parody, this method provides the client with reward relatively quickly while making the song his own. The familiarity of an existing song can also aid a client with cognitive difficulties in recognizing the song and participating, responses that may be more difficult to achieve with an unfamiliar, newly composed song.

Research Evidence

Receptive Music Therapy

Research investigating the effects of songs on mood states with neurological populations indicates that song-singing programs can effect significant change in a range of mood states (Baker & Wigram, 2004; Haneishi, 2001; Magee et al., 2006; Magee & Davidson, 2002) for both immediate and longer-term effects. Familiar precomposed songs have also been noted to promote coping and adaptation to chronic illness through enhancing a patient's sense of self and control (Steele, 2005) and have long been used as a catalyst for discussion and emotional expression with people with LTNC (Curtis, 1987; Dawes, 1985; O'Callaghan, 1996). Although this method has been described previously as "music-supported counseling" (O'Callaghan, 1993), the method described here encompasses the use of songs for explicit and implicit mood exploration. For some people, and at some times during an individual's coping process, the person may not be able to make explicit his feelings which are embodied in the songs chosen. At other times, verbal exploration might be possible. For adults with acquired chronic conditions, precomposed songs of personal meaning possess associative and temporal properties that enhance their emotional meaning (Magee, 2007). Through these properties, songs can help an individual to explore nonverbally his deeper emotional state and start to express feelings that are difficult to express explicitly in words. Songs, therefore, are useful tools when working with individuals who have difficulty acknowledging and exploring intolerable feelings in the face of loss and pending death. They are also invaluable tools when working with someone who can no longer communicate verbally.

Song-based sessions that include family members enable a client and his family to share musically evoked memories and convey important messages which are often difficult to express verbally (O'Callaghan, 1993). Messages conveyed between the client and his family are often celebrations of the positive roles they have played in each other's lives (O'Callaghan, 1993). The temporal properties of songs enable memories stretching back an entire lifetime to be conveyed, whether this be of partner-to-partner, child-to-parent, or sibling-to-sibling. In this way, at a time when it may be difficult to find meaning in shared activities, music can engage family members and client in a shared activity which fosters emotional connections capable of healing attachment or romantic bonds (Magee & Bowen, 2008). It provides families with an action-oriented way of coping that emphasizes the social partner or family member being adaptive, creative, and meeting the patient at their level (Magee & Bowen, 2008). This way of coping has been more associated with decreased psychological distress (Blankfeld & Holahan, 1999). Furthermore, emotional connection coupled with care and compassion fosters a sense of spiritual connection that endures. This is important, as carers who view their situation as meaningful and manageable appear to cope better (Koscuilek, 1997).

Musical life review has been described with people living with chronic or terminal illness (Beggs, 1991; Bright, 1986). This may more accurately be described as biographical work when working with people with long-term conditions, as there is time to tend to the reparative and alteration elements. Because meaningful songs elicit memories, memories emerge of the person as they were before their illness and before they became disabled. Thus, songs help individuals to contextualize their illness into their biography (Magee, 2007). In particular, the temporal experience of songs prompts both conscious and subconscious associations between the past and the present, particularly in relation to relationships and life situations. Engaging in multiple reviews of one's life through imagery that recaptures the past, examines the present, and projects into the future can assist someone who is managing their biography in the context of degenerative change. Perhaps most significantly, music stimulates feelings about future events, expressed as hope. For someone living with an incurable degenerative condition, thinking about the future can be frightening and too difficult. Songs may provide a container to allow the client with an LTNC to imagine a future and fantasize about what might be.

Improvisational Music Therapy

A number of empirical investigations have explored improvisation in music therapy with people with LTNC within both the quantitative and qualitative paradigms. This affords the profession with knowledge from both outcome and process perspectives. Two themes are prevalent in the research into and evidence for improvisation with LTNC: the emergence of motor function as a central concern, and how this interfaces with the emotional experience of living with chronic illness.

Improvising is a highly physical activity, demanding that an individual negotiate his physical control, strength, and stamina through the act of playing instruments (Magee & Davidson, 2004). However, quantitative studies with people with MS examining the effects of improvisational MT on motor and functional abilities have found no discernible changes in either outcome (Schmid, Ostermann, & Aldridge, 2004; Schmid & Aldridge, 2004). Indeed, in a study with people with HD, Hoskyns (1982) aimed to reduce choreic movements during improvised duets as a measure of promoting relaxation. In fact, there was a significant increase in choreic movements due to the physical activity demanded during instrument-playing, although participants indicated that instrument-playing was pleasurable even for people in the more advanced stages of the disease (Hoskyns, 1982).

Yet, the qualitative studies exploring the experience of improvisation for people with LTNC (which all happen to be with MS) suggest that improvising impacts upon how people feel about their disability and feelings of identity. In a study with 225 MS patients, Lengdobler and Kiessling (1989) found that minimally structured improvisations in group therapy enabled exploration of feelings of disability, uncertainty, anxiety, depression, and loss of self-esteem. The authors state that anxieties about playing instruments contributed far more in limiting participation than physical disability itself (Lengdobler & Kiessling, 1989). In a research study exploring the role of improvisation for people with complex disabilities stemming from MS, Magee and Davidson (2004) found that playing instruments highlighted feelings of changed skill and ability, as individuals monitored their illness progression through their physical performance during improvisation, a process titled "physical monitoring." During physical monitoring, individuals monitor the extent and type of functional change that they perceive has occurred. That is, they compare what they could achieve physically at a previous point in time with what they can achieve at the current time. Illness monitoring helps an individual to observe subtle changes occurring, thus serving to increase self-knowledge and awareness (Magee & Davidson, 2004). This in turn gives an individual some sense of control in the face of living with an incurable degenerative illness with no clear prognosis. This phenomenon has been described in health sociology research as the dialectical self

(Charmaz, 1991), which involves appraising the body as an object and comparing it with the self in different temporal and situational frameworks. In this process, individuals make comparisons of their performance between the past, present, and future, and also with others.

The empirical inquiries into improvisation have also examined the effects on mood and emotional factors. In one randomized controlled trial comparing a group engaging in improvisation with a group not engaging in improvisation, significant differences were not found in mood states between the group receiving music therapy and the comparable group that did not receive music therapy (Schmid & Aldridge, 2004; Schmid, Ostermann, & Aldridge, 2004). So, the effects of improvisation on mood are in line with the outcomes noted for motor and functional changes after improvising. The changes in mood were not significant, but improvisation was found to have medium-size effects on changes to self-esteem, depression, and anxiety, with improvements in self-acceptance. These quantitative findings reflect findings from qualitative studies examining improvisation with people with MS. Several studies indicate that engaging in improvisation may assist with coping (Lengdobler & Kiessling, 1989; Magee & Davidson, 2004; Schmid & Aldridge, 2004; Schmid, Ostermann, & Aldridge, 2004), providing participant reports of improved feelings of well-being. Researchers have suggested that this may be due to the deep connection that can be experienced during improvisation (Schmid & Aldridge, 2004; Schmid, Ostermann, & Aldridge, 2004).

It is evident that the physical experience of improvising can elicit emotional responses around how the client feels about their body, their physical ability, and the changes that are occurring. Through sustained exploration of his own individual physical change and loss, the client's physical experience can become emotionally charged (Magee, 2007). Engaging in a physically demanding task such as improvising provides a forum for the testing and retesting of physical boundaries (Magee, 2007). Through the interaction of the physical experience and the emotional response, the individual experiences shifts to self and identity constructs (Magee, 2002, 2007; Magee & Davidson, 2004). Active participation in the music therapy session provides opportunities for a different experience of "self," in which the individual may experience feelings of success, developing skill, and increased independence (Magee, 2002).

Re-creative Music Therapy

Systematic reviews of the available research into music therapy with adults with acquired brain injury of a nondegenerative nature indicate that there is little evidence for the effectiveness of music-based treatments for neurological speech and language disorders (Bradt, Magee, Dileo, Wheeler, & McGilloway, 2010; Hurkmans, et al., 2012). This is disheartening for clinicians who witness the positive functional outcomes and enjoyment in their clients' faces while engaged in these activities. However, this "lack of evidence" is an indication of the poor methodological quality of the research that exists rather than the treatments being ineffective per se.

Although the evidence is not strong for using functional singing to enhance communication in neurocommunication disorders, these methods are highly recommended for physical, social, emotional, cognitive, and general well-being reasons. First, for many people, singing is an enjoyable activity in which they have engaged since infancy. Thus, it can be motivating. Second, singing shares the same sensorimotor processes as speaking (Özdemir, Norton, & Schlaug, 2006). It can aid with maintaining speech functions in the light of degenerating speech functions. This is important for a person who may be less motivated to attempt verbal communication as it becomes increasingly difficult and frustrating. Third, singing has been shown to have benefits to mood for people with neurological disorders (Baker & Wigram, 2005; Haneishi, 2001; Magee & Davidson, 2002; Magee et al., 2006). Fourth, singing rather than speaking has been found to activate larger networks in the brains of people with neurological damage than just speaking alone (Özdemir et al., 2006) and assists with the remodeling of neural structures and pathways after acquired brain damage (Schlaug, Marchina, & Norton, 2008; Schlaug, Norton, Marchina, Zipse, & Wan, 2010). Finally, as individuals with LTNC experience degeneration of vocal production, singing may be a means for them to enjoy the use of their voice while they still have their voice. Individuals with LTNC have been found to use singing within therapy as a forum in which to monitor the changes occurring to their voice as a consequence of disease (Magee & Davidson, 2004b).

Rhythmic articulation exercises build on respiratory control and strength with strong rhythmic pulse cues to structure vocalizations (Tamplin & Grocke, 2008). Melodic articulation exercises practice positioning of the speech apparatus and promote active movement of the facial muscles and articulators (Tamplin & Grocke, 2008a). Rhythmic speech cuing (RSC) is a rate-control technique that uses auditory rhythm (metronome form or embedded in music) to cue speech (Thaut, 2005b). There are two categories of RSC: metric, in which rhythmic beats are matched to syllables, resulting in speech in which every syllable is of equal duration, and patterned, where beat patterns simulate the stress patterns of normal speech inflection (Thaut, 2005a). Other versions of RSC are reported under alternative names such as rhythmic instruction (Cohen & Masse, 1993). Rhythm-based methods are useful for slowing the rate of speech in cases of rapid speech (Cohen, 1988), which can be typical of dysarthria in PD, and also useful in helping the client to focus on the stress of his speech in order to improve speech naturalness (Tamplin & Grocke, 2008).

Sena Moore, Peterson, O'Shea, McIntosh, & Thaut (2008) examined the effects of verbal learning and memory in people with MS who scored between 3.5 and 7 (mean = 4.6) (Thaut, Sena, & McIntosh, 2008) on a scale of 10 on the Kurtzke Extended Disability Status Scale (EDSS). They compared two groups, one that learned through musical mnemonics and one that learned through verbal means alone. They did not find any significant differences between the two learning conditions; however, the people who learned in the music condition showed a significantly better word order than those people in the spoken condition (Thaut, Peterson, Sena, & McIntosh, 2008). Also, although enhanced learning through music could not be supported (Sena Moore et al., 2008), the findings indicated that musical learning seemed to enhance the ability to retrieve the verbal material, even after a week's break from the music. Most important, it seemed that people who were less impaired in cognitive capacities gained the most benefit from using music as a learning and mnemonic device. Thaut et al., (2008) also suggest that long-term practice and repetition (i.e., over weeks or months) might benefit people with MS in encoding new verbal material, particularly if the material is introduced and learned early in the disease process. This bears relevance for using orientation songs within MT. These findings suggest that music mnemonic tasks might be useful for learning and recalling words for people with MS, but might be best used with those at the higher end of the Kurtzke EDSS.

Findings from the Sena Moore et al. (2008) study recommend that people with MS might need longer to learn and consolidate verbal material presented in songs for learning, as "the longer someone can rehearse information, the more effectively it is encoded and stored into long-term memory" (p. 322). Although Sena Moore et al. suggest that their hourlong protocol may not have been long enough for people with MS to learn, it is advised to limit the length of sessions to a one-hour maximum due to the person's fatigue levels. In this case, the length of time for learning should be ensured through the repetition of sessions over time. Most important, Sena Moore et al. (2008) suggest that music may be more useful as a mnemonic aid for those earlier in the disease process.

Compositional Music Therapy

Songwriting has been noted as a useful method with a number of populations, but in particular with people who are facing chronic degenerative illness or terminal illness. Songs enable the expression of sentiments that are difficult to state in words; the musical structure of verse and chorus allow for repetition and emphasis of primary thoughts and feelings. The lyrics of songs composed in therapy by people living with life-threatening illnesses have been found to contain themes of messages; self-reflections; compliments; reflections upon significant others, including pets; self-expression of adversity; imagery; and prayers (O'Callaghan, 1996). Reflecting these research findings, the themes of songs written by hospice patients have been described as encompassing family-related issues, closure, resolution, emotional expression, and facing death (Dileo & Magill, 2005). It is not uncommon for a client to share something that is difficult or traumatic from his life when telling his story. This can be part of biographical work where he is carrying out multiple reviews of life's experiences, reframing and recontextualizing these in order to make sense of his life.

As songwriting enables reflection on one's life, it is helpful in promoting biographical work that is so important for reviewing one's life and preparing for death. Essentially, people can tell the stories of their lives through song composition. As already discussed in the earlier section in this chapter on receptive methods, re-creative or compositional song methods can be helpful when a person's illness has progressed to the point where they are unable to move (and thus cannot play instruments) or may not be able to vocalize due to the physical effects of illness (and thus cannot sing), but are able to communicate via alternative and augmentative communication aids. Compositional methods provide another means within music therapy for emotional expression when the person may no longer be able to explore their mood state due to physical or cognitive difficulties. Most important, songs function as a legacy of the person who is dying for those left behind.

Songwriting methods can comfortably include a client's significant others, either as cocreators in the song composition or as audience members in a performance of the song. Song composition is useful in individual sessions, in dyads (with other clients or family members), or in group settings. Although less usual in group work, composing songs with others facing adversity and ill health can provide a supportive environment for expressions of the many emotional experiences of living with chronic incurable illness, such as fear, sadness, hope, and love.

Research has explored the effects of songwriting on the emotional, interpersonal, and spiritual needs of individuals living with neurodegenerative diseases. While empirical evidence is extremely limited, case reports provide useful insight into the process of songwriting and the overwhelming benefits of this technique with this population. Case studies with MS patients indicate that the process of songwriting allows exploration of interpersonal and psychosocial needs, leading to a renewed sense of hope, increased spiritual well-being, and increased quality of life (Davis, 1998; Lee, 2007). The benefits of songwriting have also been explored within HD. Forrest (2002) found that songwriting provided for individual choice and expression. It allowed patients to choose the means and medium with which to express themselves and communicate their illness to others.

Summary and Conclusions

Long-term neurological conditions (LTNC) are chronic and degenerative diseases, with no cure at the present time. Individuals living with LTNC are forced to continually adapt to change resulting from intermittent yet gradually increasing symptoms. LTNC can restrict movement, communication, and thought processes; impair sense of self; disrupt social relationships; and lead to spiritual suffering.

Music therapy is an effective intervention in neurological rehabilitation. Musical instrument can stimulate functional movement patterns in therapy to address movement disorders. Minimally structured improvisations in group therapy allow for exploration of feelings, uncertainty, anxiety, depression, and loss of self-esteem. The experience of improvising can elicit emotional responses around how the individual feels about their body, their physical ability, and the changes that are occurring. Music therapy methods can aid with maintaining speech functions in the light of degenerating speech functions. Singing songs can effect significant change in a range of mood states and provide a sense of control. Songs and songwriting can enable the expression of sentiments that are difficult to state in words. Music therapy can and does aid in fostering and maintaining the independence, identity, and quality of life of individuals living with LTNC.

References

Aarsland, D., Londos, E., & Ballard, C. (2009). Parkinson's disease dementia and dementia with Lewy bodies: Different aspects of one entity. *International Psychogeriatrics, 21*(02), 216- 219.

Arciniegas, D. B., & Topkoff, J. (2000). The neuropsychiatry of pathologic affect: An approach to evaluation and treatment. *Seminars in Clinical Neuropsychiatry, 5*(4), 290 – 306.

Baker, F. (2001). The effects of live, taped, and no music on people experiencing posttraumatic amnesia. *Journal of Music Therapy, 38*(3), 170.

Baker, F., & Wigram, T. (2004). Rehabilitating the uninflected voice: Finding climax and cadence. *Music Therapy Perspectives, 22(1),* 4–10.

Baker, F., & Wigram, T. (Eds.). (2005). *Songwriting: Methods, techniques and clinical applications for music therapy clinicians, educators and students.* Philadelphia, PA: Jessica Kingsley.

Bamford, K. A., Caine, E. D., Kido, D. K., Cox, C., & Shoulson, I. (1995). A prospective evaluation of cognitive decline in early Huntington's disease. Functional and radiographic correlates. *Neurology, 45*(10), 1867–1873.

Beggs, C. (1991). Life review with a palliative care patient. In K. Bruscia (Ed.). *Case studies in music therapy,* (pp. 611-616). Gilsum, NH: Barcelona Publishers.

Blankfeld, D. F., & Holahan, C. J. (1999). Social support, coping, and psychological adjustment among caregivers of head-injured patients. *Psychology and Health, 14,* 609–624.

Bogosian, A., Moss-Morris, R., & Hadwin, J. (2010). Psychosocial adjustment in children and adolescents with a parent with multiple sclerosis: A systematic review. *Clinical Rehabilitation, 24*(9), 789–801. Retrieved from http://search.ebscohost.com.libproxy.temple.edu/login.aspx?direct=true&db=cmedm&AN=20685724&site=ehost-live&scope=site

Bol, Y., Duits, A. A., Hupperts, R. M., Vlaeyen, J. S., & Verhey, F. J. (2009). The psychology of fatigue in patients with multiple sclerosis: A review. *Journal of Psychosomatic Research, 66*(1), 3–11. Retrieved from http://search.ebscohost.com.libproxy.temple.edu/login.aspx?direct=true&db=cmedm&AN=19073287&site=ehost-live&scope=site

Bradt, J., Magee, W. L., Dileo, C., Wheeler, B. & McGilloway, E. (2010). Music therapy for acquired brain injury. (Review). *Cochrane Database of Systematic Reviews.* Issue 7. Art. no.: CD006787. DOI: 10.1002/14651858.CD006787.pub2. http://www.mrw.interscience.wiley.com/cochrane/clsysrev/articles/CD006787/frame.html

Charmaz, K. (1987). Struggling for a self: Identity levels of the chronically ill. *Research in the Sociology of Health Care,* 6, 283-321.

Charmaz, K. (1991). *Good days, bad days: The self in chronic illness and time.* New Brunswick, NJ: Rutgers University Press.

Chaudri, M. B., Kinnear, W. M., & Jefferson, D. (2003). Patterns of mortality in patients with motor neurone disease. *Acta Neurologica Scandinavica, 107*(1), 50–53. Retrieved from http://search.ebscohost.com.libproxy.temple.edu/login.aspx?direct=true&db=cmedm&AN=12542513&site=ehost-live&scope=site

Cohen, N. (1988). The use of superimposed rhythms to decrease the rate of speech in a brain-damaged adolescent. *Journal of Music Therapy, 25(2),* 85–93.

Cohen, N. (1992). The effect of singing instruction on the speech production of neurologically impaired persons. *Journal of Music Therapy, 29(2),* 87–102.

Cohen, N. (1994). Speech and song: Implications for therapy. *Music Therapy Perspectives, 12,* 8–14.

Cohen, N. S., & Ford, J. (1995). The effect of musical cues on the nonpurposive speech of persons with aphasia. *Journal of Music Therapy, 32*(1), 46-46.

Cohen, N., & Masse, R. (1993). The application of singing and rhythmic instruction as a therapeutic intervention for persons with neurogenic communication disorders. *Journal of Music Therapy, 30(2),* 81–89.

Corbin, J., & Strauss, A. L. (1987). Accompaniments of chronic illness: Changes in body, self, biography, and biographical time. *Research in the Sociology of Health Care, 6*(3), 249-281.

Curtis, S. (1987). Music therapy: A positive approach in Huntington's disease. *Proceedings of the 13th National Conference of the Australian Music Therapy Association Incorporated* (page numbers unknown). Melbourne: AMTA Inc.

Davie, C. (2008). A review of Parkinson's disease. *British Medical Bulletin,* 86(1), 109–127.

Davis, G., &, Magee, W. (2001). Clinical improvisation within neurological disease: Exploring the effect of structured clinical improvisation on the expressive and interactive responses of a patient with Huntington's disease. *British Journal of Music Therapy, 15*(2), 51–60.

Davis, K. (1998). "To never surrender": Music therapy in the fight against MS. *Journal of Music Therapy, 6*(1), 20–34.

Davis, S. L., Wilson, T. E., White, A. T., & Frohman, E. M. (2010). Thermoregulation in multiple sclerosis. *Journal of Applied Physiology, 109*(5), 1531–1537.

Dawes, S. (1985). The role of music therapy in caring in Huntington's disease. In E. Chiu & B. Teltscher (Eds.), *Handbook for caring in Huntington's disease* (pp. 97–103). Melbourne, AU: Huntington's Disease Clinic.

Degenhardt, A., Ramagopalan, S. V., Scalfari, A., & Ebers, G. C. (2009). Clinical prognostic factors in multiple sclerosis: A natural history review. *Nature Reviews Neurology, 5*(12), 672–682. Retrieved from http://search.ebscohost.com.libproxy.temple.edu/login.aspx?direct=true&db=cmedm&AN=19953117&site=ehost-live&scope=site

de Lau, L. M., & Breteler, M. (2006). Epidemiology of Parkinson's disease. *The Lancet Neurology, 5*(6), 525-535.

Dennison, L., Moss-Morris, R., & Chalder, T. (2009). A review of psychological correlates of adjustment in patients with multiple sclerosis. *Clinical Psychology Review, 29*(2), 141–153. Retrieved from http://search.ebscohost.com.libproxy.temple.edu/login.aspx?direct=true&db=cmedm&AN=19167801&site=ehost-live&scope=site

Department of Health. (2005). *The National Service Framework for Long-term Conditions.* Retrieved from http://dh.gov.uk/PublicationsAndStatistics/Publications/PublicationsPolicyAndGuidance/PublicationsPolicyAndguidanceArticles/fs/en?CONTENT_ID=4105361&chk=jl7dri

de Sa, J. C. C., Airas, L., Bartholome, E., Grigoriadis, N., Mattle, H., Oreja-Guevara, C., ... Kieseier, B. C. (2011). Symptomatic therapy in multiple sclerosis: a review for a multimodal approach in clinical practice. *Therapeutic advances in neurological disorders, 4*(3), 139-168. Retrieved from http://search.ebscohost.com.libproxy.temple.edu/login.aspx?direct=true&db=cmedm&AN=21694816&site=ehost-live&scope=site

Dileo, C, & Magill, L. (2005). Songwriting with oncology and hospice adult patients from a multicultural perspective. In F. Baker & T. Wigram (Eds.), *Songwriting: Methods, techniques and clinical applications for music therapy clinician's educators and students* (pp. 226–245). Philadelphia, PA: Jessica Kingsley.

Elefant, C., Baker, F., Lotan, M., Krogstie Lagesen, S., & Skeie, G. O. (In press). The effect of group music therapy on mood, speech and singing in individuals with Parkinson's disease —A feasibility study. *Journal of Music Therapy.*

Folstein, S. E. (1989). *Huntington's disease: A disorder of families* (pp. 1-64). Baltimore, MD: Johns Hopkins University Press.

Forrest, L. (2002). Using music therapy in the symptom management of patients with MND. (Conference Proceedings). *Music Therapy in the 21st Century: A Contemporary Force for Change, 10th World Congress of Music Therapy,* 583–601.

Genova, H. M., Sumowski, J. F., Chiaravalloti, N., Voelbel, G. T., & Deluca, J. (2009). Cognition in multiple sclerosis: A review of neuropsychological and fMRI research. *Frontiers in Bioscience: A Journal and Virtual Library, 14,* 1730–1744. Retrieved from http://search.ebscohost.com.libproxy.temple.edu/login.aspx?direct=true&db=cmedm&AN=19273158&site=ehost-live&scope=site

Goldenberg, M. M. (2012). Multiple sclerosis review. *P & T: A Peer-Reviewed Journal of Formulary Management, 37*(3), 175–184. Retrieved from http://search.ebscohost.com.libproxy.temple.edu/login.aspx?direct=true&db=cmedm&AN=22605909&site=ehost-live&scope=site

Haneishi, E. (2001). Effects of a music therapy voice protocol on speech intelligibility, vocal acoustic measures, and mood of individuals with Parkinson's disease. *Journal of Music Therapy, 38(4),* 273–290.

Harper, P. S. (1992). The epidemiology of Huntington's disease. *Human Genetics, 89*(4), 365-376.

Hoskyns, S. (1982). Striking the right chord. *Nursing Mirror, June 2,* 14–17.

Hurkmans, J., de Bruijn, M., Boonstra, A. M., Jonkers, R., Bastiaanse, R., Arendzen, H., & Reinders-Messelink, H. A. (2012). Music in the treatment of neurological language and speech disorders: A systematic review. *Aphasiology, 26*(1), 1-19.

Hustad, K., Beukelman, D., & Yorkston, K. (1998). Functional outcome assessment in dysarthria. *Seminars in Speech and Language,* 19(3), 291–302.

Jankovic, J. (2008). Parkinson's disease: Clinical features and diagnosis. *Journal of Neurology and Neurosurgical Psychiatry,* 79(4), 368–376.

Koscuilek, J. F. (1997). Relationship of family schema to family adaptation to brain injury. *Brain Injury, 11,* 821–830.

Kurtzke, J. F. (1983). Rating neurologic impairment in multiple sclerosis an expanded disability status scale (EDSS). *Neurology, 33*(11), 1444-1452.

Lee, J. (2007). Music therapy with a women who was hurt by a cowboy. *Canadian Journal of Music Therapy, 13*(1), 30–37.

Lengdobler, H. & Kiessling, W. R. (1989). "Gruppenmusiktherapie bei multipler Sklerose: Ein erster Erfahrungsbericht." *Psychotherapie, Psychosomatik, Medizin und Psychologie, 39,* 369–373.

Lillo, P., & Hodges, J. R. (2009). Frontotemporal dementia and motor neurone disease: Overlapping clinic-pathological disorders. *Journal of Clinical Neuroscience: Official Journal of the Neurosurgical Society of Australasia, 16*(9), 1131–1135. Retrieved from http://search.ebscohost.com.libproxy.temple.edu/login.aspx?direct=true&db=cmedm&AN=19556136&site=ehost-live&scope=site

Lillo, P., & Hodges, J. R. (2010). Cognition and behaviour in motor neurone disease. *Current Opinion in Neurology, 23*(6), 638–642. Retrieved from http://search.ebscohost.com.libproxy.temple.edu/login.aspx?direct=true&db=cmedm&AN=20962641&site=ehost-live&scope=site

Lindeck, J. (2005). Music technology—a tool for clinician and community. (Abstract). In *Handbook and Abstracts, 11th World Congress of Music Therapy: From Lullaby to Lament, Brisbane, 2005* (p. 98).

Magee, W. (1999). Music therapy within brain injury rehabilitation: To what extent is our clinical practice influenced by the search for outcomes. *Music Therapy Perspectives, 17*(1), 20-26.

Magee, W. L. (2002). Identity in clinical music therapy: Shifting self-constructs through the therapeutic process. In R. MacDonald, D. J. Hargreaves, & D. Miell (Eds.), *Musical Identities* (pp. 179–197). Oxford: Oxford University Press.

Magee, W. L. (2005). Music therapy with patients in low awareness states: Approaches to assessment and treatment in multidisciplinary care. *Neuropsychological Rehabilitation, 15*3–4), 522–536.

Magee, W. L. (2013). *Music Technology in Therapeutic and Health Settings*. Philadelphia, PA: Jessica Kingsley.

Magee, W. L., & Bowen, C. (2008). Using music in leisure to enhance social relationships with patients with complex disabilities. *NeuroRehabilitation, 23*(4), 305–311.

Magee, W. L., Brumfitt, S. M., Freeman, M., & Davidson, J. W. (2006). The role of music therapy in an interdisciplinary approach to address functional communication in complex neuro-communication disorders: A case report. *Disability and Rehabilitation, 28*(19), 1221–1229.

Magee, W. L., & Davidson, J. W. (2002). The effect of music therapy on mood states in neurological patients: A pilot study. *Journal of Music Therapy, 39*(1), 20–29.

Magee, W. L., & Davidson, J. W. (2004a). Music therapy in multiple sclerosis: Results of a systematic qualitative analysis. *Music Therapy Perspectives, 22*(1), 39–51.

Magee, W. L., & Davidson, J. W. (2004b). Singing in therapy: Monitoring disease process in chronic degenerative illness. *British Journal of Music Therapy, 18*(2), 65–77.

McIntosh, G. C., Brown, S. H., Rice, R. R., & Thaut, M. H. (1997). Rhythmic auditory-motor facilitation of gait patterns in patients with Parkinson's disease. *Journal of Neurology, Neurosurgery & Psychiatry, 62*(1), 22-26.

McLeod, J. E., & Clarke, D. M. (2007). A review of psychosocial aspects of motor neurone disease. *Journal of the Neurological Sciences, 258*(1–2), 4–10. Retrieved from http://search.ebscohost.com.libproxy.temple.edu/login.aspx?direct=true&db=cmedm&AN=17445834&site=ehost-live&scope=site

Millman, R., & Jefferson, R. (2000). *Music Therapy within the multi-disciplinary team: Different approaches—shared goals*. Paper presented at The Annual Conference, British Society for Music Therapy and Association of Professional Music Therapists, 2000.

Nagler, J. (1998). Digital music technology in music therapy practice. In C. Tomaino (Ed.), *Clinical Applications of Music in Neurologic Rehabilitation* (pp. 41–49). St. Louis, MO: Magnamusic-Baton.

Novak, M. J., & Tabrizi, S. J. (2010). Huntington's disease. *British Medical Journal, 340*, c3109.

O'Callaghan, C. (1993). Communicating with brain-injured palliative care patients through music therapy. *Journal of Palliative Care, 9*(4), 53–55.

O'Callaghan, C. (1996). Lyrical themes in songs written by palliative care patients. *Journal of Music Therapy, 33*(2), 74–92.

Oddy, M. (1984) Head injury and social adjustment. In N. Brooks (Ed.), *Closed head injury: Psychological, social and family consequences* (pp. 108–122). Oxford: Oxford University Press.

Özdemir, E., Norton, A., & Schlaug, G. (2006). Shared and distinct neural correlates of singing and speaking. *Neuroimage, 33*(2), 628-635.

Parvizi, J., Arciniegas, D. B., Bernardini, G. L., Hoffmann, M. W., Mohr, J. P., Rapoport, M. J., ... Tuhrim, S. (2006). Diagnosis and management of pathological laughter and crying. *Mayo Clinic Proceedings, 81*(11), 1482-1486.

Poewe, W. (2006). The natural history of Parkinson's disease. *Journal of Neurology, 253*(Suppl 7), VII2–6.

Richards, C. L., Malouin, F., Bedard, P. J., Cioni, M. (1992). Changes in L-dopa and sensory cues on the gait of Parkinsonian patients. In M. Woollacott & F. Horak (Eds.), *Posture and Control Mechanisms, Vol. 2,* 126–128. Eugene, OR: University of Oregon Books.

Samii A., Nutt J.G., & Ransom B.R. (2004). Parkinson's disease. *Lancet, 363*, 1783–1793.

Sathasivam, S. (2010). Motor neurone disease: Clinical features, diagnosis, diagnostic pitfalls and prognostic markers. *Singapore Medical Journal, 51*(5), 367–372. Retrieved from http://search.ebscohost.com.libproxy.temple.edu/login.aspx?direct=true&db=cmedm&AN=20593140&site=ehost-live&scope=site

Sena Moore, K., Peterson, D. A., O'Shea, G., McIntosh, G. C., &Thaut, M. H. (2008). The effectiveness of music as a mnemonic device on recognition memory for people with multiple sclerosis. *Journal of Music Therapy, 45*(3), 307–329.

Schlaug, G., Marchina, S., & Norton, A. (2008). From singing to speaking: Why singing may lead to recovery of expressive language function in patients with Broca's aphasia. *Music Perception, 25*(4), 315 – 323.

Schlaug, G., Norton, A., Marchina, S., Zipse, L., & Wan, C. Y. (2010). From singing to speaking: Facilitating recovery from nonfluent aphasia. *Future neurology, 5*(5), 657-665.

Schmid, W., & Aldridge, D. (2004). Active music therapy in the treatment of multiple sclerosis patients: A matched control study. *Journal of Music Therapy, 41*(3), 225–240.

Schmid, W., Ostermann, T., & Aldridge, D. (2003). Functionality or aesthetics? Music therapy as a component in an integrated medicine approach to the treatment of multiple sclerosis patients. *Music Therapy Today* (online), *6*(5), November 2003. Available at http://musictherapytoday.net

Shoulson, I. (1990). Huntington's disease: Cognitive and psychiatric features. *Cognitive and Behavioral Neurology, 3*(1), 15-22.

Sloboda, J. A. (1991). Music structure and emotional response: Some empirical findings. *Psychology of Music, 19*, 110–120.

Steele, M. (2005). Coping with multiple sclerosis: A music therapy viewpoint. *Australian Journal of Music Therapy, 16*, 70–87.

Tamplin, J. (2006). *Song collage technique: A new approach to songwriting*. Norway: GAMUT, The Grieg Academy Music Therapy Research Centre. DOI: 10.1080/08098130609478164.

Tamplin, J., & Grocke, D. (2008). A music therapy treatment protocol for acquired dysarthria rehabilitation. *Music Therapy Perspectives, 26*(1), 23–29.

Thaut, M. H., & Abiru, M. (2010). Rhythmic auditory stimulation in rehabilitation of movement disorders: A review of current research. *Music Perception, 27*(4), 263-269.

Thaut, M., McIntosh, D., Miltner, R., Lange, H., Hurt, C., & Hoemberg, V. (1999). Velocity modulation and rhythmic synchronization of gait training in Huntington's disease. *Movement Disorders, 14*(5), 808–819.

Thaut, M. H. (2005a). *Rhythm, music and the brain: Scientific foundations and clinical applications.* New York: Taylor & Francis.

Thaut, M. H. (2005b). *Medical coding and records manual: Neurologic music therapy.* Fort Collins, CO: Robert F. Unkefer Academy of Neurologic Music Therapy.

Thaut, M. H., Peterson, D. A., Sena Moore, K., and McIntosh, G. C. (2008). Musical structure facilitates verbal learning in multiple sclerosis. *Music Perception, 25*(4), 325–330.

Tyerman, A. (1996). The social context. In F.D. Rose & D.A. Johnson (Eds.), *Brain injury and after: Towards improved outcome* (pp. 97–118). Chichester, UK: Wiley & Sons.

Chapter 10

Adults with HIV/AIDS

Douglas R. Keith

Diagnostic Information

Acquired Immune Deficiency Syndrome (AIDS) is a potentially fatal, transmittable disease of the human immune system. It is caused by the Human Immunodeficiency Virus (HIV), which attacks the immune system, making it susceptible to infections and cancers. In advanced stages of AIDS, these secondary diseases eventually cause the death of the infected person (www.aids.org).

The Human Immunodeficiency Virus (HIV) is difficult to transmit; casual contact with a person who has HIV does not lead to infection. Instead, HIV is transmitted through body fluids such as blood, semen, vaginal fluid, and breast milk. The virus typically enters the body through mucous membranes, sores, or open wounds, during sexual contact, prenatally, through breast milk, or when using shared needles to inject drugs (www.aids.gov).

People can be tested for HIV at a medical office and in clinics in most cities; in recent years, tests have come on the market for testing at home. Testing positive for HIV, however, does not mean that the person has AIDS. The disease goes through multiple stages, from initial infection to what is commonly referred to as "full-blown AIDS" (Progression from HIV to AIDS, 2007). Medical professionals identify the different stages of AIDS by measuring the level of cells that fight infections (CD4 cells) or, in places where this is not possible, by reviewing the patient's current and past health history (www.aidsetc.org). This process of clinical staging gives a sense of the health problems that occur in the phases of HIV/AIDS.

The World Health Organization (WHO) measures the progression of AIDS according to measures of CD4+ T cells (cells that fight infections) and viral load (density of HIV particles in the blood). When the number of CD4 cells drops below a critical level (often around or below 200 CD4+ T cells per microliter (μL)), symptoms of opportunistic infections will appear (World Health Organization, 2010). While different organizations use different categories or levels of disease, the following list gives a sense of the trajectory of the disease from primary infection through the end of life.

Stages of HIV/AIDS

Primary HIV Infection: During the first four to eight weeks after infection, the body has not yet developed antibodies to reduce the amount of HIV in the body. Patients may develop flu symptoms such as fever, headache, and sore throat, but also enlarged lymph nodes and skin rash. These symptoms do not last long. During this phase, patients are highly infectious.

Silent Stage: During this stage, patients are typically asymptomatic. Although patients may not have many symptoms, the virus continues to attack the immune system. This phase can last several years, especially if the patient is undergoing antiretroviral treatment.

Minor Phase: Here, the weakened immune system allows minor conditions and complications to appear. For example, some patients experience swelled lymph nodes. Other symptoms include:

- Lack of energy
- Frequent fevers and sweats
- Persistent or frequent thrush infections (mouth or genital areas)
- Persistent skin rashes
- Recurrent mouth ulcers

Symptomatic Phase: The immune system finds it more and more difficult to defend against HIV. The viral load increases. Symptoms are more severe, including more serious and persistent infections listed above, as well as:

- Constant occurrence of herpes sores
- Fungal diseases of the tongue
- Chronic bacterial skin infections
- Chronic diarrhea and weight loss (more than 10% of body weight)

Full-Blown AIDS: With full-blown AIDS, patients are vulnerable to opportunistic infections and cancers. Symptoms of previous phases continue and become more severe, chronic, or persistent. Brain damage can occur, causing severe headaches, poor concentration, and memory loss. Many patients go blind at this stage.

Terminal and Final Stage: Here, patients alternate between short periods of relative health and severe illness. However, death typically occurs within three years of developing full-blown AIDS. In most cases, patients die of AIDS-related diseases, not of AIDS itself (Progression from HIV to AIDS, 2007).

In addition to the symptoms listed above, HIV can affect the central nervous system (CNS) directly. There, it may cause damage while leaving other body systems relatively intact. In the CNS, HIV can cause dysfunctions of motor, cognition, and behavior, but disease patterns are difficult to predict. Some of the symptoms include:

- Motor Dysfunction
    - Unsteady gait
    - Tremors
    - Poor hand coordination
    - Balance instability
- Cognition
    - Short attention span
    - Memory loss
    - Poor judgment
    - Slowed thinking
- Behavioral
    - Slowed task completion
    - Social withdrawal
    - Depression
    - Mood swings
    - Psychosis (in late stages)

Because of the way HIV affects the CNS, some patients with HIV/AIDS need mental health care across the entire span of the disease.

History of the Disease

Most research points to Africa as the "ground zero" of HIV/AIDS. Researchers have discovered an HIV sequence in a sample taken from a patient living in the Congo in 1959 (Zho, Korber, Nahmias, Hooper, Sharp, & Ho, 1998). The first patients with symptoms of AIDS in North America appeared in 1981. Doctors treated numbers of gay men with Kaposi's Sarcoma and pneumonia (Centers for Disease Control, 1981), diseases that are either rare or easily cured in otherwise healthy adults. Soon thereafter, intravenous drug users (Masur et al., 1981), people from Haiti (Centers for Disease Control, 1982a), and hemophiliacs (CDC, 1982b) also sought treatment with the same symptoms. In 1982, the name "AIDS" was created (CDC, 1982c). Around this time, women and heterosexual men also became ill, indicating the limitless potential threat of the disease.

Recognizing the need for a means of treating this disease, or at least identify it, researchers began studying its symptomology, transmission patterns, and disease progression. It became apparent that a virus was the root of the problem in the early 1980s. Worldwide, multiple instances of the virus were isolated, and in 1985 a screening test for blood supplied became available (Pear, 1985). In 1986, the International Committee on the Taxonomy of Viruses ruled that HIV was the official name of the virus that causes AIDS (Coffin et al., 1986). In the same year, the first drug that showed any effectiveness, azidothymidine (AZT), was tested and brought to market.

While HIV causes AIDS, other factors affect the disease trajectory from infection onward, including socioeconomics. When the first medications for HIV/AIDS became available, they were expensive, and many insurance plans did not cover them. As a result, a significant number of people with HIV/AIDS became homeless.

In the early 1990s, new antiretroviral drugs were brought to market for patients who did not tolerate the original drug (Food & Drug Administration, n.d.). The disease continued to spread worldwide, and in 1995, a cumulative total of one million cases had been reported to the World Health Organization (1995). In the US, the CDC announced that AIDS was the leading cause of death for adults ages 25 to 44 (Altman, 1995). In the same year, the first protease inhibitor, saquinivir, came to market (Schwartz, 1995). Researchers discovered that medication combinations were more effective than AZT alone at delaying disease and prolonging life (Priority Press, 1995). These combinations of antiretrovirals (and sometimes protease inhibitors) came to be called Highly Active Antiretroviral Therapy (HAART). HAART provided powerful new tools that worked together to delay disease onset and improve life dramatically for people with HIV/AIDS. These "drug cocktails" required strict adherence to be effective.

Drug treatment for AIDS was not without problems. Some people experienced side effects (diarrhea, lipodystrophy) from the drugs, and the virus continued to mutate, rendering some medications ineffective. However, other treatment approaches were discovered, including providing AZT to pregnant women at the time of birth, which dramatically reduces the spread of HIV from mother to infant, especially when the infant is delivered by caesarean section (Mandelbrot et al., 1998). People who were possibly exposed to HIV were given medications as soon as possible after exposure. This prophylaxis was determined to reduce the likelihood of seroconversion ("New experimental morning-after," 1988).

As of 2010, the World Health Organization estimated that approximately 34 million people worldwide were living with HIV. Approximately 2.5 million people were newly infected with HIV in that year, and approximately 1.7 million people died of AIDS. Statistics from the World Health Organization indicate high variation among its six world regions: the bulk of HIV infections at this time are in Africa.

This correlates with cultural behaviors and the high poverty in many African countries (World Health Organization, 2011a).

Life expectancy has changed substantially since the development of HAART, but it varies depending on several factors. Patients who are infected by intravenous drug use, in general, have a shorter life expectancy than others. Women infected with HIV have a longer life expectancy than men, and, most important, patients who maintain a high CD4 count have the highest life expectancy (The Antiretroviral Cohort Collaboration, 2008). Patients who are able to maintain a high CD4 count, and for whom effective HAART regimens can be found, can, in some cases, live a normal life span.

The causes of death for people with HIV also vary substantially worldwide. In general, they track with poverty, that is, people with HIV in poor countries tend to die of diseases or conditions that are associated with poverty, and people in wealthy countries tend to die of diseases or conditions associated with relative wealth. The top five of death for people with HIV in low-, middle-, and high-income countries are cancer, dementia, or lower respiratory infections. (World Health Organization, 2011b).

According to the National Coalition for the Homeless (2009a), HIV/AIDS is more common among people who are homeless (3.4%) than in the general population (0.4%). The elevated prevalence of infection combined with limited access to treatment and poor living conditions have contributed to HIV/AIDS becoming a leading cause of death in this population. The association between homelessness and HIV appears to be a two-way street. People with HIV are at greater risk of homelessness due to discrimination and the high costs of housing and medical care. At the same time, homeless people have an elevated risk of contracting HIV (Center for AIDS Prevention Studies, 2005). People who are homeless also commonly have other comorbidities, including psychiatric disorders such as schizophrenia, post-traumatic stress disorder, and bipolar disorder.

Applications of music therapy with AIDS have changed significantly as AIDS itself has changed. In the early years of the epidemic, music therapy predominantly addressed goals common to palliative care, i.e., those associated with the final stages of life, including emotional acceptance, pain reduction, and quality of life (Maranto, 1988). However, since the development of protease inhibitors, people with AIDS have been surviving much longer and are leading healthier lives with fewer infections. The places where music therapists work with people with AIDS have also changed; certainly music therapists still encounter people with AIDS in hospice settings, but other models of health care, including day treatment for adults (Ghetti, 2004), are now treating people with AIDS. Music therapy can now focus on long-term (mental health) goals more closely associated with chronic conditions than with terminal illness.

Needs and Resources

Because of the wide variation within the population of people with HIV/AIDS, it is impossible to describe their needs and resources in a general way. What they all have in common is the virus, and the virus does not discriminate against any group of people. Thus, music therapists working with people with HIV/AIDS should conduct as thorough an assessment as possible.

Physical

Depending on the disease stage, people with HIV/AIDS may have few or many physical needs and symptoms. Shortly after infection (typically before diagnosis and treatment), some people experience symptoms such as cramps, nausea, enlarged lymph nodes, fever, headache, joint pain, and weight loss. These are associated with so-called "acute retroviral syndrome," the first stage of infection. Notably, not all people experience this syndrome after being infected.

One of the most important factors affecting the health of people with HIV/AIDS is their adherence to a regimen of drugs (the so-called "drug cocktail"). After obtaining a diagnosis and beginning (and adhering to) treatment, patients typically rarely experience opportunistic infections and are able to recover well from health problems such as flu, etc. Patients who do not enter treatment (or do not adhere to the treatment regimen) eventually enter a chronic phase, where the virus continues to grow in the body and the immune system weakens. Chronic HIV disease can have various physical symptoms, often associated with opportunistic infections (e.g., thrush, cold sores, cervical cancer, swollen lymph nodes). With patients in later stages of the disease, or who are not adherent to the drug regimen, music therapists can expect to see more serious physical problems, including pneumonia and types of cancer that are common among people with weakened immune systems. Some patients experience neurological disorders, including neuropathy and, in some cases, dementia.

Emotional

The diagnosis of HIV, for most people, comes as a surprise. This new reality affects many areas of people's lives, including some of the most intimate ones, and carries implications for the rest of the patient's life and for the patient's family. Emotional reactions can include shock, anger, fear (of isolation, of death), denial, and worries about infecting others. Because of the combined stress of diagnosis and (frequent) social marginalization, HIV-positive patients show a greater prevalence than other populations of psychosocial adjustment reactions and psychiatric problems such as depression and anxiety (Chesney & Folkman, 1994; Levine, Bystritsky, Baron, & Jones, 1991). Patients with HIV/AIDS are at high risk for suicide (www.hivguidelines.org) due to isolation, depression, and despair, and psychosocial factors may contribute to progression of HIV-related infections (Kemeny, 1998; Soloman, Temoshok, O'Leary, & Zich, 1987). An additional concern regarding "coming out" as HIV-positive: "Whom do I tell?" Emotional support (in the form of counseling) for people who test positive for HIV has two main foci: prevention of further infections and support of the patient (Chippendale & French, 2001). Emotional support for patients is linked with improved health, in terms of both medical adherence and psychological well-being (Horberg et al., 2007).

Social

The "face of AIDS" has changed substantially since the disease first came into public awareness. During the early 1980s, the majority of persons who had HIV/AIDS were gay men and intravenous drug users, groups who were already marginalized in society. Since then, HIV/AIDS has affected a much broader swath of society, reducing the marginalization effect to some degree. Since the development of HAART in the mid-1990s, more and more people have had access to treatment, including those from traditionally hard-to-reach client groups, including the inner-city poor. In 2009, nearly 65% of all new HIV infections in the US affected African-Americans and Hispanics (Centers for Disease Control, 2011a, 2011b). There is a higher rate of poverty among these populations, and correlations between poverty and risk of HIV risk have been documented (Denning & DiNenno, 2010). In Canada, indigenous people (First Nations, Inuit, Métis) are similarly disproportionately represented (Canadian Aboriginal AIDS Network, 2009).

In other areas of the world (e.g., sub-Saharan Africa), people with HIV/AIDS are often still stigmatized and outcast from their communities. This may lead to far poorer health prognoses, as patients are reluctant to obtain a formal diagnosis and seek medical care because of the stigmatization that is associated with HIV (Mbonu, van den Borne, & De Vries, 2009).

People who are socioeconomically marginalized often do not have access to regular medical care until they test positive for HIV. They may encounter music therapy when in hospice (Bunt, 1994), in day treatment (Ghetti, 2004), in street outreach programs (Smith, 2007), or in other settings. These new clients present new challenges to music therapists, some of which seem less related to their diagnosis of HIV/AIDS than to other comorbidities, including drug use and psychiatric problems. However, it is usually HIV/AIDS that brings these clients to treatment.

Given the current demographics of HIV/AIDS, music therapists should take cultural differences into consideration. Persons with HIV/AIDS may come from complicated family histories, involving neglect or abuse, or they may come from relatively intact and safe households. It is likely that many persons with HIV/AIDS did not have access to as much formal education; they may distrust institutions and persons in authority and have had little health care knowledge and practice. Many people with HIV/AIDS have a history of homelessness; given that 20%–25% of people who are homeless also have a diagnosed mental illness (National Coalition for the Homeless, 2009b), it is common to work with clients who also have a psychiatric disorder.

Spiritual

The emotional adjustment that follows diagnosis of HIV often brings up spiritual issues for patients. Many patients experience feelings of guilt about becoming infected, and some may experience social isolation from their communities of support and families. At this time, they may need to draw on spiritual resources to cope with this change.

Through the course of the disease, patients may have spiritual needs, but these come up more frequently in later disease stages, when patients are near the end of their life. Some patients experience loss of support from family, friends, and loved ones, and will need substantial spiritual support in end-of-life care. However, in some cities the legacy remains of the support that the gay and lesbian community showed during the early years of the epidemic. There and elsewhere, it is just as common for people with HIV/AIDS to experience great spiritual support throughout the disease process.

Musical Resources and Needs

Like any clients, persons with HIV/AIDS bring their own cultural influences to music therapy, including music traditions and styles common in their cultural communities. Music therapists are well advised to be familiar with a broad range of musical styles, performers, and genres when working with such a variable population, because it can make demands on the musical resources of any person. Some patients enjoy playing music, while others do not. Some enjoy listening to music of a particular genre, while others do not. It is simply impossible to generalize, even based on ethnic background, because making assumptions about clients' musical preferences based on ethnicity is bound to lead to misunderstandings. Again, however, given the current demographics, many people with AIDS whom music therapists encounter will have little formal musical training, because of the low educational attainment associated with homelessness and poverty. Informal musical training, however, may be quite common even in disadvantaged communities.

Referral and Assessment

Referral and assessment procedures differ substantially depending on the treatment setting in which people with HIV/AIDS receive music therapy services. In the first years of the disease, patients with AIDS were treated in hospitals and in hospices. At that time, medical treatment focused on the secondary infections that inevitably attacked the patient, bypassing the compromised immune system. In many large cities in the developed world, citizens banded together to support and care for people living with the disease and to protest government inaction in the face of a growing crisis. In the US, these groups included Act Up (nationwide), the Gay Men's Health Crisis (New York), Project Inform (San Francisco), the AIDS Foundation of Chicago, AID Atlanta, and the AIDS Project of Los Angeles. In Great Britain, the Terrance Higgins Trust and AVERT took on a similar function, while in Germany, a series of health education centers called "AIDS-Hilfe" (AIDS Assistance) developed in cities across that country. There is scant record of music therapists working with people with AIDS from the early years of the AIDS epidemic, but they would likely have used assessment and referral procedures of the settings where they worked. Bruscia's case study of a client with AIDS (1991) took place in an outpatient music therapy practice. The client was self-referred, and Bruscia's assessment procedures were based in the practice of GIM.

After the introduction of antiretroviral medications, when people with AIDS began to survive for longer periods, treatment shifted to outpatient and medical day treatment programs, designed to meet the changing needs of clients, including housing, educational, and long-term health care needs. There are no standardized assessment tools for music therapists working with people with AIDS. Instead, music therapists should assess these patients or clients according to the standards of the setting where music therapy treatment takes place. These settings correspond roughly to the stage or phase of the disease. In all cases, comorbidities should be assessed.

In the time directly after infection, emotional and social needs are prominent, and music therapists may encounter patients in mental health care and assess patients accordingly, focusing on emotional and social needs. Comorbidities here may include mood disorders, adjustment disorders, and other similar problems associated with significant life change.

During times where HIV is relatively latent, adherence issues may be prominent, and music therapists may encounter patients in outpatient or drop-in centers, where they should assess issues that affect adherence, such as substance use and social support. Comorbidities here may include those associated with homelessness and social marginalization.

Later, when patients have developed more physical symptoms associated with HIV/AIDS, medical needs become prominent, and music therapists may encounter patients in inpatient or community medical settings, where they may assess things such as pain management and quality of life.

Overview of Methods and Procedures

This chapter addresses music therapy for adults who have HIV/AIDS. Therapists should realize, though, that not every technique is equally useful for each individual or group. These methods and procedures have not been sequenced to reflect relative significance, effectiveness, or complexity. General procedures for presenting each of the methods will be described along with the methods. It is important to follow the protocols of the treatment team or facility.

Receptive Music Therapy

- Lyric Analysis: Clients listen to recorded music and examine its lyrical content and their own responses to it.
- Music Listening for Relaxation: Clients listen to selected music for purposes of relaxation, usually preceded by a progressive relaxation experience of some kind.
- Unguided Music and Imagery: The client listens to music in a relaxed state. At the beginning, the therapist works with the client to choose a focus or theme, but does not interact with the client during the music imagery.

- Guided Imagery and Music: The client listens to music in a relaxed state while the therapist and music work together to support the client's imagery experience throughout.

Improvisational Music Therapy

- Drum Circle: Clients play percussion instruments together to a basic beat or "groove."
- Individual Improvisation: The client creates improvisations using instruments, the voice, or other sound sources (e.g., body percussion). The therapist may or may not improvise with the client.
- Group Instrumental Improvisation: Clients improvise together as a group, in dyads, or as soloists within a group. The therapist typically provides an idea or theme for the improvisations.

Re-creative Music Therapy

- Jam Session: Small groups of clients function like a band, using instruments and vocal styles appropriate to different genres (R&B, heavy metal, hip-hop, etc.) to make music. Often, the therapist may play a significant role in leading.
- Group Singing: Clients sing songs together as a group. These are frequently well-known songs, without a steep learning curve. The therapist typically plays a significant role in providing accompaniment and other structure (e.g., guiding the song selection process).
- Talent Show: Clients showcase their musical (and possibly other) skills in front of groups of peers or the public.

Compositional Music Therapy

- Song Parody: Clients write their own lyrics to pre-existing songs, which may be familiar or unfamiliar.
- Song as Life Story: Clients develop the lyrics and/or musical materials to wrong songs about their lives. The therapist provides structural and organizational support as needed.

Guidelines for Receptive Music Therapy

In receptive music therapy, the therapist engages clients in any kind of listening experience. The experience may focus on physical, emotional, intellectual, aesthetic, or spiritual aspects of the music, and the client may respond through activities such as relaxation or meditation, action sequences, structured or free movement, perceptual tasks, free association, storytelling, drawing or painting, dramatizing, reminiscing, imaging, etc. The music used for such experiences may be live or recorded improvisations, performances or compositions by the client or therapist, or commercial recordings of music literature in various styles (e.g., classical, popular, rock, jazz, country, spiritual, New Age, etc.) (Bruscia, 1998, p. 121).

Lyric Analysis

Overview. In lyric analysis, clients listen to recorded music and examine its lyrical content and their own responses to it. Lyric analysis represents a spectrum of receptive music therapy experiences used with clients with many different diagnoses. These experiences all focus on the lyrics of songs, but music therapists can implement them in a variety of ways, depending on the needs of clients. In terms of use with people with HIV/AIDS, lyric analysis is indicated for clients with good receptive and expressive language skills, particularly for those who need to adjust to reality, attain self-awareness, or learn to relate to others. Ideally, clients should be literate, but this is not a requirement for all versions of lyric analysis.

Goals of lyric analysis include improving reality orientation, identifying problems, improving social skills, and increasing emotional awareness. Depending on the focus of the experience, lyric analysis may occur on the augmentative or intensive level of music therapy.

Clients with very concrete language and little symbolic thought (typically correlated with lower intellectual capacity or severe mental illness) may become confused during lyric analysis experiences. The symbolic language of song lyrics may confuse clients with cognitive limitations. Lyric analysis experiences may be adapted for these clients, but the music therapist should consider these factors carefully, especially in music therapy groups.

Preparation. Prepare for a lyric analysis session by reviewing any information available on the client(s). Lyric analysis is most commonly used in group settings, and while it is not always possible to predict who will attend, it is helpful to have a series of songs and lyrics appropriate for different themes and different purposes.

Provide high-quality stereo equipment to listen to the music. Clients should be able to hear and understand the song and its lyrics. Prepare lyric sheets for all group members or use a projector. Often, lyric sheets are useful tools for clients to write down thoughts.

What to observe. Observe body language, affect, and interactions by clients. Can the clients understand the song lyrics of the recorded music? How are they reacting to the lyrics? What is happening among clients in the group during music listening?

Procedures. The essential steps in lyric analysis include selecting song(s) for focus, providing lyric sheets, asking clients to read lyrics, listening to song(s), and discussion. The order of these steps depends to some degree on the version of lyric analysis being practiced.

In some versions, music therapists may choose to listen to the song without asking clients to read the lyrics first. The order will depend on the purpose or goals of this music therapy experience. When clients look at lyrics first, the experience can become more concrete and cognitive, because clients may listen to see if the lyrics they hear match those that they are reading. By contrast, when clients listen first, the experience may access emotional content more readily.

Adaptations. This section includes descriptions of several adaptations or versions of lyric analysis. It is possible to shift from one adaptation to another in the course of a single music listening experience, depending on the needs of the client or group.

1) *Topic Discussion:* A topic discussion of lyrics is indicated for clients who are new to a group, or a new group entirely. It is a less personal approach to lyric analysis, and encourages discussion of an external topic, rather than personal issues. Goals include improving reality orientation, encouraging group cohesion, and developing trust. Topic discussions are commonly on the augmentative level of therapy. Prepare by developing lists of songs around specific topics. Topics may be physical and external (e.g., the seasons) or emotional and internal (e.g., a feeling). Bring lyric sheets and recordings of one or more songs around a specific topic for discussion. During the session, shift

between phases of listening and reading/discussion lyrics. In each phase, the focus is on the topics in the song(s), with questions such as "What is this song about?" Sample song lists are:

- Topic: Seasons
  - "California Dreamin'" (The Mamas and the Papas)
  - "Hazy Shade of Winter" (Simon & Garfunkel)
  - "In the Summertime" (Mungo Jerry)
  - "On This Winter's Night" (Lady Antebellum)
  - "See You in the Spring" (Courtyard Hounds)
- Topic: Happiness
  - "Beauty in the World" (Macy Gray)
  - "Pursuit of Happiness" (Kid Cudi)
  - "Happiness" (Alexis Jordan)
  - "Promise of a New Day" (Paula Abdul)
  - "Uptight" (Stevie Wonder)

2) *Keywords:* This experience is indicated for clients who are ready for a slightly more personal and self-revealing experience. Goals include increasing emotional awareness and self-confidence. Keywords may take place on the augmentative or intensive level of therapy. To prepare, select a song that is appropriate for the group and provide lyric sheets and pens or pencils to the clients. During the session, play a recording of the song and ask the clients to underline or circle any words or phrases that stand out to them or that mean something significant to them. After hearing the recording, ask clients to take turns stating which words or phrases they identified. The music therapist can begin to generate a discussion about what the clients identified and whether these words or phrases reveal anything. A natural progression from this point might lead to the music therapist asking clients to connect these keywords to their own lives.
3) *Compare and Connect:* This adaptation involves listening to and comparing song lyrics of two or more songs. Goals include increasing emotional awareness and enhancing trust among group members. "Compare and Connect" is likely on the augmentative level of therapy, but in some cases may move into the intensive level. Listen to one song, with lyrics, then another, ideally with a related theme. For example, the songs "Landslide" (Fleetwood Mac) and "Day After Day" (Julian Lennon) both contain themes about changes in close relationships. The group can discuss similarities and differences in the music content and emotional content of the two songs. This can lead to a fruitful discussion that may identify different ways of expressing emotions.
4) *What Is the Singer Saying?* This adaptation is indicated for clients who are able to understand not only their own attitudes and feelings, but also those of others, which is the focus of this experience. Goals include developing empathy and improving self-awareness. "What Is the Singer Saying?" is likely practiced on the augmentative or intensive level of therapy. Select a song appropriate for the group and provide lyric sheets for the clients. For example, in the song "Somewhere I Belong" (Linkin Park), the lyrics are about belonging. Listen to the song together and ask the clients to write down their comments or reactions to the song. Afterward, discuss with the clients what the singer or songwriter was saying and what that might say about any people depicted in the song. What is their world like? An

extension of this experience could involve clients and therapist together researching the history of a song, to gain a better understanding of its origins and potential meanings.

Music Listening for Relaxation

Overview. With this technique, clients listen to selected music for purposes of relaxation, usually preceded by a progressive relaxation experience of some kind. Depending on the needs of the clients, its contraindications will differ. Generally, this type of practice is on the augmentative level. This section contains general guidelines for using music listening for relaxation, with adaptations of specific types.

There are few strict contraindications for music listening for purposes of relaxation. Most people listen to music for this purpose on their own; the music therapist, in this case, adapts the experience to the needs of the clients in the group.

One of the first steps in determining what type of relaxation experience is appropriate for the clients has to do with clients' reality orientation. Clients with weak reality orientation or who are actively psychotic should participate only in a highly structured, concrete type of music relaxation experience. Focus on concrete elements of the experience, such as breathing and tensing/releasing muscle groups. Do not let the music play for long times without accompanying the client verbally.

Another consideration is level of pain. If clients are experiencing pain, make adjustments during the progressive muscle relaxation as needed. This might mean that it would be better to use a relaxation protocol that does not include tensing and releasing the muscles, but instead uses imagery of light or of the breath helping every part of the body to relax.

One possible true contraindication is for some clients on methadone treatment, because these clients often simply fall asleep during the experience. Relaxation experiences are not indicated for these clients, because they do not need to relax.

Preparation. Prepare for relaxation experiences by choosing a progressive (muscle) relaxation and music that are appropriate for the group. Typically, instrumental music without the human voice is preferred, because people tend to focus more on a singer and the lyrics being sung, instead of focusing on their body and state of relaxation. Choose music with few dynamic, tempo, or timbre changes for the same reason: helping clients focus on themselves. "New Age" music may be a preferred style for many clients. In terms of the space, provide comfortable areas for the client(s) to sit or lie down and a quality stereo system. The room should be free of outside distractions.

What to observe. Observe individual and social behavior by clients.

1) What is their affect?
    - When clients have a neutral or negative affect, consider including positive messages in the progressive muscle relaxation, such as "Notice how good it feels when your muscles relax" or "Feel the support of the floor beneath you and know that it will continue to support you."
    - Does the music selected reinforce negative fillings? For example, is it in a mode that clients associate with sadness? What is the tempo? Does the instrumentation include elements that suggest sadness, such as bells tolling?
2) Do clients interact with one another verbally or nonverbally?
    - Consider how well they know you and each other. Is the atmosphere one of trust?
    - Establish trust during the initial moments of the session.
    - Speak in a way that engenders confidence in what the clients are about to experience.

3) How are clients responding to familiar and unfamiliar elements of the experience.
    - During the music, observe their physical posture and body movements for signs of the relaxation response.
    - After the music experience, is there any observable change in their affect, body posture, or behavior?

Procedures. Music for relaxation experiences generally include the following steps

1) Check-in
    - Ask clients how they are doing that day.
    - Ask clients about their stress levels. If helpful, use a simple stress scale to increase awareness.
    - Ask if clients are experiencing pain.
    - Remind group that they can participate on the level they feel comfortable.
    - Remind group to be respectful toward members of the group.
2) Relaxation Experience
    - Begin the music chosen for the experience.
    - Ask clients to close their eyes, if they are comfortable
    - Ask clients to focus on their breathing.
    - Step by step, ask clients to focus their attention on areas of the body.
        - Option 1: Focus only on large sections of the body (limbs, torso, head).
        - Option 2: Focus on midsize sections of the body (foot, lower leg, upper leg, waist, chest, upper arm, etc.).
        - Option 3: Focus on small sections of the body (toes, foot, ankle, calf, thigh, etc.).
    - Allow the music to continue playing and observe the clients.
3) Closure. When the music ends, allow a short time for the clients to realize the music has ended and then bring them back to normal consciousness. For clients who do not respond on their own, a countdown may be helpful. For example, say, "I will count down from 5 to 0."

    5: "Notice how you feel in this relaxed state."
    4: "Gently move your fingers and toes."
    3: "Begin to become more aware of the room where we started."
    2: "Gently move your arms, legs, and head."
    1: "Open your eyes."
    0: "Come to full awareness."

Adaptations. There is not one way to use music for relaxation experiences in music therapy sessions. Below are several possible adaptations that therapists may use, dependent on the settings, needs of the client, and clinical goals.

1) Visualization: The goal of visualization is to enhance relaxation, and it is usually practiced on the auxiliary or augmentative level. Grocke and Wigram (2007) include a thorough explanation of this approach, including sample materials. Begin the visualization experience with a short relaxation induction, focusing on the breath and rhythm of breathing. Play the selected music along with this induction. In some cases, the music may follow the induction (e.g., if the clients have difficulty hearing the music therapist, or the music is too short to cover the induction as well). Next, speak the visualization image

chosen for the session. For example: *"Imagine one of your favorite places in nature. This could be a beach, a forest, a mountain, a field—anywhere you want to go. Allow the music to take you there. While you are there, look around and see what you can see. Be sure to find a comfortable place to sit down and enjoy the view. The music will accompany you while you are there, and at the end I will bring you back to the room."* After presenting the image, allow the music to continue and observe the clients. When the music ends, bring the visualization to an end. For example, say, "The music has ended; allow your image to fade, and come back to the room where we started." For clients who do not respond to this open invitation, try counting down from 10 or 5 to 0, gradually bringing clients back to normal consciousness. When clients have all returned to normal consciousness, some may want to discuss the experience. If there is time, and if this is appropriate, do so. If the music therapy session includes further experiences, transition to them at this point. If the session is over, the clients may leave in a relaxed state.

2) Directed Music Imaging (Bruscia, 1998; Grocke & Wigram, 2007) is a lengthier imagery experience that could be considered an adaptation or extension of visualization. Whereas visualization uses a brief, static image, directed music imaging uses a lengthier script that takes the client on a journey, guided by the therapist. In individual cases, the music therapist may write an individualized script for the client. Music for directed music imaging should be longer and appropriate for the script selected.

Unguided Music and Imagery

Overview. Unguided music and imagery occurs as a client listens to music in a relaxed state. At the beginning, the therapist works with the client to choose a focus or theme but does not interact with the client during the music imagery. Unguided music and imagery (Bruscia, 1998; Grocke & Wigram, 2007) is indicated for clients who are capable of symbolic thinking, who can distinguish between symbolic thinking and reality, who can communicate symbolic inner experiences, and who would benefit from imagery experiences (Grocke & Wigram, 2007, p. 136). Goals of unguided music and imagery include accessing unconscious material and achieving personal insight. This practice is on the augmentative or intensive level of therapy. Like most imagery experiences, unguided music and imagery is contraindicated for clients with weak reality orientation and clients who are actively psychotic.

Preparation. Unguided music and imagery is an approach suitable for individual therapy. Prepare by becoming familiar with the background and current health status of the client. Unguided music and imagery can take place in many types of settings, from hospital rooms to private practice, but the client needs to be in a comfortable seated or reclining position. In all cases, quality music playback equipment is required.

What to observe. Observe the client's emotional state, as indicated by facial affect, body posture, and any communication. Observe the client's physical state during imagery for any signs of discomfort, fear, or other negative emotional experiences that may occur as a result of the imagery.

Procedures. First, discuss a focus or theme for the imagery experience; a focus often helps clients engage in imagery and helps the music therapist proceed with the next steps. Next, decide what music to use. The client may state a preference, or the therapist may make a selection based on discussion up to this point.

Conduct a relaxation induction. For most unguided imagery experiences, a short induction is appropriate. At the end of the induction, transition the client verbally into the imagery experience. For example, the therapist may say "... and now, focus your attention on ________ and allow the music to guide you." During the music imaging experience, attend to the client's body movements or changes in facial expression.

When the music has finished, allow a moment and then bring the imagery experience to an end by using language such as "the music has ended ... allow your consciousness to return to the room ...." Bring the client out of the relaxed state gently, by encouraging gentle stretching.

Finally, discuss the imaging experience with the client, allowing a few minutes before beginning this discussion. Use open-ended questions, focusing on the experience and possibly how the music affected the experience. Some music therapists ask clients to create a drawing of the imaging experience.

Adaptations. Group music and imagery (Bruscia, 1998; Grocke & Wigram, 2007) can be considered an adaptation of unguided music and imagery. Unguided group imagery experiences are typically designed for a group with a shared identity; certainly this adaptation is possible for adults with HIV. The procedures include the following specific adaptations:

1) Assess the suitability of group members for this method, particularly focusing on the ability to respect others and not be disruptive.
2) Start with a group discussion and determine a theme for the group session. Facilitate a discussion of the theme, summarize the views of the group, and suggest a focus for imagery.
3) During the induction, ask clients to focus on their own feelings, reminding them to let others take care of any distractions.
4) Because the music cannot be adjusted to individuals, bring the attention of group members to the focus and ask them to allow the music to enter the image and to allow the image to change as needed.
5) After the music ends, gently bring group members back to a normal waking state, possibly reminding some members of the physical and social location (e.g., in a group meeting room).
6) Monitor the group's experience and check in after imagery to be sure the clients are leaving the session in a "safe" state of mind.
7) In some cases, discuss the imagery or allow the clients to draw (e.g., mandala drawings) from their imagery (Grocke & Wigram, 2007, pp. 140–141).

Guided Imagery and Music (GIM)

Overview. In GIM, a client listens to music in a relaxed state while the therapist and music work together to support the client's imagery experience throughout the listening experience. Guided imagery and music (GIM) is typically an individual music therapy approach, indicated for music therapy clients who wish to pursue a form of music psychotherapy. Summer (1988) described the characteristics of clients suitable for GIM: capable of symbolic thinking, able to differentiate between symbolic thinking and reality, able to relate experiences to the therapist, and likely to achieve positive growth as a result of GIM therapy (Summer, 1988, p. 32).

The goals of GIM are those typically associated with (music) psychotherapy and may include "greater self-awareness, the resolution of inner conflicts, emotional release, self-expression, changes in emotions and attitudes, improved interpersonal skills, the resolution of interpersonal problems, the development of healthy relationships, the healing of emotional traumas, deeper insight, reality orientation, cognitive restructuring, behavior change, greater meaning and fulfillment in life, or spiritual development" (Bruscia, 1998, pp. 1–2). Specific goals in Guided Imagery and Music are typically determined in conjunction with the client.

Because GIM is a form of psychotherapy, it is typically practiced at the intensive level, although in some cases, it may function at the primary level of therapy. On both of these levels, GIM is offered in an individual setting, and is not typically part of a group treatment program. Music therapists should be aware of the important differences between GIM and other similar receptive music therapy practices. Music therapists working with clients with HIV/AIDS should consider carefully the suitability of this approach for the setting in which they work. Possible GIM goal areas for people with HIV include identity issues, identifying internal and external supports, and improving mental health.

Clients who have severe personality disorganization or who have a diagnosis of schizophrenia or another disorder that severely affects their relationship to reality should not participate in GIM because it is dangerous for their psychological health. In general, GIM is indicated for clients who are relatively healthy, psychologically speaking.

Preparation. GIM requires advanced training. Information on training is available from the Association for Music and Imagery (www.ami-bonnymethod.org).

Adaptations. Guided Imagery and Music is practiced on a spectrum, and its practice varies according to therapeutic goals, client functioning levels, level of therapy, and individual vs. group setting. It is worth mentioning that music imagery experiences can be very beneficial and appropriate for small groups. Music therapists should bear in mind that it is more difficult to manage and contain client behaviors in a group. Therefore, it is even more important to assess clients' emotional status during the initial check-in with a group.

Guidelines for Improvisational Music Therapy

In improvisational music therapy, clients "make up" music while playing or singing, extemporaneously creating a melody, rhythm, song, or instrumental piece. Clients may improvise "solos" or participate in a duet, trio, or ensemble, which also includes the therapist, relatives, or other clients. Clients may use their voice or any musical instrument of choice within their capability (e.g., drums, cymbal, xylophone, autoharp, melodica, piano). The therapist helps clients to improvise by creating an ongoing musical accompaniment that stimulates or guides clients' sound productions; presenting clients with a musical theme or structure upon which to base the improvisation (e.g., a rhythm, melody, scale, form); or presenting a nonmusical idea to express through the improvisation (e.g., an image, feeling, story, movement, dramatic situation) (Bruscia, 1998, p. 116).

Drum Circle

Overview. In drum circles, clients play percussion instruments together to a basic beat or "groove." Drum circles serve the needs of clients who need to function in groups. For purposes of working with people with HIV/AIDS, this often translates into clients who are in residential, day treatment, or drop-in programs and who need to engage in the treatment process. The primary therapeutic goal of a drum circle is to help clients develop group skills; secondary goals include providing positive emotional experiences, reducing isolation, promoting engagement in treatment, and developing self-awareness.

A drum circle is typically practiced on the auxiliary level of therapy, because in most cases, drum circle facilitators do not assess clients and develop and work toward individualized goals. However, in some cases, music therapists may use drum circles in a more clinically focused way; in these cases, drum circles are on the augmentative level of music therapy.

Drum circles may be contraindicated for clients who are actively hallucinating or experiencing a loss of reality. Clients with sociopathic tendencies require close observation, so that they do not take advantage of weaker group members. Correspondingly, vulnerable group members may need protection from people who may take advantage of them.

Preparation. Because drum circles are often informal experiences, it may be difficult to learn specific information about the clients who attend. The music therapist should provide adequate numbers of percussion instruments for the expected size of the group. These instruments should require little instruction and represent a broad spectrum of the different types of percussion instruments: those played by scraping, striking, and shaking. The space where the session is held should ideally be acoustically isolated from other nearby spaces, because drum circles can be loud.

What to observe. One can say that the benefits of drum circles are the same as their essential characteristics: participating in an aesthetic musical experience. Thus, the music therapist should observe primarily musical behavior. Naturally, musical behaviors are often seen as representative of other, nonmusical behaviors. Because drum circles are always group experiences, it is useful to observe how individuals behave in a group, particularly the roles that players take on.

Procedures. Introduce all instruments to the clients. Gardstrom (2007) provides an excellent process called "sound vocabulary" for introducing instruments to clients. Ask clients to select instruments that they can play while seated.

While drum circles can proceed in many different ways, the therapist often begins by assessing the listening and playing skills of the clients by playing a short rhythm and asking the clients to play it back. Often the music therapist develops a basic beat or pulse and asks clients to join in. During the next phase, the therapist may ask clients to take turns playing their own rhythms while the basic beat continues.

A drum circle may take up part of a session or its entirety, and may come to a natural closing or require intervention from the music therapist. Often, drum circles may see the emergence of natural leaders, whose leadership may encourage other group members to take ownership of the group and engage more actively. As mentioned earlier, some clients may attempt to control others during drum circles; the music therapist must remain aware of these tendencies. For example, the writer once led a drum circle with a group of clients that included former prostitutes, along with other men and women. Some of the women who had been prostitutes had been victimized by men many times. Some of the women had been on the street with each other. The dynamics of the group were very complicated. The women were alternately competitive and supportive of each other, and the men had a tendency to objectify the women. In this situation, the structure of the music helped to build and maintain some sense of group cohesiveness, but the experience required vigilance in order to keep it safe for all members.

Adaptations. A drum circle is typically structured around aesthetic and interpersonal concerns; music therapists can use the entire spectrum of aesthetics and interpersonal interactions to adapt the experience to a given group or setting. Bruscia (1987) describes various *givens* (essentially play rules) that can be used to structure improvisations, including procedural, interpersonal, and musical givens. Many of these adaptations can be shaped to fit the less formal nature of drum circles and can serve to provide different forms of structure when needed.

Individual Improvisation

Overview. With the techniques, the client creates improvisations using instruments, the voice, or other sound sources (e.g., body percussion). The therapist may or may not improvise with the client. Individual improvisation sessions are indicated for clients who wish a more individualized approach to therapy. These clients may not be ready for group sessions, or they may have concerns or issues that they wish to explore more deeply than is possible in a group. These indications are closely related to the goals, which are either musical or psychotherapeutic, depending on the approach of the music therapist

(Ansdell, 1995; Gardstrom, 2004; Lee, 1996; Pavlicevic, 1997). For patients with HIV/AIDS, common goal areas include self-awareness and behavioral change. The goals are also closely related to the type of improvisational music therapy practiced. This practice is on the intensive level of therapy.

Individual improvisational music therapy is a flexible and advanced practice; it has few direct contraindications for trained practitioners. The only general contraindication would be for those clients who are unable or unlikely to benefit from individual work.

Preparation. Improvisational music therapy is practiced on a spectrum, and some approaches [e.g., Creative (Nordoff-Robbins) Music Therapy, Analytical Music Therapy] are considered forms of advanced practice, requiring extensive training beyond professional-level competencies. Music therapists who wish to practice improvisational music therapy at an advanced level should seek training in the approach that interests them.

To prepare for individual improvisational music therapy sessions, review client records and conduct an assessment of the client. In Creative Music Therapy, the therapist often begins by directly engaging the client in music-making, and the musical information that emerges from the first encounters is a key part of the assessment process. In Analytical Music Therapy, the assessment and preparation process typically includes a more formal review of client records, as well as some improvising by the client and/or therapist. The key difference here is the prominence given to nonmusical information.

The session should be held in a room that includes an adequate and appropriate instrumentarium, typically, a piano (or two) and pitched and nonpitched percussion instruments. These instruments should be of high quality and age-appropriate. Some music therapists make video recordings of their sessions; this provides additional information for documenting the session.

What to observe. At all times, music therapists practicing improvisational music therapy must observe the musical and "perimusical" actions (i.e., any actions peripherally involved in making or responding to music) of the client. These include all musical and extramusical elements, such as language and/or affect, or lack of any of these.

Procedures. Improvisational music therapy is both an empirical and intuitive practice. It is empirical in that the therapist implements musical interventions, observes what happens, and adjusts accordingly. It is intuitive in that the music therapist intuitively draws on his or her own experience and musical knowledge in the whole process.

The basic procedures of improvisational music therapy sessions have been described in detail by Bruscia (1987). However, depending on the approach taken, these procedures will differ. For example, Creative Music Therapy procedures engage the client in a therapeutic music-making experience; all else is optional. The therapist typically plays with the client in this form of improvisational music therapy, but in some cases may listen empathically (Lee, 1996). The client or the therapist may initiate the music. The session may begin with music or with discussion or some other form of interaction, though this is not typical. The therapist and client may share an instrument (e.g., piano) in some cases, or may play different instruments (e.g., therapist at piano, client on percussion instruments).

In other improvisational approaches, the therapist and client may alternate between music and other activities, such as talking or exploring other media (e.g., movement, visual art). Bruscia has developed a taxonomy of "givens" or play rules that music therapists can use effectively (both in individual and group improvisational music therapy) to structure the experience (Bruscia, 1987, pp. 413–414).

Group Instrumental Improvisation

Overview. Group instrumental improvisation consists of clients improvising together as a group, in dyads, or as soloists within a group. The therapist typically provides an idea or theme for the improvisations. Group instrumental improvisation is indicated for clients who wish to pursue goals such as improving self-awareness, improving social skills, building community, and increasing engagement in the treatment process (e.g., establishing or increasing access to medical/nursing care). These are important goals for clients who are not accessing care. It is typically at the augmentative level.

Preparation. Prepare by becoming familiar with client treatment records, if these are accessible. While it may be difficult to predict which clients will attend a group, depending on the type of treatment facility, it is good to be familiar with clients who are likely to attend and common issues they face. For example, at a drop-in center, the music therapist may encounter many clients whose lives are unpredictable and difficult (e.g., homeless persons). At a more structured facility, the music therapist may have full access to medical records and be able to predict which specific clients will attend.

Specific preparation for the session and environment may be of greater importance, because this type of experience is improvisational. Make sure the room has instruments and seating appropriate to facilitate a group improvisation. The instruments should be of diverse types, including shakers, scrapers, and strikers (Gardstrom, 2007), and be adequate in number for the expected group size.

What to observe. In group improvisations, the music therapist should observe all musical and nonmusical behaviors of the clients: instrument choices, individual clients' music (intramusical aspects), musical interactions between clients (intermusical), actions by individual clients relating to themselves only (intrapersonal), and interactions between clients (interpersonal). All of these are important aspects of improvisational music therapy, and all provide information and possibilities for further exploration. However, music therapists will make different choices about what is most important to observe, based on their training, the goals of therapy, the setting, and other factors. For example, if a prominent goal is to engage clients in the treatment process, the music therapist may be less interested in musical observations than in other observations, such as interaction among group members. On the other hand, if goals are more psychotherapeutic in nature (e.g., to promote self-expression; to increase self-awareness), the music therapist may choose to observe both musical and nonmusical behavior equally.

Procedures. In nearly all cases, the therapist presents the clients something to stimulate an improvisation. The stimulus may consist of an idea, an instrument, a specific instruction, an image, a mood, etc., and the improvisation that follows may involve the whole group, subgroups, or individuals; the therapist may or may not improvise, depending on the stimulus.

The flow of the session will also differ, depending on the degree of structure the therapist provides and to some degree on the degree of structure the clients create. Sessions may be relatively free-flowing or may have a clearer structure. In most cases, more structure is helpful for group improvisations, especially with clients who need structure. Many (not all) clients with HIV/AIDS are in this category.

Procedurally, a more structured session should begin with a preparatory experience, move toward a more focused experience, and end with some kind of closure. For example, the group might begin by exploring the instruments available. The music therapist may need to demonstrate the instruments or allow the clients to explore them on their own. Next, the music therapist could choose a simple given, such as "take turns improvising alone." By beginning this way, this section of the session feels like a preparation for more serious work.

The main focal improvisation will probably be different in nature and more intense. Here, givens of different types will be very useful. Clients may be asked to play an image, a relationship, or an idea—individually, in dyads, or as a group. For example, the current author has used the idea "making changes" with groups of this type. Alternately, clients may be asked to play using a particular procedure. For example, asking clients to enter the music one at a time can encourage listening and cooperation.

Closure occurs in different ways during improvisational music therapy. Sometimes clients talk about their music. Sometimes the music therapist may choose to conduct a simple improvisation experience at the end. Sometimes the group may choose to listen to a recording of an improvisation. The music therapist can make choices based on the perceived needs of the group, the treatment setting, and their own training and preferences.

Guidelines for Re-creative Music Therapy

In re-creative music therapy experiences, the therapist engages clients in vocal or instrumental tasks that involve reproducing music in some way. These may include learning how to use the voice or produce sounds on an instrument, imitating melodies or rhythms, learning to sing by rote, learning to use musical notation, participating in a sing-along, rehearsing, taking music lessons, performing a song or instrumental piece from memory, working out the musical interpretation of a composition, performing in a musical show or drama, etc.

Jam Session

Overview. In jam sessions, small groups of clients function like a band, using instruments and vocal styles appropriate to different genres (R&B, heavy metal, hip-hop, etc.) to make music. Often, the therapist may play a significant role in leading. Jam sessions are a low-barrier, nonthreatening approach to music therapy for clients with HIV/AIDS. Thus, they are ideal for clients who are not yet invested in the therapeutic process and who may be resistant to the idea of participating in therapy. It helps these clients develop a basis of trust. Jam sessions are especially appropriate for clients who know how—or who want to learn how—to play instruments commonly used in jam sessions.

Goals of jam sessions are both musical and clinical; these may be the same, in fact (Aigen, 2005). Specific clinical goals are to encourage engagement in treatment, to promote self-care, and to develop the therapeutic alliance. Jam sessions typically operate on the auxiliary or augmentative level.

Preparation. Decide what genres or styles of music the clients would enjoy. In general, popular music styles of the 20th century lend themselves well to jam sessions, especially music from the 1960s and 1970s. Choose instruments appropriate to the genre, such as guitars (lead and bass), drums, keyboards, etc. Become intimately familiar with this music, including stylistically appropriate rhythms, guitar-playing styles, riffs, songs, etc. In some cases, the clients are the best teachers. Jam sessions require enough space to move around while playing and are best held in a space where they will not disturb other clients (i.e., in an acoustically isolated room).

What to observe. Observe clients for their degree of engagement in music. Is the music of a type to which they can relate? Do they know the music? Is it within their skill level?

Procedures. The basics of the approach involve re-creating client-preferred music and using this experience as a jumping-off point. The music therapist usually plays whatever instrument is appropriate and/or needed. The clients will select instruments that they prefer or have mastered, and often one client or the music therapist will need to get the song started. Determine who will be singing.

Play the song. Observe what improvisational elements occur naturally: riffs, solo sections, etc. The group should spend enough time with the song to find their "groove," that is, to get into the natural flow of performing the song. Use the song's elements (verses, chorus, bridge, instrumental section, etc.) to encourage clients to play solos, to transition to another song, etc. Expect there to be pauses and breaks in the song or between songs. Over time, the client group can work together to develop transitions between songs.

After the song, discuss the process if appropriate. Clients often enjoy the jamming experience on its own, so discussion should be approached with care.

Adaptations. Different styles of popular music will require adaptations of instrumentation and of roles. For example, some instruments that serve a lead role in American popular music (such as guitar) may have a supportive role in other cultures.

Some groups may want to perform songs that they practice during jam sessions, e.g., in a talent show or special community concert. This can be a sign of greater engagement and may be encouraged.

Group Singing

Overview. Group singing is clients singing songs together as a group. These are frequently well-known songs, without a steep learning curve. The therapist typically plays a significant role providing accompaniment and other structure (e.g., guiding the song selection process). Group singing (e.g., sing-along) is indicated for clients who benefit from a casual and low-barrier approach to music therapy. Because most people have some history with songs, participating in a group sing-along is a relatively common approach that addresses a broad range of goals, including providing positive experiences, improving memory and affect, and improving quality of life. Depending on adaptations, sing-alongs can address many more roles. Group singing is on the augmentative level of therapy.

Preparation. Prepare for sing-along sessions by developing or purchasing songbooks. Songbooks and "fake books" are readily available, but many music therapists like to create their own songbooks that are tailored to the preferences of their clientele. In some settings, a book of song titles, with lyrics on a projector, is a good option.

Accompanying instruments are an absolute requirement: Provide a piano, guitar, or other instruments appropriate for the genres and styles that clients prefer. Sing-alongs may take place in several types of settings, from closed rooms to large, open spaces. In some cases, instruments may need amplification. Clients will need adequate seating, arranged to facilitate engagement. This often means chairs in a circle rather than in rows.

What to observe. Primarily, observe all musical and nonmusical actions and interactions of the clients, during all phases of the experience.

Procedures. A basic outline of a sing-along session follows. First, invite clients to sit down and distribute songbooks or books of song titles. If the group has a traditional opening song, sing that with the clients first. Next, ask clients to select a song. If clients do not suggest or select any, consider suggesting a song. Sing the song with the group, taking time as needed to teach the words, the melody, etc., if the group does not know the song. The teaching phase provides a wealth of information about clients. Often, after each song, clients talk about the song or a time in their lives. Encourage this when appropriate. Depending on the makeup of the client group, the therapist may suggest a theme or genre. For example, a session may focus on country songs, R&B songs, or songs on a theme like "home."

Adaptations. Because the idea of a "sing-along" is very general (essentially, people singing together), it is inherently adaptable. For example, some clients enjoy using a karaoke machine in sessions. Karaoke machines provide a more "authentic" accompaniment and can often display the lyrics on a screen for clients to read while they sing; in many cases, they also transpose to more comfortable keys. However, many people have strong associations with karaoke, and the experience of singing along with an inflexible machine is different from singing with a music therapist accompanying on piano or guitar.

In some places, music therapists cooperate with chaplains or other religious personnel to facilitate music in regular or special religious services. If religious practice is an important part of clients' lives, the music of religious services can be framed as a sing-along experience, with fairly similar goals. For example, the author frequently provided music for memorial services of people who had been clients at a community health site. In these cases, the singing was often one of the most memorable experiences from these services and served to draw the community together and provide emotional support for clients.

Talent Show

Overview. Talent shows involve clients showcasing their musical (and possibly other) skills in front of groups of peers or the public. Talent shows are indicated for clients who are interested in developing and sharing their talents with other members of the community. Goals include developing and improving self-confidence and self-esteem, building community, and enhancing existing strengths. Talent shows occur on the auxiliary level of music therapy, because the process is typically not tied to specific therapeutic goals and because they may not need the qualifications of a music therapist. However, a talent show that occurs as part of a planned therapeutic process may be on the augmentative level.

Talent shows, while an enjoyable event for many communities, can reinforce narcissistic tendencies of performers. Clients with some personality disorders, therefore, may not benefit from performing.

Preparation. A talent show requires weeks or months of preparation, and the talent show itself is not the "session," per se. The talent show is the product of many rehearsal sessions, where the therapeutic interventions may typically occur. This is not to say that the show itself cannot be a part of the therapeutic process.

The sessions will typically take the form of rehearsals, and preparation for rehearsals will depend on the types of presentations the show will include. In some cases, the music therapist may have access to the space where the performance will take place, but since space is often at a premium (especially given the urban settings of many HIV treatment centers), rehearsals may take place in the music therapy room or other space. In any case, performers (clients) will need to get used to the performance space, so the therapy room should be set up to resemble the stage, as the performance approaches.

What to observe. During sessions/rehearsals, observe the performance level of the clients. Are the clients comfortable with the quality of what they plan to perform? Pay attention to what happens during planning stages, to ensure that the clients agree with every stage of planning. For example, the order of a performance may mean a great deal to some clients.

Procedures. Conduct sessions/rehearsals like typical rehearsals for a talent show. Given that the attendance of clients in HIV treatment settings (especially loosely structured ones, such as those based on harm reduction) is unpredictable, the session should have a flexible structure. In some cases, rehearsing and performing in a talent show can be meaningful therapeutic experiences for clients, and the music therapist should be sensitive to this. Plan for a check-in at the beginning and a time for processing at the end, if possible.

Adaptations. The basic idea of a talent show is to showcase the randomly appearing talents among a group of people, talents that individual group members value. However, a talent show can easily be adapted to other types of performances, such as lip-synching shows, drag shows, etc. While these suggestions may seem unusual, community members often appreciate them for their entertainment value, if nothing else.

Guidelines for Compositional Music Therapy

In compositional music therapy experiences, the therapist helps clients to write songs, lyrics, or instrumental pieces, or to create any kind of musical product such as music videos or recordings. Usually, the therapist simplifies the process by engaging the client in the easier aspects of composing (e.g., generating a melody or writing the lyrics of a song) and by taking responsibility for more technical aspects (e.g., harmonization, notation) (Bruscia, 1998, p. 119).

Song Parody

Overview. With song parody, clients write their own lyrics to pre-existing songs, which may be familiar or unfamiliar. It is indicated for clients who have good receptive and expressive language skills, but who may need to work on skills such as cooperation with others and problem-solving. Goals for song parodies include developing organizational and planning skills, encouraging ownership, and, for group settings, improving group skills. Typically, song parodies occur on the augmentative level of therapy.

Song parodies are contraindicated for clients who are actively psychotic or who behave in ways that are not conducive to group experiences (for groups only). While song parody can be a part of individual music therapy, it is commonly a part of music therapy groups. For this reason, this description focuses on group music therapy experiences.

Preparation. Prepare by choosing a song or songs appropriate for the experience. Structural elements may include repetitive patterns in the lyrics, use of relatively predictable harmonic materials, and possibly familiarity to the clientele. The music therapist should be ready to play the song and sing it with or for the group, or provide a recording. Lyric sheets with the original lyrics and/or space for filling in new lyrics are helpful.

The music therapy space should have enough room for several clients and the music therapist; a piano or guitar and music playback equipment are required; recording equipment (e.g., a computer with a microphone and recording applications) allows the clients and therapist to record and listen to their own work.

What to observe. Observe clients' level of engagement. What do individual clients contribute to the creative process? How do they interact with other group members? While natural leaders may emerge, it is important that all group members have a voice and contribute to the process.

Procedures. Introduce a song and its lyrics. The therapist may choose to play a recording of the song or to sing it live; often, listening to the song helps clients "warm up" to the process. Familiar songs make it easier for clients to imagine how their parody will sound, but familiar songs may be so entrenched in some clients' minds that they are unable to get beyond their own musical expectations.

1) Present the lyrics to clients: In some cases, the music therapist should provide a sheet with the complete lyrics for the clients to follow while listening to the song; in others, the music therapist may wish to provide lyrics with certain phrases left blank. Clients will write their own words to these "missing parts."
2) Discuss the original song (optional): When appropriate, discuss the message of the song with clients, focusing on the "missing parts." Who is speaking? What is she or he saying?
3) Facilitate lyric writing: Some clients will develop these without prompting, while others will need the music therapist to provide more structure or prompts. The therapist can easily provide structure by leading in naturally from the previous step. Clients may write part of the lyrics or the entire song, depending on the level of structure the group needs.
4) Perform the song: The music therapist should facilitate performance of the new song (parody). Ideally, clients should sing it, but if clients do not wish to perform the song, the therapist may sing it for the group. Depending on how the music therapist structured the experience, clients may sing part of the song or the entire song. Finally, discuss the song parody (when appropriate).

Adaptations. Using computer applications and recording equipment, record the song parodies with the clients and listen to the recording. What do the clients notice, and how do they feel about the product they created?

Individual Songwriting: Song as Life Story

Overview. Individual songwriting occurs when clients develop the lyrics and/or musical materials to wrong songs about their lives. The therapist provides structural and organizational support as needed. Individual songwriting is indicated for clients who can use expressive language effectively and who need to (or like to) express themselves verbally. The goals of individual songwriting range widely, depending on the functioning level and needs of the client. Goals may include improving self-awareness, increasing self-expression, and promoting self-acceptance. In short, the goals of individual songwriting are often psychotherapeutic in nature. Because of the alignment with psychotherapeutic goals, individual songwriting can occur on the augmentative or intensive levels of therapy.

Individual songwriting is less effective for clients with rudimentary language skills and the tendency to think very concretely. Clients on this level may benefit more from a group songwriting experience, carefully structured to facilitate expression in a group setting.

Preparation. The client should have writing tools and paper or a white board. The music therapist needs instruments for developing the music for the lyrics the client writes; this may be a keyboard instrument, guitar, or percussion. Clients who are skilled at computers may prefer to develop the music for their songs using computer applications. At some stage of the songwriting process, a client may want to record a song, so recording equipment is ideal; again, some clients will accomplish this using computer equipment. In fact, many aspects of the songwriting process can be accomplished using computer applications and/or the Internet. In terms of the environment, the space should be safe for emotional exploration and, ideally, private, especially during the initial stages of the songwriting process.

What to observe. Observe all aspects of the client's engagement in the songwriting process, from affect to verbal contributions to musical contributions.

Procedures. First, the client and music therapist develop material for lyrics. This can be accomplished in several ways. For example, Hatcher (2007) asked a client to write a letter to the world about himself and then worked with the client to select specific words and phrases to use as lyrics. Other music therapists will develop their own approaches, tailored to the setting and the needs of the client. The purposes of this stage are to initiate an exploration of the client's inner world and to encourage verbal self-expression.

Next, the client and therapist develop musical materials for the lyrics. Some clients may develop only rhythmic materials to support the lyrics, while others will go further to generate tonal materials. The music therapist should take the cultural background of the client into consideration when developing these materials, so as not to impose his or her own musical styles on the client. The purposes of this step are to explore specific aspects of the lyrics the client initiated and to promote decision-making.

Next, the client performs the song, as a solo or with the therapist. In some cases, the client may ask the therapist to perform the song. This is a private performance at this stage, and not meant for the broader community. The client may choose to record the song for later listening. The purposes of recording are many: developing mastery of the technical side of recording, maintaining a record of one's work, sharing one's inner world with others, etc.

Adaptations. In some cases, the client may wish to start with music rather than lyrics. Many common genres (e.g., 12-bar blues) provide a natural structure for writing original songs. Starting with music often affects the lyrical content of songs, whereas starting with lyrics often affects the musical content.

Research Evidence

The research evidence on music therapy with HIV/AIDS is weak; readers are advised to consult the literature on music therapy for palliative care, psychiatry, chronic illnesses, or substance abuse, depending on the setting and needs of clients. In an early article on music therapy and AIDS, Maranto (1988) informed music therapists about issues that they may encounter when working with people with AIDS. Maranto focused on the stigma associated with the disease, as well as its means of transmission, symptoms, and prognosis. She also discussed the relevance of psychoneuroimmunology, which looks at the relationship between the central nervous system and the immune system. Given the effects of stress on the immune system and the established record of stress reduction by music therapists, this was a promising area of research and practice for music therapists working in the field of HIV/AIDS. However, little music therapy research specific to HIV/AIDS has focused on psychoneuroimmunology since.

Receptive Music Therapy

Bruscia (1991) treated a client using the Bonny Method of Guided Imagery in Music (GIM), and described the profound impact that music had on his client's imagery and on his process in therapy. AIDS patients in GIM often report experiencing a "visit" from a deceased loved one. These "visits" are unexpected and are always beneficial to the patient, usually bringing an important message or sense of peace. Music plays multiple roles in this phenomenon: First, it deepens the altered state in GIM; second, it provides the emotional and spiritual environment for the client to receive the "visitor." This phenomenon can be understood as an attempt by the psyche to return to sources of unconditional love that the client once knew; the status of that source—i.e., alive or deceased—is irrelevant to the psyche (Bruscia, 1992).

GIM also seems to bring forth certain images with AIDS patients. Bruscia (1995) found several thematic areas in the imagery patients experienced: Being in Limbo, Releasing Feelings, Finding Love, Emotional Healing, and Embracing Life and Death. The themes that emerge depend on the physical and emotional state of the client. GIM seems to be suited for clients addressing issues associated with living with a terminal illness because its main goal is "healing," not in the literal sense of being cured of an incurable disease, but in the sense of emotional or spiritual healing, or of healing broken relationships (p. 122).

Another way of responding to music is movement. In one study, persons with AIDS participated in a six-week Dalcroze Eurhythmics program (Frego, 1995). Dalcroze Eurhythmics is an approach that teaches music concepts through movement. Each session or lesson focused on a single music concept (e.g., melody), which participants explored with movement experiences, followed by a closing, music-assisted relaxation experience. At the end of each session, clients received a summary of the music concept explored during that session and suggestions for continued exploration outside of the session. Participants were interviewed throughout the six-week session. The researcher/instructor observed less inhibition and greater fluidity of movement, as well as increased emotional support among group members and a quicker relaxation response. Initial interviews revealed feelings of anger, frustration, despair, and helplessness, but later interviews reported benefits of nonverbal communication through eye contact and physical touch. This study, while not based in music therapy, suggests the power of listening experiences for groups.

Improvisational Music Therapy

Colin Lee (1992, 1996) studied the use of improvisation with AIDS patients. In his doctoral dissertation (1992), he presented a case study of his work with a client diagnosed with AIDS. This client worked closely with Lee to explore the personal and musical meanings in the music. Lee described the different stages the client and therapist went through in their relationship and included many musical excerpts, both transcribed and on CD.

A significant focus of Lee's approach is the connection between the music—its qualities and changes—and the client's verbal commentary and discussion. During the course of therapy, Lee asked his client to listen to the recorded improvisations. While listening, he was invited to stop the tape at any time—when he felt something meaningful was happening in the music or whenever he felt like it. The comments were recorded, and the places where he stopped the tape were correlated and used to determine which sections of the improvisations would be analyzed musically. This being a qualitative case study, Lee does not draw any conclusions of efficacy. Instead, the main thrust of the study lies in the connections between changes in the music and changes in the way the music was talked about.

Re-creative Music Therapy

In countries from Uganda to China to the US, re-creative music (i.e., singing) functions to educate people about HIV. Because music involves the audience, engages the emotions, is culturally relevant, is therapeutic and empowering, and enhances memory, it is considered an effective tool for a public health approach to AIDS prevention (MacKinnon, 2005). Little research exists on re-creative methods with adults with HIV.

Compositional Music Therapy

Songwriting (Cordobés, 1997; Hatcher, 2007) is a relatively common approach with many clients, including adults with HIV. Cordobés (1997) found that participating in songwriting increased the use of emotion-related words among patients. Songwriting also helped patients to stay focused on treatment issues better than a control condition. The strong presence of emotional words in group songwriting supported its usefulness as a form of group psychotherapy.

Hatcher (2007) described a case study with a client who had a history of complex trauma. This therapeutic songwriting process had goals based in music psychotherapy, such as promoting emotional investigation and integrating the personality. For this client, HIV was only one of several complex factors affecting his well-being, including a history of sexual abuse, incarceration, and illicit drug use. The case study focuses on the songwriting process and describes key lyric themes and the new roles that the client explored through the music psychotherapy process.

Summary and Conclusions

Acquired Immune Deficiency Syndrome (AIDS) is an infectious disease, caused by the Human Immunodeficiency Virus (HIV). AIDS attacks the immune system, making it vulnerable to infections and cancers. Music therapists have treated people with HIV/AIDS since the mid-1980s, shortly after it emerged as a public health issue in the United States. During those years, the focus of music therapy with AIDS was palliative, because no medications were available to improve long-term survival rates.

After the development of improved medications in the mid-1990s, treatment shifted from palliative care to chronic care. Since this shift, less attention has been paid to research into and the practice of music therapy with people with AIDS. Currently, few music therapists work in settings specific to HIV/AIDS care, and these are in urban centers. Instead, music therapists treat people with HIV/AIDS in other settings, such as psychiatric clinics, drop-in centers, and substance use programs. In general, music therapists work to improve clients' engagement in the treatment process and to improve access to medical care. In South Africa and other countries with high infection rates, music therapists work with adults with HIV/AIDS using a community music therapy approach, with goals of building community and improving quality of life.

References

AIDS Dementia Complex. (n.d.). Retrieved October 15, 2012, from http://www.webmd.com/hiv-aids/aids-dementia-complex.

AIDS Education & Training Centers National Resource Center. (2012). HIV Classification: CDC and WHO Staging Systems. http://www.aidsetc.org/aidsetc?page=cg-205_hiv_classification.

Aigen, K. (2005). *Music-Centered Music Therapy*. Gilsum, NH: Barcelona Publishers.

Altman, L. K. (January 31, 1995). AIDS is now the leading killer of Americans from 25 to 44. *The New York Times*. Retrieved from http://www.nytimes.com

Ansdell, G. (1995). *Music for life: Aspects of creative music therapy with adult clients*. Philadelphia, PA: Jessica Kingsley.

The Antiretroviral Cohort Collaboration. (2008). Life expectancy of individuals on combination antiretroviral therapy in high-income countries: a collaborative analysis of 14 cohort studies. *Lancet, 372*(9635), 293–299. DOI:10.1016/S0140-6736(08)61113-7.

Bunt, L. (1994). *Music Therapy: An Art Beyond Words*. London: Taylor and Francis.

Bruscia, K. E. (1987). *Improvisational Models of Music Therapy*. Springfield, IL: Charles C. Taylor.

Bruscia, K. E. (1991). Embracing life with AIDS: Psychotherapy through Guided Imagery and Music (GIM). In K. E. Bruscia (Ed.), *Case Studies in Music Therapy*, (pp. 581–602). Gilsum, NH: Barcelona Publishers.

Bruscia, K. E. (1995). Images of AIDS. In C. Lee (Ed.), *Lonely Waters: Proceedings of the International Conference of Music Therapy in Palliative Care* (pp. 119–124). Oxford, UK: Sobell Publications.

Bruscia, K. E. (1998). *Defining Music Therapy* (2nd ed.). Gilsum, NH: Barcelona Publishers.

Canadian Aboriginal AIDS Network. (2009). Aboriginal strategy on HIV/AIDS in Canada II. Retrieved from http://caan.ca/new/wp-content/uploads/2010/03/ASHAC-2009-English.pdf

Center for AIDS Prevention Studies. (2005). What are homeless persons' HIV prevention needs? (Fact sheet). Retrieved from http://caps.ucsf.edu/factsheets/homeless-persons/

Centers for Disease Control and Prevention. (1981). *Kaposi's sarcoma and Pneumocystis pneumonia among homosexual men—New York City and California*. Retrieved from http://www.ncbi.nlm.nih.gov/pubmed/6789108

Centers for Disease Control and Prevention. (1982a). *Opportunistic infections and Kaposi's sarcoma among Haitians in the United States*. Retrieved from http://www.cdc.gov/mmwr/preview/mmwrhtml/00001123.htm

Centers for Disease Control and Prevention. (1982b). *Epidemiologic notes and reports pneumocystis carinii pneumonia among persons with hemophilia A*. Retrieved from http://www.cdc.gov/mmwr/preview/mmwrhtml/00001126.htm

Centers for Disease Control and Prevention. (1982c). *Current trends update on Acquired Immune Deficiency Syndrome (AIDS)—United States*. Retrieved from http://www.cdc.gov/mmwr/preview/mmwrhtml/00001163.htm

Centers for Disease Control and Prevention. (2012). HIV in the United States: At a glance (Fact sheet). Retrieved from http://www.cdc.gov/hiv/resources/factsheets/PDF/HIV_at_a_glance.pdf

Chesney, M. A., & Folkman, S. (1994). Psychological impact of HIV disease and implications for intervention. *Psychiatric Clinics of North America, 17*(1), 163–182.

Chippendale, S., & French, L. (2001). HIV counseling and the psychosocial management of patients with HIV or AIDS. *British Medical Journal, 322*(7301). 1533–1535. Retrieved from http://www.ncbi.nlm.nih.gov/pmc/articles/PMC1120575/

Coffin, J., Haase, A., Levy, J. A., Montagnier, L., Oroszlan, S., Teich, N., ... & Vogt, P. (1986). What to call the AIDS virus? *Nature, 321*(6065), 10. Retrieved from http://www.ncbi.nlm.nih.gov/pubmed/3010128

Cordobés, T. (1997). Group songwriting as a method for developing group cohesion for HIV-seropositive adult patients with depression. *Journal of Music Therapy, 34*(1), 46–67.

Denning, P., & DiNenno, E. (2010). Communities in crisis: Is there a generalized HIV epidemic in impoverished urban areas of the United States? Retrieved from www.cdc.gov/hiv/topics/surveillance/resources/other/pdf/poverty_poster.pdf

Department of Health and Human Services. Fluids of transmission. Revision Nov. 1, 2011. Retrieved from http://aids.gov/hiv-aids-basics/prevention/reduce-your-risk/fluids-of-transmission/

Food & Drug Administration. (n.d.). HIV/AIDS historical timeline 1991–1994. Retrieved from http://www.fda.gov/ForConsumers/ByAudience/ForPatientAdvocates/HIVandAIDSActivities/ucm151078.htm

Frego, R. J. (1995). Music movement therapy for people with AIDS: The use of music movement therapy as a form of palliative care for people with AIDS. *International Journal of Arts Medicine, 4*(2), 21–25.

Ghetti, C. M. (2004). Incorporating music therapy into the harm reduction approach to managing substance abuse problems. *Music Therapy Perspectives, 22*(2), 84–90.

Grocke, D., & Wigram, T. (2007). *Receptive Methods in Music Therapy*. Philadelphia: Jessica Kingsley.

Hatcher, J. (2007). Therapeutic songwriting and complex trauma. *Canadian Journal of Music Therapy, 13*(2), 115–131.

Horberg, M. A., et al. (2007). Effects of depression and selective serotonin reuptake inhibitor use on adherence to Highly Active Antiretroviral Therapy and on clinical outcomes in HIV-infected patients. *Journal of Acquired Immune Deficiency Syndrome, 47*(3), 384–390.

Horwath, E. (2002). Psychiatric and neuropsychiatric manifestations of HIV infection. *Journal of the International Association of Physicians in AIDS Care, (Suppl. 1),* S1–S15.

Kemeny, M. E. (1994). Psychoneuroimmunology of HIV infection. *Psychiatric Clinics of North America, 17*(1), 55–68.

Lee, C. (1992). *The analysis of therapeutic improvisatory music with people living with the virus HIV and AIDS*. Unpublished doctoral thesis. City University, London.

Lee, C. (1996). *Music at the edge: The music therapy experiences of a musician with AIDS*. London: Routledge.

Levine, S. H., Bystritsky, A., Baron, D., & Jones, L. D. (1991). Group psychotherapy for HIV-seropositive patients with major depression. *American Journal of Psychotherapy, 45*(3), 413–424.

MacKinnon, E. M. (2005). Music as an educational tool for HIV/AIDS: A comparative study. Unpublished bachelor's thesis. University of Ottawa, Ottawa, Canada.

Mandelbrot, L., Le Chenadec, J., Berrebi, A., Bongain, A., Bénifla, J. A., Delfraissy, J. F., Blanche, S., & Mayaux, M. J. (1998). Perinatal HIV-1 transmission: interaction between zidovudine prophylaxis and mode of delivery in the French perinatal cohort. *Journal of the American Medical Association, 280*(1), 55–60.

Maranto, C. D. (1988). AIDS: Information for music therapists. *Music Therapy Perspectives, 5,* 78–81.

Masur, H., Michelis, M. A., Greene, J. B., Onorato, I., Stouwe, R. A., Holzman, R. S., ... & Cunningham-Rundles, S. (1981). An outbreak of community-acquired pneumocystis carinii pneumonia: Initial manifestation of cellular immune dysfunction. New England Journal of Medicine, 305(24), 1431–1438. Retrieved from http://www.ncbi.nlm.nih.gov/pubmed/6975437

Mbonu, N. C., van den Borne, B., & De Vries, N. K. (2009). Stigma of people with HIV/AIDS in Sub-Saharan Africa: A literature review. *Journal of Tropical Medicine, 2009,* 1–14. Retrieved from http://www.hindawi.com/journals/jtm/2009/145891/. DOI:10.1155/2009/145891.

National Coalition for the Homeless. (2009a). HIV/AIDS and Homelessness. Retrieved from http://www.nationalhomeless.org/factsheets/hiv.html

National Coalition for the Homeless. (2009b). Mental illness and homelessness (Fact sheet). Retrieved from http://www.nationalhomeless.org/factsheets/Mental

New experimental morning-after HIV treatment. (1988, June 30). *CNN.com.* Retrieved Nov. 1, 2012, from http://articles.cnn.com/1998-06-30/health/9806_30_aids.morning.after_1_hiv-infections-hiv-virus-aids-virus?_s=PM:HEALTH

Pavlicevic, M. (1997). *Music Therapy in Context: Music, Meaning and Relationship.* Philadelphia, PA: Jessica Kingsley.

Pear, R. (March 3, 1985). AIDS blood test to be available in 2 to 6 weeks. *The New York Times.* Retrieved from http://www.nytimes.com/1985/03/03/us/aids-blood-test-to-be-available-in-2-to-6-weeks.html

Power, C., & Johnson, R. T. (1995). HIV-1 associated dementia: Clinical features and pathogenesis. *Canadian Journal of Neurological Sciences, 22*(2), 92–100.

Priority Press. (1995). *Update on combination antiretroviral therapy: results of the Delta study.* The Fifth European Conference on clinical aspects and treatment of HIV Infection, Copenhagen, Denmark, September 26–29, 1995. Retrieved from http://www.mednet.ca/html/ppaids07.htm

Progression from HIV to AIDS. (December 5, 2007). Retrieved from http://www.skillsportal.co.za/page/training/training_companies/hiv_aids_awareness_training/705542-Progression-from-HIV-TO-AIDS#.UKAkoOOe-z5

Schwartz, J. (December 8, 1995). FDA approves first in new family of AIDS drugs, saquinavir is most hopeful news in years for victims, Shalala says. *The Washington Post.* Retrieved from http://washingtonpost.com

Smith, J. (2007). Creating a "circle of song" within Canada's poorest postal code. *Canadian Journal of Music Therapy, 13*(2), 103–114.

Solomon, G. F., Temoshok, L., O'Leary, A., & Zich, J. (1987). An intensive psychoimmunologic study of long-surviving persons with AIDS: Pilot work, background studies, hypotheses, and methods. *Annals of the New York Academy of Sciences, 496,* 647–655.

Summer, L. (1988). *GIM in the Institutional Setting.* St. Louis, MO: Magna Music Baton.

World Health Organization. (1995). *Global Programme on AIDS: The current Global Situation of the HIV/AIDS Pandemic,* Presented at the World Health Organization Conference, Geneva, Switzerland, January 1995.

World Health Organization. (2007). *WHO Case Definitions of HIV for Surveillance and Revised Clinical Staging and Immunological Classification of HIV-Related Disease in Adults and Children.* Retrieved from http://www.who.int/hiv/pub/guidelines/HIVstaging150307.pdf

World Health Organization. (2010). International Statistical Classification of Diseases and Related Health Problems (10th Revision). Retrieved from http://apps.who.int/classifications/icd10/browse/2010/en

World Health Organization. (2011a). *Annex 8: HIV and AIDS statistics by WHO and UNICEF region, 2010.* Retrieved from http://www.who.int/entity/hiv/data/tuapr2011_annex8_web.xls

World Health Organization. (2011b). *The ten leading causes of death by income group (2008).* (Fact sheet). Retrieved from http://www.who.int/mediacentre/factsheets/fs310/en/

Zho, T., Korber B., Nahmias, A., Hooper, E., Sharp, P., and Ho, D. (1998). An African HIV-1 sequence from 1959: Implications for the origin of the epidemic. *Nature, 391* (6667), 594–597.

Chapter 11

Adults with Cancer

Joy L. Allen

Our bodies are made up of trillions of living cells. Normally, these cells grow, divide, and die in a systematic process to allow for growth, replacement of worn-out cells, or injury repair. Problems arise when the DNA, present in all cells, becomes damaged and the cell does not repair itself or die off like it should. Instead, the damaged cell continues to divide, growing out of control, replicating damaged DNA, and invading healthy tissues (National Cancer Institute, 2013). This is how cancer forms; if it is not controlled, it can result in death.

Diagnostic Information

Cancer is the general name for a group of more than 100 diseases. Although there are many different types of cancer, all are characterized by abnormal cells that grow out of control (National Institutes of Health, 2013; World Health Organization, 2013). Most cancers are named for the organ or type of cell in which they start. In addition to abnormal cell growth, cancer cells have the ability to travel through a body's bloodstream or lymphatic system. This process allows cancer cells to spread and invade healthy tissues throughout the body, a process referred to as metastasis (National Cancer Institute, 2013). Metastases are the major cause of death from cancer. Additional terms used to describe cancer include malignant tumors and neoplasms.

Cancer is the leading cause of death, accounting for 7.6 million deaths, or 13% of all deaths worldwide (Ferlay et al., 2008). Cancer deaths are projected to continue to arise, with as estimated 13.1 million deaths in 2030 alone (Ferlay et al., 2008). However, cancer deaths can be reduced and controlled by implementing evidenced-based strategies for cancer prevention, early detection, and management of cancer treatment. Many cancers have a high chance of cure, if detected early and treated adequately. While the most frequent types of death differ between men and women, the most common forms of cancer are lung, stomach, liver, colorectal, breast, and cervical (World Health Organization, 2013).

Cancer is caused by both external and internal factors that may act together or in sequence to initiate or promote damaged cell DNA. Evidence indicates that more than 30% of cancer deaths could be prevented by modifying key risk factors, including tobacco use, obesity, limited consumption of fresh fruits and vegetables, limited physical activity, alcohol use, sexually transmitted diseases, urban air pollutions, and assimilation of known carcinogens such as asbestos, arsenic, and aflatoxins (World Health Organization, 2013). The greatest internal risk factor for cancer development is age. In economically developed countries, 78% of all newly diagnosed cancer cases occur at age 55 and older (American Cancer Society, 2011). Genetic predisposition does play a role in some cancers. About 5% of all cancers are strongly hereditary (American Cancer Society, 2011).

Once cancer is suspected, proper diagnosis is essential. Initial symptoms and signs are investigated, and tests (including blood, urine, and/or tissue), diagnostic imaging, and pathology reports are ordered to identify the type and stage of cancer (National Cancer Institute, 2012). Stage describes how far the cancer has spread, as each stage of cancer may be treated differently. While many staging systems exist, TNM is the most common. "T" refers to the size of the tumor, "N" to the number of lymph nodes involved, and "M" to metastasis. TNM measures the extent of disease by evaluating the above and assigning a stage, usually from 0–4. Generally, the lower the stage, the better the prognosis (Edge et al., 2012).

- Stage 0—Precancer
- Stage 1—Small cancer found only in the organ where it started
- Stage 2—Larger cancer that may or may not have spread to lymph nodes
- Stage 3—Larger cancer that is also in the lymph nodes
- Stage 4—Cancer in a different organ from where it started

Cancer survival rates vary by the type of cancer, stage at diagnosis, treatment given, and a multitude of other factors. They are based on research that comes from information gathered on hundreds of thousands of people with a specific cancer, which includes people of all ages and health conditions, including those diagnosed early and those diagnosed late. Cancer survival rates often use a five-year survival rate. Overall survival rates don't specify whether cancer survivors are still undergoing treatment at five years or if they have become cancer-free, or in remission (Mayo Clinic, 2011). In general, survival rates are improving, secondary to early prevention and screening. Cancers with high survival rates include breast, prostate, testicular, and colon cancer. Those with low survival rates include brain and pancreatic cancer (Ferlay et al., 2008). In addition to differences in screening and treatment, international, ethnic, and racial differences impact cancer survival rates (World Health Organization, 2011). This is largely due to variances in detection, practice, awareness, and overall health care spending.

Cancer Treatment

Specific cancer treatments are determined by cancer type, a patient's overall health, the extent of the disease process, treatment tolerance, and the patient's preference. Primary methods of treatment for cancer include surgery, radiation, chemotherapy, targeted therapies, immunotherapies, and stem-cell transplants (National Cancer Institute, 2012).

Surgery is the oldest form of cancer treatment. Additionally, surgery plays a key role in diagnosing and staging cancer growth (National Cancer Institute, 2012). Most individuals with cancer will have some type of surgery, either to remove part or all of a tumor, obtain tissue for biopsy, or determine if cancer cells have spread. Side effects of surgery include significant blood loss, damage to internal organs and vessels, pain, infection, blood clots, and slow recovery of activity level. Today, surgery offers the greatest chance for cure for many types of cancer, especially those that have not spread (Fleming, 2001).

Radiation therapy uses high-energy radiation to shrink tumors and kill cancer cells. The radiation used may be delivered by a machine outside the body, from radioactive material placed in the body near tumor cells, or from injection into the bloodstream. The most common side effects include skin irritation, damage to regions exposed to the radiation beams, fatigue, and decreased appetite. Potential long-term side effects include memory loss, infertility, fibrosis, and the chance of secondary cancer development. About half of all cancer patients receive some type of radiation therapy during the course of cancer treatment (American Cancer Society, 2012a).

Chemotherapy is the use of medications or drugs to stop or slow the growth of cancer cells. Chemotherapy is often used in conjunction with surgery and radiation therapy. This includes using chemotherapy to shrink a tumor before surgery or radiation, after radiation or surgery to kill any remaining cells, or if the cancer returns. The most common side effects include nausea and vomiting, hair loss, bone marrow changes that lead to anemia, increased risk for infection, risk for bleeding, sores in the mouth and throat, itching skin, hives, and lowered libido. Long-term side effects of chemotherapies can include fertility problems, memory changes, and emotional changes (American Cancer Society, 2013).

Targeted therapies are drugs that attack cancer cell inner workings, while doing little damage to normal cells nearby. These drugs tend to have different and less severe side effects than chemotherapy drugs, warranting a separate treatment category. Common side effects of targeted therapies include skin problems (rashes, hand-foot syndrome, changes in hair growth, skin turning yellowish), changes in or around eyes, high blood pressure, problems with bleeding or clotting, and problems with wound healing. Most of these side effects are temporary; however, given how new targeted therapies are, long-term side effects are unknown at this time. Currently, targeted therapies are a major focus of cancer research (American Cancer Society, 2012b).

Immunotherapy uses certain parts of the immune system to fight the cancer by stimulating the immune system to work harder to attack cancer cells or giving it components, such as man-made immune system proteins. Side effects of immunotherapies are usually mild and are often similar to an allergic reaction. Additional side effects include flulike symptoms, fatigue, loss of appetite, and low blood pressure (Restifo, Robbins, & Rosenberg, 2008).

Stem cell transplants are used to restore the stem cells when the bone marrow has been destroyed by cancer, chemotherapy, or radiation. Depending on the source of the stem cells, this procedure may be called a bone marrow transplant, a cord blood transplant, or a peripheral blood stem cell transplant. Common side effects that occur shortly after transplant include infections, bleeding, lung inflammation, graft-vs.-host disease (donor immune cells attack certain organs), and graft failure. Potential long-term side effects include organ damage, abnormal growth of lymph tissue, infertility, hormone changes, and cataracts (National Cancer Institute, 2012).

Advances in medical technology and public health programs focused on screening and prevention have led to earlier diagnoses and improved treatment of many cancers.

NEEDS AND RESOURCES

Cancer Survivor

Many cancers have changed in definition from incurable diseases to chronic illnesses, and so has the definition of a cancer survivor. The National Coalition for Cancer Survivorship (2012) embraces a broader definition, proposing that cancer survival begins at the moment of diagnosis and proceeds along the continuum through and beyond treatment to remissions, recurrences, cure, and the final stages of life. The National Cancer Institute (2012) further expanded this definition to include caregivers and family members of individuals diagnosed with cancer. Today, many health providers differentiate between survivors who are receiving therapy of any kind and survivors who have completed treatment (Leigh & Clark, 2002). Mullan (1985) outlined a model of life after a cancer diagnosis that consists of three stages: acute, extended, and permanent stages. Each of these stages will be defined, along with potential need areas.

Acute Stage. The acute stage of life after cancer begins at the moment of diagnosis and extends through the initial treatments such as surgery, chemotherapy, and/or radiation. Those newly diagnosed may be dealing with a fear of dying, treatment-related side effects, and disruption in family and social roles (Leigh, 2005). Mullan (1985) describes fear, anxiety, and pain resulting from both illness and treatment as common characteristics of individuals within this stage.

Music therapists working with survivors in this stage should take a supportive and re-educative role. Interventions should be directly aimed at the physiological effects of cancer and/or cancer treatment as well as addressing coping skills. When appropriate, music therapists should involve caregivers in this process. This can be done by having caregivers participate in music therapy–based interventions and/or by teaching them techniques to use during episodes of increased discomfort.

Extended Stage. Once the initial crisis of diagnosis and treatment has subsided, cancer survivors enter a new crisis—the crisis of returning to a "normal" life. Survivors in the extended stage may be in remission or receiving maintenance therapy. Issues that generally arise during this stage include the severing of treatment-based support systems, feelings of ambiguity related to the joy of being alive and fear of recurrence, adjusting to physical or psychosocial changes, reintegrating and reorganizing individual and family concerns, isolation secondary to external or self-imposed forces, and seeking community-based support groups (Christ, 1991; Fredette, 1995; Leigh, 2005; Rowland & Massie, 1998). Specific questions and dilemmas that often arise may include identity issues ("Am I a cancer patient and/or survivor?"), changes in relationships, changes in appearance, reprioritization of daily activities, control issues, and questions of whether personality or behavior affects their health. This all occurs while the patient is living with the possibility of recurrence and death (Spira & Reed, 2003).

The therapeutic goals for extended-stage cancer survival include developing and implementing active, emotion-oriented coping strategies; reexamining life values, beliefs and priorities; mediating the expectations of others; offering support to others; and confronting mortality (Carter, 1993; Pelusi, 1997; Spira & Reed, 2003; Westbrook, 2006). When therapeutic goals are addressed, cancer survivors can find renewed meaning in their lives, build stronger connections with others, and foster a commitment to give back to others going through similar experiences (National Cancer Institute, 2002).

Permanent Stage. The permanent stage of survival represents a time of diminished probability for disease recurrence. Permanent survivors may still be adapting to a number of physical and psychosocial changes not limited to lowered self-esteem, diminished social support, and workplace discrimination (Leigh, 2005).

The ultimate therapeutic goal of extended-stage survival is adjustment and acceptance of the condition and its associated limitations, along with a realistic appraisal and implementation of strengths (Falvo, 2005). Integrating the cancer experience into one's self-concept is vital to an improved quality of life for extended and permanent survivors of cancer (Zebrack, 2000). Individuals who are able to minimize disruptions to life roles, regulate emotional distress, and remain actively involved in aspects of life that continue to hold meaning and importance are most likely to successful navigate a cancer diagnosis (Spencer, Carver, & Price, 1998).

Need Areas

Diagnosis of cancer is a threat to a person's physical, psychological, social, spiritual, and economic well-being. Specific symptoms in each of these areas will be provided. The severity of each symptom is related to the specific cancer and related treatment as well as to the individual's personality and coping skills. It is important to remember that symptoms can occur at any stage and, when left untreated, can lead to unnecessary trauma and suffering.

Physical. Physical symptoms of cancer can be acute or chronic and occur during and after treatment. The most common physical symptoms include pain, fatigue, nausea, and hair loss. When severe, these symptoms can be quite debilitating and lead to bed rest. Long-term physical effects of cancer and/or its treatment can include decreased sexual functioning, loss of fertility, persistent edema, fatigue, chronic pain, and major disability. These side effects can lead to loss of mobility, changes in bodily functions, and changes in body appearance (Kroenke et al., 2010).

Psychological. Psychological issues associated with cancer include fear, stress, depression, anger, and anxiety. Emotional impacts include feelings of helplessness, lack of self-control, changes to self-esteem, changes in self-image, and added stress and anxiety for caregivers (National Cancer Institute, 2002).

Social. Social well-being is affected when physical and psychological issues associated with cancer impact an individual's well-being. Survivors often experience increased difficulties in school or work when treatment interrupts day-to-day activities. During treatment, survivors may have had to change or forgo customary roles and/or duties within the family, at work, or in relation to their friends. Once treatment has been completed, survivors then face the challenge of reintegrating back into family, educational, work, and social environments (President's Cancer Panel, 2003/2004).

Spiritual. Research indicates the importance of religious and spiritual factors in adjustment to cancer, throughout the course of the illness, for both patients and caregivers (McCullough, Hoyt, Larson, Koenig, & Thoresen, 2000). It is not uncommon for cancer survivors to struggle with spirituality as part of their cancer experience. While some survivors question their faith, others gain support from their faith. Some struggle with the question of "Why me?," while others experience survivor's guilt. Additional struggles related to spirituality may include unresolved grief, reevaluation of life and its meaning, and reprioritization of goals and ambitions.

Economic. Economic costs incurred by survivors are important to consider, as it can impact all of the above areas of concern. Cost implications of cancer are related to accessing quality care and related health care cost and income loss resulting from work limitations. With job changes, survivors may not be able to qualify for health insurance or obtain life insurance after diagnosis. Furthermore, family members may experience significant financial burdens while serving in the role of caregiver. Research indicates that lack of money and/or the loss of health insurance may contribute to worse outcomes for medical treatment, putting the survivor at higher risk for illness, disability, and death (Adler & Page, 2008).

Resources

It is difficult to predict how individuals will cope with cancer, making it important to recognize those factors that influence adjustment. In general, persons who adjust well remain committed and actively engaged in the process of coping with cancer and continue to find meaning and importance in their lives (Spencer, Carver, & Price, 1998). They are able to balance positive expectations with the realities of ongoing fears and apprehensions. They are more likely to be comfortable expressing a wide variety of positive and negative emotions, including being honest with themselves about their feelings, articulating those feelings, and working through those feelings. Finally, research indicates that those who adjust well to a cancer diagnosis have support from others who are willing to listen and accept the wide range of positive and negative feelings and emotions related to a cancer diagnosis. Conversely, survivors who have poorer adjustment tend to have greater medical problems, fewer social supports, poorer premorbid psychosocial adjustment, and fewer economic resources (Kornblith, 1998).

Adjustment or psychosocial adaptation to cancer is an ongoing process in which survivors try to manage emotional distress, address specific cancer-related problems, and gain mastery over cancer-related life events (Brennan, 2001; Folkman & Greer, 2000; Nicholas & Veach, 2000). Adjustment involves a series of ongoing coping responses to multiple challenges that vary with the clinical course of the disease as well with the intra- and interpersonal resources of the cancer survivor. The role of treatment professionals is to continue to assess a survivor's coping responses, providing appropriate resources and interventions as needed. Despite the challenges inherent with a cancer diagnosis, studies of cancer survivors and healthy comparison groups have found no significant differences in measures of psychological distress, marital and sexual adjustment, social functioning, and overall psychosocial functioning (Kornblith, 1998).

The purpose of music therapy with cancer patients is to address those factors impairing physiological and/or psychological adjustment to cancer and cancer-related treatment. Physically, the music therapist might design interventions to address pain, fatigue, and nausea. Emotionally, the music therapist may focus on interventions to address feelings of helplessness, lack of a fighting spirit, and emotions, including anger, anxiety, distress, and/or depression. Socially, the music therapist may address support systems and patterns of communication. Spiritually, the music therapist might explore life's meaning, connection to a higher power, or reaffirmation of one's faith.

REFERRAL AND ASSESSMENT

Oncology is the branch of medicine that specializes in the diagnosis and treatment of cancer (National Cancer Institute, 2013). A doctor who specializes in the treating of individuals with cancer is called an oncologist. In most situations, a clinical oncologist manages the care and treatment once a person is diagnosed with cancer. Within the field of clinical oncology, there are three primary disciplines: medical oncology (the use of chemotherapy, hormone therapy, and other drugs to treat cancer), radiation oncology (the use of radiation therapy to treat cancer), and surgical oncology (the use of surgery and other procedures to treat cancer), (National Cancer Institute, 2013). Other medical professionals involved in an individual's care usually include a pathologist (a physician who specializes in interpreting laboratory tests and evaluates cells, tissues, and organs to diagnose disease), a diagnostic radiologist (a doctor who uses radiological techniques, such as X-rays or ultrasound tests, to diagnose disease), an oncology nurse, an oncology social worker, and an expressive arts therapist. Depending on the setting and type of cancer being treated, all or some of these medical personnel may be part of an individual's treatment team.

The treatment setting and related policies and procedures determine the referral process for music therapy services. In some settings, any member of the treatment team, including the patient and family members, may make a referral for music therapy services. In other settings, referrals may be automatically generated based on established criteria. For example, a setting may have computer-generated referrals for anyone being treated for chemotherapy-related nausea and emesis, receiving palliative care services, experiencing pain, and/or showing signs of psychological distress. Regardless of the setting, it is important for the music therapist to establish consistent criteria for referral and educate treatment team members on such criteria.

Once a referral is made for services, it is important for the music therapist to gather information in a short amount of time. It is not unusual for a therapist to have to assess and treat patients within one session, particularly in the acute stage of survivorship. It is very important for the therapist to be educated on the various types of cancer and associated symptomology as well as common treatment protocols and related side effects. For example, high levels of pain are associated with pancreatic cancer and cervical cancer. Breast cancer is associated with body image struggles. Stage 4 lung cancer has a high mortality rate. Brain tumors can lead to confusion, hallucinations, and memory struggles. While it is not possible to discuss in detail specific cancers and related symptomology within the scope of this chapter, music therapists working in oncology are encouraged to seek additional education through local, regional, and/or national cancer associations, professional conferences, and continued education seminars and workshops.

Currently, a standardized music therapy assessment for use in cancer care or medical settings does not exist. Thus it is important for the therapist to establish a working assessment model based on facility guidelines and protocols, music therapy standards of clinical practice, and common symptoms addressed within music therapy and cancer care. Assessment data should be collected through therapist observation, communication with the treatment team, engagement in music experiences, medical charts, and/or communication with the patient. Music therapy interventions may need to be initiated prior to a complete assessment taking place, particularly if the patient is in crisis. Reassessment will be necessary at crisis points throughout the course of the disease. Finally, as with all medical patients, there is an inherent hierarchy of needs for assessment and treatment purposes. Physical needs should be addressed and treated first, followed by establishing a sense of safety and comfort and a sense of belonging, and then exploring a sense of self or individual identity. Listed below are suggested areas of assessment under each domain area.

- Physical/physiological
    - Type of cancer, functional status, symptom profile, disease stage, impact of current treatment
    - Pain, including identification of variables contributing to the pain (e.g., tumor pressing against nerve cells)
    - Any nausea
    - Procedural support that may be needed
- Psychological/emotional
    - Overall mood
    - Anxiety levels
    - Locus of control
    - Signs of depression, distress, fear
    - Expression of emotions
    - Feelings of hopelessness/helplessness
- Social/communication
    - Communication patterns
    - Current support systems
    - Knowledge of available support systems
    - Strengths, weaknesses of identified support systems
- Spirituality
    - Religious beliefs
    - Practices that impact disease management
    - Religious affiliation(s) and level of importance
    - Involvement of members from a religious community
    - Spiritual distress
    - Basic questions on meaning of life: What did I come here to do? Why am I here?
- Musical
    - Previous and current musical involvement
    - Role of music in their lives, including various stages of life
    - Preferences
    - Adaptations necessary for successful engagement in music experiences

Overview of Methods and Procedures

The following methods and procedures are most commonly implemented in cancer care. These have not been sequenced to reflect relative significance, effectiveness, or complexity. Throughout the course of cancer, patients often experience procedural, acute, and/or chronic pain. The reader is referred to chapter 3, *Adult Pain Management*, for methods and procedures to address cancer related pain, including advanced cancer pain. Lastly, while science has made great advances in cancer treatment, not all cancers go into remission. The reader is referred to chapter 12, *Palliative Care and Hospice,* for methods and procedures to address cancer care at the end of life.

Receptive Music Therapy

- Music Listening: The individual listens to self-selected music during treatment and/or medically necessary procedures.
- Lyric Analysis/Song Discussion: The therapist engages the client in analysis of a song based on the client or the client's life.
- Song Communication: The client selects songs based on themes, thoughts, and/or wishes they would like to express.
- Music-Assisted Relaxation: The therapist designs and guides the patient through music-centered relaxation routine.
- Bonny Method of Guided Imagery and Music: Individual form of psychotherapy in which the client images to specifically designed music programs while in an altered state/
    - Group Music Psychotherapy: The therapist continuously guides the imagery of group members while listening to selected music programs in an altered state.

Improvisational Music Therapy

- Song Improvisation: The client creates lyrics and or melody in the moment, musically supported by the therapist.
- Referential Improvisation: The client explores musical sounds to express an experience, feeling, idea, event, or relationship.

Re-creative Music Therapy

- Cancer Choirs: Group of survivors, treatment team members, and/or families bonded by cancer diagnoses that perform for community events.

Compositional Music Therapy

- Lyric Substitution: The therapist supports the client in changing the lyrics to a precomposed song.
- Songwriting: The therapist provides appropriate structure to engage the client in the writing of original lyrics and/or accompaniment

GUIDELINES FOR RECEPTIVE MUSIC THERAPY

Music Listening

Overview. Listening to self-selected music during treatment and/or medically necessary procedures is a relatively common application of music for cancer care. The goal of this method is to decrease any treatment-related distress as well as diminish hospital-related noises. Treatment related distress might include anxiety levels before and during radiation therapy as well as effects of chemotherapy-related nausea and emesis.

Depending on the facility or treatment setting, the music therapist might play an auxiliary or consultant role in the establishment of a listening library. This includes selecting music from various genres that are conducive to a relaxation experience. In other facilities, the music therapist might serve as a preprocedure consultant who meets with patients considered at high risk of anxiety. During this time, they work with the patient to develop a program of familiar, relaxing music to play during the medical procedure.

Preparation. Create a listening library or a list of music suggestions to present to clients. Either one should be broken down by genres. Songs should be chosen for their therapeutic value, focusing on tempi close to that of the natural heartbeat and supportive themes. Efforts should be made to include selections from a wide variety of genres. Additionally, the facility will need to provide appropriate listening devices or encourage patients to bring in personal audio equipment. It may be necessary to have personal audio equipment checked by appropriate staff to ensure it meets safety and infection control requirements.

What to observe. The therapist and/or staff should watch for any visible signs of decreased distress and/or increased relaxation. This includes changes in affect, muscle tension, heart rate, respiratory rates, and breathing patterns.

Procedures. Approach the patient and assess music preferences. Helpful questions may include the following: What types of music do you listen to for pleasure? Is there a particular style of music that you find relaxing? Is/are there particular artist(s) or song(s) that you enjoy listening to? Are there any songs that you listen to when you need comfort or reassurance? If the patient has time and resources, it is beneficial to encourage them to bring in personal selections. During the music listening experience, the patient should be encouraged to listen to the music, breathing in time to the beat, if appropriate. After the music listening experience, the music therapists should follow up with the patient to determine the success of this experience, noting any changes that might be helpful in future situations. This is particularly true if music listening is being used during medical procedures such as radiation or chemotherapy infusions.

Song Communication

Overview. Song communication focuses on the patient selecting songs for the therapist to play and sing with them. Depending on implementation procedures, this method can be useful to promote a sense of control, enhance decision-making opportunities, or provide an outlet for self-expression. At a more advanced level, this technique can be used as a way to communicate feelings, wishes, emotions, or messages to others. Song communication is also a great technique to use for assessment purposes, as choices can be directed toward emotional, social, and spiritual coping mechanisms (Dileo, 1999).

This technique is contraindicated for patients experiencing high levels of fatigue or pain. If the therapist is intending to use this technique for insight-oriented experiences, a comfort level with the implementation of verbal processing techniques is necessary.

Preparation. The therapist should have a wide repertoire of songs, from a variety of genres. It is helpful to provide the patient's with a list of potential songs, categorized by genres, as a starting point. Additionally, when possible, it is helpful to provide patients with lyric sheets, allowing them to hear and see the lyrics simultaneously. Several resources provide the therapist with song titles matched to specific themes. While this might be helpful for a beginning therapist or a starting point for creating a songbook, the risk is the development of preconceived notions of a song and subsequent patient meanings to a song. It is important to remember that songs hold different meanings for every individual based on the situation. Engaging the patient in a discussion regarding their choice opens the therapeutic space for accessing, exploring, and connecting.

What to observe. The therapist should watch for signs of fatigue or increased discomfort, particularly if the patient is currently admitted to the hospital. Additionally, the therapist should watch the patient's body language and facial expressions for any visible reactions to the lyrics, message, mood, or emotions portrayed in the song. Lastly, the therapist should be mindful of any emerging themes or messages.

Procedures. The first step is directing the patient to choose a song. This can be done in a number of different ways, depending on the overall goal of the experience. On a more supportive level, the therapist might ask the client to choose something they would like to hear or enjoy hearing. On a deeper level, they might be asked to choose a song that captures how they feel in the moment, what they need in the moment, or what has meaning to them in the moment. Next, the therapist plays the song chosen. It is okay to invite the patient to participate in any way they feel comfortable—some patients may choose to sing with the therapist, while others might enjoy a more passive role. After the song has concluded, the therapist can engage the patient in a discussion, being mindful to balance supportive questions/reflection with more probing questions. Grocke and Wigram (2007) suggest the following order of questions:

- First-level questions: Ask about the music to gain information about the patient's preferences as well as if the patient is open to exploring specific lyrics or overall themes. Examples include "What did you like about the song?" "What do you like about the composer?"
- Second-level questions: Probe the meaning of the song to the patient to uncover parallels with the client's current life situation. Examples include: "Do any lyrics stand out to you?" "Does the song remind you of anything significant to you?"
- Third-level questions: Connect the meaning of the song with what is happening in the patient's life at the moment. Examples include "How did that song make you feel?" "Is there something in your current situation that is described in that song?"

It is important to remember that some patients might immediately open up to the song choice and its connection to their current life situation, while others might feel vulnerable. At the end of the discussion, the therapist can choose, depending on the client's presenting state and available time, to continue the experience with another song or end the session by thanking the patient for sharing with them.

Adaptations. Song communication can be used to spur reminiscence as well as to establish a life review. For reminiscence purposes, the memory evoked by the music should be explored, including feelings, emotions, and important persons pertinent to that memory. Using song communications for life review helps the patient to reaffirm significant memories and experiences, and their overall uniqueness. It is helpful to record the chosen songs, in a patient-directed sequence.

Music-Assisted Relaxation

Overview. In music-assisted relaxation, the therapist designs and guides the patient through a music-centered relaxation routine. The purpose might be to address physical needs, including nausea, or emotional needs such as anxiety and distress. A psychoeducational approach should be applied; with emphasis on working with the patient to create a routine they will be able to independently implement in time of need. While advanced training is not needed to implement this technique, it is essential that the therapist have supervision during the learning process.

Preparation. The therapist should be familiar with a variety of recorded music suitable for relaxation experiences. Individual preferences can and should be taken into account when choosing suitable music. The most effective music for relaxation experiences is characterized by a steady pulse; supportive base line; predictability in melodic, harmonic, and rhythmic elements; few dynamic changes; and repetition. The therapist should take the length of the music experience into consideration. In acute care settings, it is very difficult to have uninterrupted sessions for more than 15–20 minutes. Given the procedural steps that need to be implemented within this time frame, it is suggested that selections average from 4–6 minutes in length. Finally, based on the experience level and training level of the therapist as well as the potential association with voices, it is recommended that the therapist choose instrumental as opposed to vocal pieces. This eliminates any concerns over a patient projecting a human persona onto the music. Several suitable pieces can be found within classical, New Age, and jazz music.

In addition to appropriate music selections, the therapist should be prepared to implement a variety of relaxation experiences, including, but not limited to, progressive muscle stretching, breathing exercise, autogenics, and imagery. Each of these will be briefly described below.

Progressive muscle stretching focuses on physically stretching large muscle groups throughout the body. It is recommend for patients who need to experience a physically active form of relaxation, those who have pent-up energy, and those who respond best to concrete instructions. This technique is similar to progressive muscle relaxation; however, it is more suitable for medical patients for whom tensing muscles is contraindicated. In this technique, the therapist leads the patient through body stretches, beginning with the feet/ankles and finishing with the neck and/or jaw muscles.

Breathing exercises focus on encouraging deep breathing, set to a tempo close to that of the natural heart rate. Breathing exercises are particularly helpful for those patients who are anxious and taking shallow breaths, those who have no prior experience with relaxation methods, or those with short attention spans. During implementation, it is helpful for the therapist to model breathing patterns by exaggerating their own breath for the patient to hear.

Autogenics is a method that emphasizes awareness of one's autonomic nervous system. The goal is to teach the patient to become more aware of their physiological responses and to direct those responses to change into a relaxed state. This is accomplished through a series of "I" or "my" statements. This technique is great for establishing a sense of control. It is contraindicated for those with an underlying cardiac condition.

Imagery uses the patient's imagination to "escape" the current situation and transport them to a place, time, or experience that is more pleasant. In acute care settings, it is best that the therapist solicit information from the client about where they go to relax, a favorite place to visit, or a time in their life when they remember feeling peaceful. From this information, the therapist can direct an imagery experience to re-create the experience for the patient. It is important to keep the images simple and uncomplicated, as well as incorporate the various senses. Common experiences include oceans, open field with sun shining, and meadows. Imagery is contraindicated for those patients who experience periods of confusion.

What to observe. Physiological responses need to be monitored at all times. For those patients with medical monitoring equipment, this would include heart rate, respiratory rate, and pulse. Additional physiological responses include muscle tension, facial grimaces, and vocalizations.

Procedures. The therapist begins with assessing the patient's needs, resources, preferences, and preferred outcome. This includes having the patient rate their pain and/or anxiety level on a scale of 1–10. Next, the therapist determines what type of music and relaxation experience to implement. For those patients with advanced knowledge of relaxation techniques, it may be helpful to include them in the decision-making process. This information will direct the therapist to the type of relaxation experiences and corresponding music selections to use. With medical patients, it is helpful to inform them of the experience that will be implemented. For example, "I will lead you through a progressive muscle stretching experience, followed by listening to a selection of music. The entire time, I will be monitoring you for relaxation responses, and I will process with you afterward as to what worked for you." Next, an environment conducive to a relaxation experience should be established, using the following guidelines:

- Uninterrupted space: The therapist should inform the nursing staff and, if possible, place a sign on the door stating that a session is in progress. If the patient is in a semiprivate room, the roommate should be informed of the session and asked to minimize interruptions. If appropriate, they may be invited to join the experience. Phones should be disconnected or silenced, as well as all electronic equipment.
- Comfortable position for the patient: The therapist should help the patient get in as comfortable a position as possible. To foster this, it may be necessary to lower the bed, adjust pillows and blankets, reposition the patient's body, and reposition any tubes pulling on the patient.
- Darkening room: It is helpful to turn off overhead lights, particularly if they are fluorescent. If natural light is too bright, closing curtains might be beneficial.
- Setting up music: When using recorded music, it is imperative to check the reproductive quality and volume prior to starting the music-assisted relaxation experience. This includes making sure that a specific track is cued and ready to be played when needed.

Once the environment is established, the therapist is ready to start the music-assisted relaxation experience. Start by verbally reassuring the client that they are in a safe place and that this time is just for them. Then, invite the patient to close their eyes and begin the relaxation experience. While directing the relaxation experience, the therapist should be mindful that the voice is midrange, at a volume the patient can hear, and that the pace is consistent and at a tempo close to that of the natural heartbeat. It is important that the therapist sound natural and not as though they are reading off a script. At the end of the relaxation induction, the therapist should direct the client to listen to the music and allow it to bring to them what it is that they need. After the music listening experience, the therapist will need to bring the patient back to the here-and-now, slowly reacclimatizing them back into the environment. This may include bringing their awareness back to the sounds in the environment and physical sensations such as the support of the bed against their back. Once they are acclimatized, the therapist should process the music-assisted relaxation experience with the patient.

In processing the experience, the therapist should ask the patient to once again rate their pain and/or anxiety level. They should inquire as to any feelings, sensations, and/or images the patient experienced as well as their reactions to such. Did they find the relaxation experience helpful? Was the music helpful? All of this can help the therapist and patient determine any changes that might need to be made to the protocol. Finally, the therapist should determine if a relaxation routine may be established for self- or family implementation.

Adaptations. Several variances can be made to the music-assisted relaxation routine, based on the therapist's level of experience. These include choreographing music to the relaxation experience, separate selections of music for the relaxation experience and music listening experience, and more advanced imagery techniques. It is possible to use this technique with family members present as well as train them on how to implement aspects of this technique for their loved ones.

Bonny Method of Guided Imagery and Music

Overview. This is an individual form of psychotherapy in which the client images to specifically designed music programs while in an altered state. The Bonny Method of Guided Imagery and Music (BMGIM) refers to the specific method developed by Helen Bonny (Bruscia, 2000). It is a form of therapy that allows one to imagine, explore, and more fully experience possible life choices in a safe and supportive environment. Short (2002) suggests that guided imagery and music with medical patients typically includes ventilation of emotions, insight into problem relations or negative patterns of behaviors, symbolic transformation of body parts, and increased feelings of physical and mental health, in addition to emotional reactions related to self-concept. BMGIM is an advanced practice technique that requires specialized training. Additional information, including information on training programs, can be found through the Association for Music and Imagery.

BMGIM is contraindicated for those who are not medically stable. This includes those in active treatment. As such, it should be considered only for those in the extended or permanent stages of cancer survivorship. Additionally, BMGIM is contraindicated for patients with challenges related to reality orientation or appropriate interpersonal boundaries. Other methods need to be considered for those with intellectual impairments.

Preparations. BMGIM sessions require the therapist to have necessary music programs as well as quality audio equipment, including speakers, for playing the selected program. Clients are generally encouraged to lie in a flat position, with their head elevated on a pillow. BMGIM fellows may have use futons, couches, or reclining chairs to accomplish this. BMGIM sessions require uninterrupted space over a 45 – 120 minute time frame. For this reason, may fellows have specialized office space for conducting sessions.

What to observe. Throughout the session, BMGIM practitioners position themselves in a way that ensures their ability to observe the clients physiological, affect related, and verbal responses as well as connections to the music experience. These responses help guide the therapist in their response to the client.

Procedures. Sessions involve a preliminary conversation, a relaxation induction, guided music imaging, return to an alert state, and a postlude discussion. Given the advanced nature of this technique, an overview of each of these steps will be provided; however, specific instructions on how to implement them will not be.

The preliminary conversation serves to identify the goal, concern, theme, and/or conflict that is relevant to the individual for that session. Once the overall theme is decided upon, the type of listening experience, the induction and focus, and the music program are selected.

The purpose of the relaxation induction is to prepare the individual physically and emotionally for the imagery experience. The type of induction for each session is based on the nature of the presenting problem, theme, and music selection. Inductions may include breathing exercises, progressive body stretches, autogenics (repeating verbal phrases focused on a particular effect to facilitate a deeper state of relaxation), and/or directed imagery (e.g., ball of energy massaging each part of your body). The induction concludes with the therapist providing a starting image based on the theme and chosen music.

During the music imaging experience, an individual images while listening to music in a relaxed state, assisted by verbal interventions by the therapist, all aimed at helping each individual to explore and work through the selected theme. As the music imaging experience comes to a close, the therapist helps the individual return to the here-and-now and the session transitions into the postlude discussion.

The purpose of the postlude is to process, work through, and/or consolidate the music imaging experience. The therapist works with individual to process and reflect on the experience in an effort to find connections and meaning. Alternatively, the therapist explores the experience even further or consolidates the experience to closure. The specific approach taken during the postlude is based on the overall direction of the session as decided on in the prelude.

Adaptations. Group music and imagery is an adaptation of BMGIM and is used for groups that have a common purpose or identity (Grocke & Wigram, 2007). Short (2002) identifies many advantages of group GIM work, including the exertion of less energy, the diffusion of fears about the nature of therapy, and the opportunity to connect to others with similar medical problems. This, in turn, may enhance therapeutic development.

Group music psychotherapy is a specific group adaptation of BMGIM. Within this method, the therapist continuously guides the imagery of group members while listening to selected music programs in an altered state. Note that within group music psychotherapy, the therapist continuously guides the clients through the music imagery experience; other forms of group GIM allow the clients to image without verbal intervention by the therapist.

Like BMGIM, the format for group music psychotherapy includes a preliminary conversation; relaxation induction, music imaging experience, return to alerted state, and postlude discussion. However, within each, variations are made to incorporate group members and foster the group experience.

The preliminary conversation serves to identify the goal, concern, theme, and/or conflict that is relevant to the group or any of its members for that session. This may be determined by the therapist, based on assessment of group needs or wants, or based on what members presented in the opening discussion. Alternatively, group members may have determined the theme based on a group discussion of concerns.

During the music imaging experience, group members image while listening to music in a relaxed state, assisted by verbal interventions by the therapist, all aimed at helping each individual to explore and work through the selected theme. Based on the preliminary conversation, group members may have interacted within the imagery independently, as a group, or within subgroups. Additionally, the image may have been directed (participants image what the therapist presents so that the entire group has a very similar inner experience), unguided (each participant images to music separate from one another and without direction from the therapist), progressive (each participant takes a turn in contributing to an evolving image or story), and/or interactive (the therapist guides as participants co-image to music) (Bruscia, 2004).

During the postlude, the therapist works with the group to process and reflect on the experience in an effort to find connections and meaning. Alternatively, the therapist explores the experience even further or consolidates the experience to closure.

GUIDELINES FOR IMPROVISATIONAL MUSIC THERAPY

Song Improvisation

Overview. Song improvisation is when the therapist musically supports the client in creating lyrics or melody lines, in the moment. This technique usually occurs spontaneously and is not preplanned by the therapist. It is particularly useful for clients who need to access, explore, or fully experience an emotion and/or reaction. It is an inherently creative process, allowing the client to connect to their emotional, creative self vs. their cognitive self. It shares comparisons with free association. However, unlike as in free association, the therapist provides musical direction to keep the client within the experience. This technique requires advanced clinical skills, particularly in clinical improvisation.

This technique has several potential counterindications. It is contraindicated for clients not comfortable with using their voice, as this is a particularly intimate part of their being. It is also contraindicated for patients who have difficulty using their voice or supporting their breath or voice secondary to medical procedures or precautions. Precautions should be taken with clients exhibiting disorientation or confusion. Lastly, it is contraindicated for those patients who are not medically stable to explore emotions, feelings, or reactions. This technique is most effective when used in individual versus group or family sessions.

Preparations. The therapist will need to have a quality guitar or keyboard available to musically support the client during the song improvisation. If the client expresses the desire to play as well as sing, a quality percussive instrument or instrument of patient's choice may be provided. The therapist may choose to have recording equipment available, however, this is not necessary.

What to observe. The therapist should be aware of emotional and physiological reactions during the experience. This will help direct musical responses of the therapist. Additionally, the therapist needs to watch for signs of fatigue, increased discomfort, or exhaustion, particularly if using this technique with hospitalized patients.

Procedures. With cancer patients, song improvisation generally begins one of two ways. The first is when the therapist enters a patient's space and, during the assessment process, determines the patient is "stuck" on a particular experience, feeling, or emotion. This may present as the patient perseverating on few words or a few key words. This is an opportunity for the therapist to musically support the client by vocally reflecting those words and/or musically reflecting the portrayed emotions or feelings. This process of musical support and/or reflection continues, with the therapist offering musical empathy, structuring, redirection, and/or elicitation in direct response to the patient's musical offerings. The song improvisation ends when it appears as though the patient has expressed or explored what they needed to and is ready to end.

The second way song improvisations can begin is when, through the assessment process, the therapist determines the client is open to using musical creativity to freely explore what needs to be said or heard. This type of song improvisation may start with the client choosing a musical accompaniment that matches their current emotions and/or feelings. The therapist can explore several patterns and styles of chordal accompaniments with the client, with the goal of finding one that resonates with them. The therapist would then improvise with this pattern. If needed, the therapist might start with just having the client freely explore vocal sounds. This can help the client get into the experience before adding words. During this process, the therapist should musically support the client, offering musical reflection, empathy, structuring, elicitation, or redirection, as appropriate. If the client chooses to add words, the therapist would continue musical support. The song improvisation ends when the client has explored and expressed what they needed to, or when fatigue prevents continuation.

Gardstrom (2007) provided several examples of music facilitation skills to use during improvisation experiences. A selection of these is listed below:

- Empathy Techniques
    - Imitate a client's response
    - Synchronize with a client's playing
    - Incorporate a musical motif of the client into one's improvising

    - Pace one's improvising with the client's energy level
    - Reflect the moods, attitudes, and feelings exhibited by the client
- Structuring Techniques
    - Establish and maintain a rhythmic ground
    - Establish and maintain a tonal center
- Elicitation Techniques
    - Use repetition as an invitation for the client to respond
    - Model desired musical responses
    - Make spaces in one's improvising for the client's improvising
    - Interject music into the spaces made by the client
- Redirection Techniques
    - Introduce musical change to redirect the client's playing
    - Intensify elements within the improvisation

After the song improvisation ends, the therapist will need to decide whether verbally processing the experience is necessary. In many cases, the experience speaks for itself, and additional processing is not necessary.

Referential Improvisation

Overview. In referential improvisation, the client explores musical sounds to express an experience, feeling, idea, event, or relationship. This type of music experience can foster self-expression and identity exploration, as well as exploration of self in relation to others. The therapist can have cancer survivors explore referents and continuums based on emotions, feelings, and/or experiences related to a diagnosis of cancer, treatment of cancer, and/or related life changes. Creating and hearing these emotions and/or experiences provides a different sensory experience for the survivor, which can open the door for healing to occur. The music therapist should have advanced training in improvisational techniques, including improvisation assessment and evaluation.

Instrumental improvisation is not recommended for cancer survivors admitted to the hospital. The energy level required to play as well as the potential volume of the experience are of great concern for inpatient medical settings. Additionally, most facilities prefer that a bare minimum of musical instruments be transported to patient rooms, as infection control procedures are usually in place.

Preparation. The therapist should have a selection of quality rhythm and melodic percussive instruments for the patient to select from. Recording equipment is also helpful, for playback of the improvisation to the client.

What to observe. The therapist should be aware of emotional and physiological reactions during the experience, including changes in affect, energy level, and body positioning. This will help direct musical responses of the therapist. Additionally, the therapist needs to watch for signs of fatigue, increased discomfort, and exhaustion, particularly if using this technique with patients receiving medical treatment.

Musically, the therapist should be aware of instrument choices, the playing of the instruments, and the interplay of various musical elements and relationships in the improvisational experience.

Procedures. The improvisational experience should begin with the therapist selecting instruments to present to the client. The client should be given ample time to explore each instrument, encouraging characteristic and non-characteristic playing of the instruments. This allows the patient to experience the variety of sound potentials for each instrument. Once this is done, the therapist and client will have to decide the individual roles within the improvisation. Considerations include solo, duo, or group play. The therapist and/or client deciding on a specific theme for the improvisation follows this. Possibilities include specific emotions (nervousness, apprehension, grieving, confident, comforted, etc.), events (celebrations, appointments, procedures, etc.), relationships (with children, spouse, significant other, friends, etc.), or ideas (winning a battle, invasion, peacefulness, healing, etc.). The improvisation experience is ready to begin, and if possible, the therapist should record this experience for later playback. During the improvisation, the therapist should engage in musical facilitation skills, as appropriate.

After the improvisation ends, the therapist should process with the client. This should begin with a focus on the musical sounds created and corresponding reactions. Next, the therapist should work with the client to make any connections between the client's interpretation of the musical sounds and the referent provided at the beginning of the improvisation. During this time, if appropriate, the therapist can replay the improvisation for the client. The therapist should support the client in making any connections to the musical sounds and referent given, and the client's current life situation.

Adaptations. Song portraits are a specific type of instrumental improvisation, beneficial for increasing locus of control and internalization of sound. One type of sound portrait beneficial for cancer survivors is creating a sound portrait of healing music. Another example may be a sound portrait related to the invasion of cancer cells. Sound portraits can be recorded and played back by the patient, as appropriate, during times of need and is an excellent way to increase a sense of control.

GUIDELINES FOR RE-CREATIVE MUSIC THERAPY

Cancer Choirs

Overview. A cancer choir is a group of survivors, treatment team members, and/or families bonded by cancer diagnoses with a goal of performing at selected community events. For members, it is a chance to connect and belong to a group composed of individuals going through similar experiences. This is particularly important for those struggling with identity issues. Cancer choirs provide an opportunity for cancer survivors to find a support system outside of the medical offices. While members may share their experiences, the focus is on growing and learning something new together, not on treatment-related issues or things that happened in the past.

Cancer choirs generally have open memberships. Previous choir, vocal, or music performance experience is not necessary. It is not uncommon for individuals to experience voice changes secondary to cancer-related treatment. For the trained vocalist, the inability to sing the same voice part or vocal range restrictions might be very disconcerting, and additional support from the therapist might be warranted as they grieve this loss and open up to a new "normal."

Preparation. The therapist will need to decide the structure of the choir. While it is certainly therapeutic to involve members in the song selection process, the therapist should be prepared to offer a selection of choices based on themes or particular performance venues/opportunities.

The therapist will have to provide copies of the selected music for all participants. Those with musical backgrounds enjoy the opportunity to read music, while those who do not might find it easier just to have the lyrics. Recordings of selected songs are also helpful. Provide a list of titles with corresponding artists for the participant to independently download or purchase or provide this via individual CDs for choir participants. It is possible that several members may have limited musical talent or experiences; therefore, the therapist should select pieces that are not overly ambitious to perform.

The therapist will need to designate rehearsal place and times. This information needs to reach potential members in a timely manner. The rehearsal room should be set up upon their arrival. Most therapists find it helpful to have an accompanist available. This allows the therapist to focus on the needs of the members without any additional responsibilities.

Performance opportunities should be decided upon in advance, when possible. This allows the therapist to involve members in the decision-making process as well as to plan song selections according to performance. Additionally, "dress uniforms" may be decided upon.

What to observe. During rehearsals, the therapist should monitor affect and affect-related changes. Additionally, the therapist should monitor and encourage proper breath support and watch for signs of fatigue. It may be necessary to alternate sitting and standing positions for some or all members to address fatigue issues.

Procedures. Begin rehearsals with a musical introduction. A familiar song can be used to solicit participant names while establishing a welcoming atmosphere for new members. After the musical opening, the therapist should consider involving participants in vocal warm-ups. Vocal warm-up suggestions include the following:

- Breath Relaxation: releases tension often associated in the breathing mechanism that can interfere with effective voice production. Participants should be directed to take a normal breath and then exhale on an "s" sound, making sure shoulders and chest are low and relaxed. This can be repeated many times, while making sure the breaths are focused low in the abdomen and there is no chest, neck, or shoulder tension while breathing. It is sometimes helpful to have participants place one hand on their abdomen to remind them to keep the focus low and away from the chest and shoulders.
- Jaw Release: reduces tension in the mouth and jaw area during speaking and singing. Participants should place the palm of each hand directly below the cheek bone and then push in and down from the cheeks to the jaw, massaging the facial muscles. This can be repeated several times.
- Lip Trills: releases lip tension and connects breathing and speaking. Participants should place their lips loosely together and exhale in a steady stream to create a trill or raspberry sound.
- Two-Octave Scales: provides maximum stretch on the vocal folds. Participants should start in a low pitch and gently glide up the scale on a "me" sound. The therapist should not push the top or bottom of the vocal range but try to increase the range gently each time the scales are repeated. The therapist can reverse and glide down the scale from the top to the bottom on an "e" or "oo" sound.

After the choir is warmed up, rehearsal should begin. To keep participants engaged, it is helpful to plan specific songs and song sections that you intend to rehearse before each practice. Always starting rehearsals at the beginning of each song can become boring, whereas rehearsing specific sections allows members to focus their practice. If feasible and desired, the therapist may record sections or entire pieces for the members to hear and comment on.

Rehearsal should conclude with an opportunity for group processing. This may be established informally and include coffee and dessert, or formally. During this time, members should be encouraged to reflect on their experiences with the music and the performance of the music, as well as on being a member of the group.

Adaptations. Cancer choirs can be adapted in several ways. Small vocal groups or ensembles can be formed or a group of amateur musicians may wish to form a survivor's band. Cancer choirs can be modified to meet the needs of staff working with cancer patients. Staff choirs can provide an opportunity for self-expression, relaxation, and increased self-control and identity for participating members. Some facilities have formed workplace choirs to address issues related to burnout with staff members working with individuals living with chronic illnesses. Performance opportunities exist at national holidays, survivor celebrations, as well as services to honor those patient's lost to the disease.

GUIDELINES FOR COMPOSITIONAL MUSIC THERAPY

Lyric Substitution

Overview. Lyric substitution is when the therapist provides the necessary support for a client to change the lyrics to a precomposed song. It is a great way of providing opportunities for self-expression, particularly when there are predetermined session time limits or when it is unknown if there will be further session opportunities. Goals of lyric substitution are focused on self-expression. While lyric substitution can be used to gather insight into coping responses and/or validate emotions and experiences, it can also be used as a fun, leisure-centered activity. Having experiences whereby the patient can "poke fun" at unpleasant situations can help decrease frustration levels while providing alternative ways of coping.

Preparation. The therapist should have a selection of songs with lyrics that can easily be substituted. Alternatively, the therapist can use a song previously used in a session with the patient with the suggestion of changing the lyrics to capture a feeling, emotion, wish, or previous/future experience. Guitar or piano is needed to facilitate live performance of the song.

What to observe. The therapist should be aware of the overall mood, style, and message of the song and how it relates to the patient's current situation. It is also good to be aware of how the patients place themselves in the music. Do they speak of themselves is first or third person? Are they more concerned about family and their needs, or their own needs in the moment? This information is valuable and can help the therapist structure the experience to meet the needs of the patients.

Procedures. First, determine the presenting mood or theme of the client and related need. This will decide what type of song might be used. Sometimes this process might be quite natural, wherein the client is sharing a part of their life story, during which a theme or a chorus of a song emerges. Alternatively, the therapist can engage the patient in free association of topics or focus on specific topics such as family support, treatment regimes, and/or a life story. Once a theme emerges, a song that musically coincides, complements, or matches that theme should be used. This can be patient-selected or therapist-suggested. Once a line and/or verse is created, the therapist should sing/play that verse to the client for feedback and/or approval. This musical engagement will also support the creative process vs. the cognitive decision-making process, which is important for emotional expression.

Adaptations. Song affirmations are a specific type of lyric substitution. With song affirmations, the therapist supports the client in changing the lyrics to a song of choice to lyrics that celebrate accomplishments, highlight strengths, and/or validate the uniqueness of the patient. Song affirmations serve to counteract critical and judgmental thoughts while creating a needed space for change. When engaging a patient in the process of writing a song affirmation, it is important to have the patient choose a familiar melody that captures their overall personality. For some, this may be a song to which they feel a connection; for others, it may be a song that reminds them of a special time, memory, or place, or it could be the first song that "pops" into their head or a song in which they like the overall beat or tempo. Once the melody is chosen, it is time to work on the lyrics. The therapist should take a supportive role in this process, providing open-ended questions for the patient to respond to. There will be times when it is difficult for the patient to think of positive traits or characteristics. When this happens, it is helpful to process the negative or challenging beliefs and/or thoughts and then gradually move into more positive or uplifting experiences. As lyrics are added, it is helpful for the therapist to play/sing what has been composed. This aids in the process, as the client is able to musically experience their creation as it unfolds. Once the song affirmation is complete, the therapist should musically support the client in singing their affirmation. Hearing the sung affirmation allows for the internalization of the experience.

Songwriting

Overview. With this technique, the therapist provides an appropriate structure to engage the patient in the writing of original lyrics and/or accompaniment. Songwriting is a great way to foster the decision-making process while providing a valuable tool for the exploration of feelings, beliefs, wishes, and emotions. It can also be used to encourage communication and reminiscence. In order to engage a patient in songwriting, the therapist should be a solid musician with the ability to play a variety of musical styles. Furthermore, they should be comfortable with changing leadership roles with the client, allowing for flexible give-and-take to ensure it is the client's experience, not the therapist's interpretation of the experience or the therapist's need for a finalized "product." The therapist should be comfortable with verbal processing techniques, particularly those needed to enhance or deepen the patient's experience. Open-ended questions, timely reflection of statements, and probing are useful verbal techniques within this experience.

Songwriting is contraindicated for those patients exhibiting or experiencing high levels of physical or emotional distress or who are disoriented or confused.

Preparation. In addition to the therapist having a guitar and/or keyboard available, it is also necessary to have something for writing down the lyrics and chords. If desired, a recording device is helpful for those opportunities when a patient may want to record the final product.

What to observe. The therapist should be mindful of the choices the patient makes during the experience, focusing on any insights and/or incongruities present.

Procedures. Wigram (2005) developed the Flexible Approach to Songwriting in Therapy (FAST). This working model outlines the possibilities within each stage of songwriting. Aspects of the FAST model are outlined below:

- Introduction to Songwriting
  - Improvising incorporating story creation or the client's life story
  - The therapist proposes idea in discussion
- Formulation of Lyrics
  - Brainstorming themes (client and therapist)
  - Words are spontaneously suggested (client or therapist)
  - Words related to client issues are suggested (client or therapist)
  - Client brings precomposed lyrics
- Development of Music
  - Improvised (client and therapist)
  - Improvised melody over structured harmonic frame (client and/or therapist)
  - Client creates melody and harmony
  - Therapist offers ideas in short fragments or chords of melody and harmony, accepted or rejected by client
- Writing Down a Song
  - Lyrics only
  - Lyrics and melody
  - Lyrics, melody, and basic guitar/piano chordal harmonic structure
- Performing a Song
  - The song is performed by client and therapist together

    - The song is performed to staff and other clients
    - The song is performed to family and friends
- Recording of Song
    - The song is recorded by client and therapist

Throughout the experience, the therapist needs to be mindful of the client's word choices, including where they place themselves within the song. Additionally, the therapist may need to shape the client's words into a verse. While doing so, they need to make sure they capture what the client communicates, not what they think the client is communicating. This can be done verbally with such statements as: "What I hear you saying is ... ?" "Do the words capture what you were communicating, or does something need to be changed?" "Would you like this to go like this or should we change the order of this?"

With hospitalized cancer patients, it is imperative that the therapist completes the songwriting experience within a single session. This is secondary to the variety of complications as well as discharge decisions that can be made or happen in a moment's notice. In these situations, the therapist should be realistic about time constraints and make necessary modifications in the decision-making process. In many cases, it might mean focusing on the lyrics and melody and saving harmony and full accompaniment for when/if the situation presents itself.

Adaptations. Story songs are a specific type of songwriting. A story song is an imaginative story created through music by a client, with the support of the music therapist, which depicts the client's situation or understanding of his or her situation. This may be done vocally, instrumentally, or through a combination of vocals and instruments. The musical structure of a story song is similar to that of a story and includes the following elements: recitation, theme, conflict, variations, and resolutions (Rubin-Bosco, 2007). The creation of story songs can take several sessions, so it is best to use this technique with outpatient survivors. Story songs are a great way to support clients in their process of accessing, exploring, and expressing their experience of cancer and can easily be adapted for group situations.

CARING FOR THE CAREGIVERS

A cancer diagnosis can have a devastating effect on the family system. Caregiving can trigger a host of difficult emotions, including anger, fear, resentment, guilt, helplessness, and grief. It's important for family members to acknowledge and accept what they are feeling, both good and bad. In addition to a host of emotions, caregivers are often physically and socially burdened by a cancer diagnosis. It is not uncommon for caregivers to forgo caring for themselves in an effort to reduce the burden of their loved one. This includes sacrificing exercise, healthy eating, sleep, and their own health needs. The responsibilities of supporting a loved one through the initial diagnosis and treatment of cancer often impinge on a caregiver's social opportunities. Many times they give up hobbies, relationships, or other things of importance secondary to time constraints, exhaustion, or feelings of guilt.

The goal of music therapy with caregivers is to bring families together to develop meaningful communication, resolve conflicts, and promote a sense of togetherness through the battle. Having separate support groups or session availability for family members is preferred. Support groups foster understanding and knowledge that the caregiver is not alone, while providing support and encouragement. Music experiences should be designed to address how the family and/or specific members are coping with cancer while encouraging creative self-expression, tension release and relaxation, and being heard by loved ones. Any of the above techniques can be modified and implemented to address the specific needs of caregivers.

RESEARCH EVIDENCE

Research on the use of music therapy has focused on the physical, emotional, social, and spiritual needs of cancer patients.

Receptive Music Therapy

Several studies were found investigating the effects of receptive music therapy methods used with cancer patients. The following review of the literature will be broken down into music listening interventions, the use of songs, the use of music and imagery, and the use of guided imagery and music in individual and group music therapy sessions.

One of the earliest studies examined live vs. tape-recorded music in reducing tension and anxiety in hospitalized cancer patients (Bailey, 1983). Results indicated that live music was significantly more successful than taped music in reducing tension and anxiety as well as in alleviating physical discomfort and negative affect. Hanser et al. (2005) investigated the effectiveness of music therapy sessions with women with metastatic breast cancer. Three individual sessions were provided, with an average of 2-3 weeks between sessions, in an effort to provide survivors an opportunity to experience and learn techniques they may use at home. Immediate improvements were found in measures of relaxation, comfort, happiness following each music listening interventions. Additionally, music therapy participants reported greater treatment satisfaction and subsequent use of music to cope. Lastly, Burns, Sledge, Fuller, Daggy, & Monahan (2005) investigated cancer survivors interest in participating in music therapy sessions while receiving chemotherapy. Results indicated a majority of survivors were interested in music therapy. Furthermore, younger age and higher levels of distress were associated with a preference for music listening experiences as compared to active music making experiences.

In addition to the above study, several studies have focused on the benefits of music listening interventions during active cancer treatments. Frank (1985), in a study investigating the effects of music therapy and guided visual imagery on chemotherapy-induced nausea and vomiting, found that state anxiety, length of nausea and vomiting, and perceived severity of vomiting were all significantly reduced. Standley (1992) examined the effects of music listening on frequency and degree of nausea in cancer survivors receiving chemotherapy. Survivors reported less nausea and later onset of emesis when music listening was provided during chemotherapy infusions. Additionally, survivors reported music listening was a helpful technique they would use during future chemotherapy infusions. Clark, et al. (2006) investigated the effects of music listening during series of radiation therapy. A music therapist met with participants to develop a music listening and relaxation routine that was then taped and listening to during subsequent radiation treatments. Results indicated significant reductions in treatment related anxiety and distress. Ferrer (2007) investigated the effectiveness of live, familiar music on survivors undergoing chemotherapy. Statistically significant improvements were found on measures of anxiety, fear, fatigue, relaxation, and diastolic blood pressure. Additionally, survivors reported an overall increase in quality of life during the music listening intervention. Lastly, Chaput & Silverman (2012) investigated the effects of live music on post-surgical oncological patients. Results indicated significant improvement in measures of relaxation, anxiety and pain.

Songs have long been used in work with cancer patients to address emotional, social, and spiritual needs. Bailey (1984) described the beneficial qualities of songs in providing support, acting as a tool for change, and in reducing suffering. Specifically, Bailey presents the characteristics of songs and their use in providing a framework for tension release, integration and pleasure as well as for promoting contact, awareness and resolution. Cook (1985) described numerous uses of songs in music therapy to address anxiety, increase communication, and serve as outlets for self-expression. Porchet-Munro (1995) reported on the use of songs to address coping, withdrawal, expression, anxiety, fear, anguish, confusion, boredom, loneliness, and a search for meaning in cancer patients.

Using a bio-psycho-social approach to cancer care, Dileo (1999) outlined the use of songs throughout the experience of cancer. Dileo states song choice is a valuable assessment tool in regard to patient feelings, attitudes, identity, and coping styles. Song discussion can be used to focus on models of coping and losses, as well as for empowerment, optimism, and self-esteem. Song biographies can be used to foster memories as well as explore aspects of identity. Song dedications and song communications can promote social interaction, communication, emotional intimacy, forgiveness of self and others, and acknowledgement of change. McDougal-Miller (2010) also highlighted the use of songs, including relevant song titles, across the cancer continuum. Specific phases of the cancer experience are aligned with potential music therapy goals and corresponding interventions to address physical, emotional, social, cognitive, and spiritual need areas.

Music listening has also been used in group situations. Waldon (2001) found that group music listening experiences resulted in significant improvements in self-reported mood states in adult oncology patients. Burns, Harbuz, Hucklebridge, & Bunt (2001) investigating the effects of group music listening in a relaxed state on increases in positive emotions and the immune system of patients attending a cancer help center. Results indicated increased feelings of well-being and relaxation, decreased tension, decreased levels of cortisol, and increased levels of SigA in patients participating in group music listening experiences.

A few studies have investigated music and imagery techniques with cancer survivors. Logan (1998), in an investigation of music-evoked imagery with cancer survivors, found this combination useful in promoting insight and healing. She found this experience allowed the client to generate imagery based on his or her needs and desires which, in turn, could provide comfort, a sense of control, a means of self-expression, and reduce anxiety. Burns (2002), in an overview of guided imagery and music with in the treatment of individuals with chronic illness, stated the music played in music and imagery techniques provides structure for breathing and relaxing while encouraging peaceful feelings and images that promote comfort and relaxation. Allen (2008), examined the application of music and imagery in the management of advanced cancer pain. Results found that music-evoked imagery decreased pain perception and addressed the captioned emotional components of the pain experience in individuals with advanced cancer.

Guided imagery and music is often reported as an effective technique to address the emotional and spiritual needs of cancer survivors. Burns (2001) investigated the effects of ten weekly individual GIM sessions on mood and quality of life indicators in female cancer patients. Results indicated increases in positive mood, improvement in tension, fatigue, and confusion, as well as changes in depression and anger. Furthermore, at six weeks after follow-up, participants continued to have a better quality of life in comparison to wait-list control. McKinney and Clark (2003) investigated the effectiveness of six BMGIM sessions on distress, life quality, and relevant endocrine markers in women recovering from treatment for non-metastatic breast cancer. Results demonstrated that six BMGIM sessions significantly reduced levels of depressed mood and total mood disturbance, increased emotional and social well-being and well-being associated with breast cancer concerns, and decreased intrusive thoughts and avoidance behaviors related to cancer. Bonde (2005) explored the influence of guided imagery and music sessions on mood and quality of life indicators. Results indicated that after ten individual sessions, survivors reported improved mood and quality-of-life. Additionally, Bonde reported that imagery within sessions was not cancer specific; instead, participant-directed imagery focused on general issues of self-understanding and coping during periods of transition.

In addition to the above studies, several case studies examined guided imagery and music sessions with cancer survivors. Hale (1992) presented a case study on a women recovering from a mastectomy. She found that individual GIM sessions, over a 1 ½ year period, resulted in a more positive self-image, an improved ability to trust, and that fear of recurrence no longer dominating the survivor's life. Cadrin (2005–2006) examined the process of BMGIM in addressing the psychosocial, spiritual and existential issues of a breast cancer survivor. Cadrin found the process of GIM allowed the survivor to move forward toward her goal of reclaiming her identity. Lastly, Marr (1998–1999) reported the benefits of BMGIM with a breast cancer survivor. Results highlighted the ability of GIM to enhance spirituality, express strong emotions, and re-evaluate identity.

Guided imagery and music has also been used in group sessions. Pienta (1998) examined the effects of group music and imagery on the self-esteem and well-being of breast cancer survivors. After six group sessions, results indicated an increase in self-esteem and overall well-being for study participants. Allen (2011) examined the effectiveness of group music psychotherapy, a modified form of guided imagery and music, on the self-concept of breast cancer survivors. Results indicated significant improvement in measures of identity, family role relationships, self-esteem, and body image after 10 weeks of group guided imagery and music sessions. Furthermore, group music and imagery was significantly more effective compared to a standard cognitive-behavioral based breast cancer support group on measures of identity, role relationships, and body image.

Improvisational Music Therapy

Despite being documented and researched less frequently, improvisational methods have an important role in meeting the emotional, social, and spiritual needs of cancer survivors. This includes song improvisation and referential improvisation methods used in individual and group music therapy sessions.

Song improvisations can serve as a starting point for exploring meaning and spirituality, when the therapist sets specific themes or questions for the patient to musically explore (Dileo, 1999). Furthermore, song improvisations are beneficial during the difficult process of forgiveness of self and/or others. Aldridge (1996), in a case study with a survivor of breast cancer, reported the benefits of melodic improvisation for self-expression. More specifically, he explored the benefits of creating for accessing feelings into the conscious without the need for verbal labels. Turry and Turry (1999) reported that song improvisations can be used with cancer survivors to gain awareness of, explore, and express feelings. Furthermore, it is a tool to integrate fragmented parts of self; serve as a catalyst for self-discovery; foster hope; and cultivate the desire to re-establish meaningful relationships with others.

Referential improvisations with cancer survivors have been used to meet the emotional, spiritual, and social needs of cancer survivors. Dileo (1999) highlighted the benefits of referential improvisation for identifying and expressing emotions. She stated, "Themes of these improvisations often involve how the patient is experiencing living with, living against, or living through the illness" (Dileo, 1999, p. 160). In discussing improvisation as a tool to explore meaning and spirituality, she described a musical "Orpheus" experience. With this technique, a patient is directed to select a group of preferred instruments with which to engage in free improvisation. As the improvisation continues, they must gradually "surrender" instruments, one by one. The proceeded discussion focuses on the metaphorical connection of the improvisation to life.

A few studies have investigated group improvisation with cancer survivors. Bunt and Marston-Wyld (1995) reported that improvisation was beneficial in identifying and expressing emotions, achieving new awareness, and developing group cohesion. Burns, Harbuz, Hucklebridge, & Bunt (2001) investigated group improvisation within the context of a cancer help center. Participation in group improvisation resulted in increased well-being, increased energy, and decreased tension, as well as increased levels of SigA and decreased levels of cortisol. Rykov (2008), in research describing a music therapy–based support group, reported that the experience of improvisation was particularly empowering to group members. Specifically, improvisation provided opportunities for experiencing feelings of control during a time of loss of control inflicted by the cancer experience. Lastly, Daykin, McClean, & Bunt (2007) examined patients perception of group music improvisation. The authors note themes of choice and enrichment counteracted themes of limitation and restriction commonly experience by cancer survivors.

Re-creative Music Therapy

The prevalence of cancer choirs is increasing across the globe. These choirs are composed of survivors, family/friends, and/or health care professionals. Research on the effectiveness of these choirs is extremely limited. O'Callaghan, Hornby, Pearson, and Ball (2009) reported increased positive emotions and memories and validation of the importance of enjoying the moment in a study investigating the benefits of listening to a cancer center staff choir. At this time, no research studies have investigated the impact of participation in a cancer choir.

Anecdotal evidence does support the emotional, physical, and social benefits of cancer choir participation. Moorer (2004), in a report on a local cancer choir, reported that members benefited from shared experience, enhanced mood, social networking, increased activity tolerance, and reaffirmation of life after cancer. Similar results have been reported in news articles of local cancer choirs across the globe.

Compositional Music Therapy

Songwriting is a technique often used with adult cancer survivors. Several early studies reported songwriting fostered self-expression, increased self-esteem, enhanced quality of life, reduced isolation, and opportunities for sensory stimulation (Lane, 1992; Nolan, 1992; O'Callaghan, 1996; Robertson-Gillam, 1995) in hospitalized cancer survivors. O'Brien (1999) interviewed cancer patients about their songwriting experience. She found that songwriting was a calming, pleasurable, and unique experience for hospitalized patients that fostered self-expression, helped to clarify thoughts, and acted as a timekeeper in a patient's life. Finally, O'Brien (2003) explored the nature of the interactions between therapist and patient during the songwriting experience. She found that songwriting fostered self-expression while facilitating communication with bone marrow transplant patients.

Songwriting has been reported to be beneficial for improving interpersonal relationships in cancer survivors. O'Callaghan, O'Brien, Magill, and Ballinger (2009) engaged hospitalized parents with cancer in songwriting directed toward their children. This process was found to promote the parent-child connection and emotional expression, and convey a sense of the emotional availability of the parent. Lastly, lyrics within the songs addressed issues of spirituality, memories, meaning, hope, and direction.

In regard to spiritual needs, Dileo (1999) reported that song affirmations are beneficial for inspiring hope. Furthermore, the act of creating and listening to the song affirmation is affirmation of self for the survivor. Dileo further advocated the use of songwriting as a final part in the process of forgiveness. Accordingly, the therapist can support the process of writing a song to the person needed to be forgiven or as a way to acknowledge forgiveness of self.

Songwriting has been used in group therapy with cancer survivors. O'Brien (2006) described the process before, during, and after creating and performing an opera with cancer survivors. Overall themes of anger, fear, humor, suffering, and peace were present, leading O'Brien to conclude that the experience of writing and performing an opera was a transformative method of self-expression for cancer survivors.

Lastly, Dileo and Magill (2005) explored songwriting with oncology and hospice adult patients from a multicultural perspective. They report songwriting provides the patient and family members opportunities to enhance communication, regain a sense of control, and gain or regain fulfillment and purpose in their lives. More specifically, multicultural songwriting aims to address the following need areas: self-expression, relationship closure, life review, and enhanced spirituality. Dileo and Magill conclude by offering ways a music therapist may offer cultural sensitivity. Cultural sensitivity can be enhanced by the therapist having a working knowledge of and skills in variety of ethnic song forms, knowledge of cultural characteristics and awareness of personal culturally based biases and attitudes.

Summary and Conclusions

Cancer temporarily or permanently disrupts lives, hopes, careers, aspirations, integrity, dreams, and sense of security. If the crisis of cancer is successfully managed, patients and families can experience psychological growth and maturity. Music therapists use music and the relationship that develops between the client and therapist through the music to promote healing and enhance quality of life. When used in conjunction with other cancer treatments, music therapy has the potential to help patients cope mentally and physically with their diagnosis.

Music therapists work with cancer patients in a variety of treatment settings, during various stages of survivorship. Music therapy sessions may involve creating music, improvising, listening to music, and/or performing music. After a thorough assessment of patient needs, the music therapist will design treatment sessions using any of these methods to induce change. What makes music therapy such a unique treatment modality is that music allows one to access what is still healthy, creative, and expressive, no matter how ill the patient may be. Through the client/therapist relationship that develops with and through the music, a healthy space is created that allows for needed physical, emotional, and/or spiritual change to take place, which, in turn, allows for the patient to live their life without giving in to the illness.

References

Adler, N., & Page, A. (Eds.) (2008). *Cancer care for the whole patient: Meeting psychosocial health needs* (pp. 55–56). Washington, DC: National Academies Press.

Aldridge, G. (1996). "A Walk through Paris:" The development of melodic expression in music therapy with a breast cancer patient. *The Arts in Psychotherapy,* 23(3), 207–223.

Allen, J. (2008). Music imagery in the exploration of oncological pain. Unpublished manuscript.

Allen, J. (2011). Group music psychotherapy in improving the self-concept of breast cancer: survivors. Conference proceedings. *Music Therapy Today, 9*(1), 100–101.

American Cancer Society. (2011). *Global cancer facts & figures,* 2nd ed. Atlanta, GA: American Cancer Society. Retrieved from http://www.cancer.org/acs/groups/content/@epidemiologysurveilance/documents/document/acspc-027766.pdf

American Cancer Society. (2012a). *Understanding radiation therapy: A guide for patients and families.* (Brochure). Retrieved from http://www.cancer.org/acs/groups/cid/documents/webcontent/003299-pdf.pdf

American Cancer Society. (2012b). *Targeted therapies.* (Brochure). Retrieved from http://www.cancer.org/acs/groups/cid/documents/webcontent/003024-pdf.pdf

American Cancer Society. (2013). *Understanding chemotherapy: A guide for patients and families.* (Brochure). Retrieved from http://www.cancer.org/acs/groups/cid/documents/webcontent/003321-pdf.pdf

Bailey, L. (1983). The effects of live music versus taped-recorded music on hospitalized cancer patients. *Music Therapy, 3*(1), 17 – 28.

Bailey, L (1984). The use of songs in music therapy with cancer patients and their families. *Music Therapy, 4*(1), 5–17.

Bonde, L. (2005). *The Bonny Method of Guided Imagery and Music with cancer survivors: A psychosocial study with focus on the influence of music therapy on mood and quality of life.* Unpublished doctoral dissertation, Aalborg University, Denmark.

Brennan, J. (2001). Adjustment to cancer—coping or personal transition? *Psycho-oncology, 10*(1), 1–18.

Bruscia, K. (2000). A manual for level one training in Guided Imagery and Music. Unpublished.

Bruscia, K. (2004). Moving in and out of GIM. Unpublished.

Bunt, L., & Marston-Wyld, J. (1995). Where words fail music takes over: A collaborative study by music therapist and a counselor in the context of cancer care. *Music Therapy Perspectives, 13*(1), 46–50.

Burns, D. (2001). The effect of the Bonny Method of Guided Imagery and Music on the mood and life quality of cancer patients. *Journal of Music Therapy, 38*(1), 51–65.

Burns, D. (2002). Guided imagery and music (GIM) in the treatment of individuals with chronic illness. In K. Bruscia & D. Grocke (Eds.), *Guided imagery and music: The Bonny Method and beyond* (pp. 171–186). Gilsum, NH: Barcelona Publishers.

Burns, D., Sledge, R., Fuller, L., Daggy, J., & Monahan, P. (2005). Cancer patients' interest and preferences for music therapy. *Journal of Music Therapy, 42*(3), 185–199.

Burns, S., Harbuz, M., Hucklebridge, F., Bunt, L. (2001). A pilot study into the therapeutic effects of music therapy at a cancer help center. *Alternative Therapies, 7*(1), 48–56.

Cadrin, L. (2005–2006). Dying well: The Bonny Method of Guided Imagery and Music at end of life. *Journal of the Association for Music and Imagery, 10,* 1–25.

Carter, B. (1993). Long-term survivors of breast cancer: A qualitative descriptive study. *Cancer Nursing, 16,* 124–127.

Chaput, J., & Silverman, M. (2012). Effect of music therapy with patients on a post-surgical oncology unit: A pilot study determining maintenance of immediate gains. *The Arts in Psychotherapy,* 39(5), 1-27.

Christ, G. (1991). Principals of oncology social work. In A. Holleb, D. Fink., & G. Murphy (Eds)., *American Cancer Society textbook of clinical oncology.* Atlanta, GA: ACS.

Clark, M., Issacks-Downton, G., Wells, N., Redlin-Frazier, S., Eck, C., Hepworth, J., & Chakravarthy, B. (2006). Use of preferred music to reduce emotional distress and symptom activity during radiation therapy. *Journal of Music Therapy, 43*(3), 247-265.

Cook, J. (1985). The therapeutic use of music in the oncology setting. (Meeting abstract). *Oncology Nursing Forum, 12*(2), 86.

Daykin, N., McClean, S., & Bunt, L. (2007). Creativity, identity, and healing: Participants' accounts of music therapy in cancer care. *Health: An Interdisciplinary Journal for the Social Study of Health, Illness, and Medicine, 11*(3), 349-370.

Dileo, C. (1999). Songs for the living: The use of songs in the treatment of oncology patients. In C. Dileo (Ed.), *Music therapy and medicine: Theoretical and clinical Applications* (pp. 151–166). Silver Spring, MD: American Music Therapy Association.

Dileo, C., & Magill, L. (2005). Songwriting with oncology and hospice adult patients form a multicultural perspective. In T. Wigram & F. Baker (Eds.), *Songwriting: Methods, techniques and clinical applications for music therapy clinicians, educators and students.* (pp. 226 – 245). Philadelphia, PA: Jessica Kingsley.

Edge, S., Byrd, D., Compton, C., Fritz, A., Greene, F., & Trotti, A. (Eds.). (2010). *American Joint Committee on Cancer Staging manual* (7th ed.). New York: Springer.

Ferlay, J., Shin, H. R., Bray, F., Forman, D., Mathers, C., & Parkin, D. M. (2008). GLOBOCAN 2008 v2.0, Cancer incidence and mortality worldwide: IARC Cancer Base No. 10. (Internet). Lyon, France:

International Agency for Research on Cancer, 2010. Retrieved August 12, 2012, from http://globocan.iarc.frFerrer, A. (2007). The effect of live music on decreasing anxiety in patients undergoing chemotherapy treatment. *Journal of Music Therapy, 44*(3), 242-255.

Flavo, D. (2005). *Medical and psychosocial aspects of chronic illness and disability*, 3rd ed. Boston: James & Bartlett.

Fleming, I. (2001). Surgical therapy. In R. Lenhard, R. Osteen, & T. Gansler (Eds.), *Clinical oncology* (pp. 160–165). Atlanta, GA: American Cancer Society.

Folkman, S., & Greer, S. (2000). Promoting psychological well-being in the face of serious illness: When theory, research, and practice inform each other. *Psycho-oncology, 9*(1), 11–29.

Frank, J. (1985). The effects of music therapy and guided visual imagery on chemotherapy-induced nausea and vomiting. *Oncology Nursing Forum, 12*(5), 47–52.

Fredette, S. L. (1995). Breast cancer survivors: Concerns and coping. *Cancer Nursing, 18*(1), 35–46.

Gardstrom, S. (2007). *Music therapy improvisation for groups: Essential leadership competencies.* Gilsum, NH: Barcelona Publishers.

Grocke, D. & Wigram, T. (2007). *Receptive methods in music therapy: Techniques and clinical applications for music therapy clinicians, educators, and students.* Philadelphia, PA: Jessica Kingsley.

Hale, S. (1992). Wounded women: The use of guided imagery and music in recovering from a mastectomy. *Journal of the Association for Music and Imagery, 1,* 99–106.

Hanser, S., Bauer-Wu, S., Kubicek, L., Healey, M., Bunnell, C., & Manola, J. (2005). Effects of music therapy intervention for women with metastatic breast cancer. *Oncology Nursing Forum, 32*(1), 185–186.

Kornblith, A. (1998). Psychosocial adaptation of cancer survivors. In J. Holland, W. Breitbart, P. Jacobson, M. Lederberg, M. Loscaizo, & R. McCorkle (Eds), *Psycho-oncology* (pp. 223–241). New York: Oxford University Press.

Kroenke, K., Zhong, X., Theobold, D., Wu, J., Tu, W., & Carpenter. (2010). Somatic symptoms in patients with cancer experiencing pain or depression: Prevalence, disability, and health care use. *Archives of Internal Medicine, 170*(18), 1686-1694.

Lane, D. (1992). Music therapy: A gift beyond measure. *Oncology Nursing Forum, 19*(6), 863-867.

Leigh, S. (2005). Coping: Survivorship issues and financial Concerns. In J. Itano & K. Taoka (Eds), *Core curriculum for oncology nursing* (4th ed.). (pp. 80–88). Philadelphia: Elsevier.

Leigh, S., & Clark, E. (2002). Psychosocial aspects of cancer survivorship. In A. Berger, R. Portenoy, & D. Weissman (Eds.), *Principles and practice of supportive oncology,* 2nd ed. (pp. 1032–1043). Philadelphia, PA: Lippincott Williams & Wilkins.

Logan, H. (1998). Applied music-evoked imagery for the oncology patient: Results and case studies of a three-month music therapy pilot program. Unpublished manuscript.

Mar, J. (1998–1999). GIM at the end of life: Case studies in palliative care. *Journal of the Association for Mental Imagery, 6,* 37–54.

Mayo Clinic (2011). *Cancer treatment.* Phoenix, AZ: Mayo Clinic. Retrieved from: http://www.mayoclinic.org/cancer-treatment/

McCullough, M., Hoyt, W., Larson, D., Koenig, H., & Thoresen, C. (2000). Religious involvement and mortality: A meta-analytic review. *Health Psychology, 19*(3), 211–222.

McDougal – Miller (2010). Music therapy in adult cancer care: Across the cancer continuum. In D. Hanson-Abromeit and C. Colwell (Eds.), *Medical music therapy for adults in hospital settings.* (pp. 284-298). Silver Spring, MD: American Music Therapy Association.

McKinney, K., & Clark, M. (2003). *The effect of the BMGIM on distress, life quality, and endocrine hormone levels in women with non-metastatic breast cancer: Pilot study report 1998-2002.* Baltimore, MD: Center for Health Enhancement, St. Joseph Medical Center.

Moorer, T. (2004). Mass choir of breast cancer survivors sings messages of hope. *New Amsterdam News, 96*(1), 30–32.

Mullan, F. (1985). Seasons of survival: Reflections of a physician with cancer. *New England Journal of Medicine, 313,* 270–273.

National Cancer Institute. (2012a). *What is cancer?* (Fact sheet). Retrieved February 10, 2013, from http://www.cancer.gov/cancertopics/cancerlibrary/what-is-cancer

National Cancer Institute. (2012b). *Bone marrow transplantation and peripheral blood stem cell transplantation.* (fact sheet). Retrieved August 31, 2012, from www.cancer.gov/cancertopics/factsheet/Therapy/bone-marrowtransplant

Nicholas, D., & Veach, T. (2000). The psychosocial assessment of the adult cancer patient. *Professional Psychology, 31*(2), 206 –215.

Nolan, P. (1992). Music therapy with bone marrow transplant patients: Reaching beyond the symptoms. In R. Spintge and R. Droh (Eds). *MusicMedicine.* St. Louis, MO: MMB Music.

O'Brien, E. (1999). The experience of song writing and song sharing in cancer care. Paper presented at the Ninth World Congress of Music Therapy, Washington, DC.

O'Brien, E. (2003). The nature of the interactions between patient and therapist when writing a song on a bone marrow transplant unit. Unpublished master's thesis. The University of Melbourne.

O'Brien, E. (2006). Opera therapy: Creating and performing a new work with cancer patients and professional singers. *Nordic Journal of Music Therapy, 15*(1), 82–96. DOI: 10.1080/08098130609478153.

O'Callaghan, C. (2006). Clinical issues: Music therapy in an adult cancer inpatient therapy setting. *Journal for the Society for Integrative Oncology,* 4, 57-61.

O'Callaghan, C., Hornby, C., Pearson, E., & Ball, D. (2009). "The moment is all we have": Patients and visitors reflect on staff Christmas choir. *Medical Journal of Australia, 191*(11-12), 681-687.

O'Callaghan, C., O'Brien, E., Magill, L., & Ballinger, E. (2009). Resounding attachment: Cancer inpatients' song lyrics for their children in music therapy. *Supportive Cancer Care, 17,* 1149 – 1157.

Pienta, D. (1998). The effects of guided imagery and music on the self-esteem and well-being of cancer survivors: A pilot study. Unpublished manuscript.

Pelusi, J. (1997). The lived experience of surviving breast cancer. *Oncology Nursing Forum, 24,* 1343–1353.

Porchet-Munro, S. (1995). The supportive role of music. *European Journal of Palliative Care, 2*(2), 77–80.

President's Cancer Panel. (2003/2004). *Annual report. Living beyond cancer: Finding a new balance.* Bethesda, MD: National Cancer Institute, 2004. Retrieved July 11, 2012, at http://deainfo.nci.nih.gov/ADVISORY/pcp/pcp03-04rpt/Survivorship.pdf

Restifo, N., Robbins, P., & Rosenberg, S. (2008). Principles of immunotherapy. In V. DeVita, S. Hellman, & S. Rosenberg (Eds.). *Cancer: Principles and practice of oncology,* 8th ed. (pp. 351–368). Philadelphia: Lippincott Williams & Wilkins.

Robertson-Gilliam, K. (1995). The role of music therapy in meeting the spiritual needs of the dying person. In C. Lee (Ed.), *Lonely waters.* Oxford: Sobell Publications.

Rowland, J., & Massie, M. (1998). Breast cancer. In J. Holland (Ed.), *Psycho-oncology* (pp. 308–401). New York: Oxford University Press.

Rykov, M. (2008). Experiencing music therapy cancer support. *Journal of Health Psychology, 13,* 190–200. DOI: 10.1177/1359105307086708.

Short, A. (2002). Guided imagery and music (GIM) in medical care. In K. Bruscia & D. Grocke (Eds.), *Guided imagery and music: The Bonny Method and beyond (pp. 151-170).* Gilsum, NH: Barcelona Publishers.

Spencer, S., Carver, C., & Price, A. (1998). Psychological and social factors in adaptation. In C. Holland, W. Breitbart, P. Jacobson, M. Lederberg, M. Loscaizo, & R. McCorkle (Eds.), *Psycho-oncology* (pp. 211–222). New York: Oxford University Press.

Spira, J., & Reed, G. (2003). *Group psychotherapy for women with breast cancer.* Washington, DC: American Psychological Association.

Standley, J. (1992). Clinical applications of music and chemotherapy: The effects on nausea and emesis. *Music Therapy Perspectives,* 10(1), *30-40.*

Turry, A., & Turry, A. E. (1999). Creative song improvisations with children and adults with cancer. In C. Dileo (Ed.), *Music therapy & medicine: Theoretical and clinical applications* (pp. 167–178). Silver Spring, MD: American Music Therapy Association.

Waldon, E. (2001). The effects of group music therapy on mood states and cohesiveness in cohesiveness in adult oncology patients. *Journal of Music Therapy, 38*(3), 212–238.

Westbrook, J. (2006). Attachment, optimism, coping, and social support as predictors of psychosocial and psychological adjustment in women with breast cancer. *Dissertation Abstracts International: Section B: The Sciences and Engineering, 67*(2-B), 1174.

Wigram, T. (2005). Songwriting methods – Similarities and differences: Developing a working model. In F. Baker and T. Wigram (Eds.), *Songwriting: Methods, techniques, and clinical applications for music therapy clinicians, educators, and students.* Philadelphia, PA: Jessica Kingsley.

World Health Organization (2013). Fact sheet on cancer. Retrieved from: http://www.who.int/mediacentre/factsheets/fs297/en/index.html

Zebrack, B. (2000). Cancer survivor identity and quality of life. *Cancer Practice, 8*(5), 238–242. DOI: 10.1046/j.1523-5394.2000.85004.

Chapter 12

Adults in Palliative Care and Hospice

Amy Clements-Cortés

DIAGNOSTIC INFORMATION

The hospice care movement of the 19th and 20th centuries produced leaders in the medical field who wanted to share the vision of dying patients as whole persons (Watson, Lucas, Hoy, & Back, 2005). These leaders strove to connect many different treatment methods to address multiple issues that someone may face during the dying process. Cicely Saunders was a leading figure in the modern hospice movement and founded one of the first hospices in the United Kingdom, which soon became a model for other countries and medical practitioners to follow (Lawton, 2000). The modern hospice movement of the mid–20th century critiqued the impersonal, medical, and technologically based treatment of dying patients and shifted the philosophy of treatment to regard death as a normal and natural part of life. The movement also strove to emphasize the quality as opposed to the quantity of a person's life and acknowledge how personalization, family involvement, and decision-making were all key elements of patient care (Lawton, 2000). It is through this movement that the modern view of palliative care and treatment of the dying has emerged.

The need for palliative care services throughout the globe is growing due to the increasing aging population and the upsurge in disease and terminal disorders. In 2010, an estimated 1.58 million patients received services from hospice in the United States (National Hospice and Palliative Care Organization [NHPCO], 2012), and in the same year, NHPCO estimated that approximately 41.9% of all deaths in the United States were under the care of a hospice program (National Hospice and Palliative Care Organization [NHPCO], 2012). Statistics Canada projected that the rate of deaths in Canada would escalate by 33% in the year 2020 to over 330,000 deaths per year (Statistics Canada, 2004). Further, the Canadian Hospice Palliative Care Association (CHPCA) estimated that more than 160,000 (or approximately 62%) of the annual deaths in Canada require access to hospice palliative care services (CHPCA, 2011), and Rachlis (2006) acknowledges chronic diseases account for 70% of all deaths. Multiple resources and a variety of treatment options are essential for the care and treatment of current and future patients diagnosed with chronic or terminal illnesses. The World Health Organization (WHO, 2011a) defines palliative care as an approach that improves the quality of life of patients and their families facing the problems associated with life-threatening illness, through the prevention and relief of suffering by means of early identification and impeccable assessment and treatment of pain and other problems, physical, psychosocial, and spiritual. (para. 1)

The WHO also describes that care in palliative settings affirms life and regards dying as a normal process, integrates the psychological and spiritual aspects of patient care, offers a support system to help the family cope during the patient's illness and in their own bereavement, uses a team approach to address the needs of patients and their families, including bereavement counseling in conjunction with other therapies that are intended to prolong life, such as chemotherapy or radiation therapy, and includes those investigations needed to better understand and manage distressing clinical complications. (para. 2)

The terms palliative care and hospice care are often used interchangeably in the medical field, although the CHPCA distinguishes the two terms by affirming that in Canada, medical professionals use both terms to refer to the same subject, which is the specific approach to care described in the definition. However, some professionals use hospice care to describe care that is offered in the community rather than in hospitals, maintaining that palliative care may be received in many settings, including in-home services, hospitals, hospices, and long-term care facilities.

Palliative Care Australia recently released a glossary of palliative care terms. They describe end-of-life care as follows: "Combines the broad set of health and community services that care for the population at the end of their life. Quality end-of-life care is realized when strong networks exist between specialist palliative care providers, primary generalist providers, primary specialists and support care providers, and the community—working together to meet the needs of people requiring care." (Palliative Care Australia, 2008)

Typical Diagnoses

Definitions from various health organizations list the possible illnesses that fall under the scope of palliative care. Patients in palliative care suffer life-threatening illnesses, which may include: cancer, cardiovascular disease, chronic respiratory diseases, kidney disease, liver disease, spinal cord injuries, Amyotrophic Lateral Sclerosis (ALS), Multiple Sclerosis (MS), Alzheimer's Disease, and Acquired Immunodeficiency Syndrome (AIDS)/Human Immunodeficiency Virus (HIV) (Canadian Hospice Palliative Care Association, 2011; National Consensus Project for Quality Palliative Care, 2009). These will each be briefly defined below.

Cancer: A large group of diseases that can affect any part of the body; a rapid growth of abnormal cells that can then invade adjoining parts of the body and/or spread to other organs (WHO, 2011b, para. 2).

Cardiovascular Disease: Disorders of the heart and blood vessels, including coronary heart disease (heart attacks), cerebrovascular disease (stroke), raised blood pressure (hypertension), peripheral artery disease, rheumatic heart disease, congenital heart disease, and heart failure (WHO, 2011c, para. 1).

Chronic Respiratory Diseases: Diseases of the airway and other structures of the lung, including: asthma, chronic obstructive pulmonary disease, occupational lung diseases, and pulmonary hypertension (WHO , 2011d, para. 2).

Kidney and Liver Disease: The presence of kidney damage, or a decreased level of kidney function, for a period of three months or more (The Kidney Foundation of Canada, 2011, para. 2); cirrhosis, which is the end stage of many different forms of liver disease and is known to cause a number of additional health problems, including variceal bleeding, ascites, and hepatic encephalopathy (The Canadian Liver Foundation, 2011, paras. 1, 2).

Neurological Diseases: Disorders that affect brain and nervous system development and/or function are also typical diagnoses in palliative/hospice care. These include: spinal cord injuries, Amyotrophic Lateral Sclerosis, Muscular Dystrophy, and Alzheimer's Disease (National Institute of Neurological Disorders and Stroke, 2011).

Spinal Cord Injury: An injury [that] usually begins with a sudden, traumatic blow to the spine that fractures or dislocates vertebrae. Some injuries will allow almost complete recovery.

Others will result in complete paralysis (National Institute of Neurological Disorders and Stroke, 2011, para. 1).

Amyotrophic Lateral Sclerosis (ALS): A chronic, progressive disease marked by gradual degeneration of the nerve cells in the central nervous system that control voluntary muscle movement. The disorder causes muscle weakness and atrophy; also called Lou Gehrig's Disease or Motor Neuron Disease (The ALS Society of Canada, 2011, para. 8).

Multiple Sclerosis: Disease of the central nervous system, which is composed of the brain and spinal cord (The Multiple Sclerosis Society of Canada, 2011, para. 1).

Alzheimer's Disease: A progressive, degenerative disease. Symptoms include loss of memory, judgment, and reasoning; difficulty with day-to-day tasks; and changes in communication abilities, mood, and behavior (The Alzheimer Society of Canada, 2009, paras. 1, 2).

Immune System Disorders: Retrovirus that infects cells of the immune system, destroying or impairing their function. The most advanced stage of HIV infection is Acquired Immunodeficiency Syndrome (AIDS) (WHO, 2011, para. 1e).

The large variety of the disorders and illnesses that fall within the scope of palliative care demonstrates the need for individualized care and a variety of therapies to address numerous issues among patients.

Needs and Resources

The needs of patients in palliative care vary depending on the individual strengths and resources of the patient. However, there are common issues that patients in palliative care might present, including pain management, symptom control, anxiety, maintaining dignity, and cultural, spiritual, and emotional needs (Halpin, Seamark, & Seamark, 2009; Higginson, Wade, & McCarthy, 1990; McKinnon & Miller, 2002).

Physical Needs

Patients receiving palliative or hospice care have a range of physical complications and needs. These include managing the effects of pain, nausea, vomiting, constipation, dry mouth, and fatigue. Additional medical complications such as intestinal obstruction, opioid toxicity, dermatologic problems, and disease-specific symptoms may occur (Mount, Hanks, & McGoldrick, 2005). Respiratory and respiratory system complications include dyspnea (difficult or labored respiration [Merriam-Webster, 2012a]), congestive heart failure, respiratory infections, superior vena cava syndrome (restricted blood flow to the heart caused by compression from tumors or blood clots, which creates increased pressure in the veins in the face and arms, causing fluid buildup [Wedro, 2012]), pleural effusion, ascites (abnormal accumulation of serous fluid in the spaces between tissues and organs in the abdominal cavity [Merriam-Webster, 2012b]), cough, hemoptysis, and lymphangitic carcinomatosis (a condition characterized by the presence of carcinomas, the most common type of cancer, that have metastasized through the lymphatics of the lung [American Heritage, 2008; Ikezoe, Godwin, Hunt, & Marglin, 1995]) (McKinnis, 2002). Neurological complications consist of delirium, dementia, and seizures (Maluso-Bolton & Schlecter, 2002). Physical symptoms are often the main foci in palliative care; however, when medical staff and the patient are primarily focused on physical needs, psychosocial needs may remain unmet, which in turn may cause a multitude of problems and prove antiproductive in the patient's care (Mount, Hanks, & McGoldrick, 2005).

Emotional/Psychological Needs

Common emotional/psychological needs consist of adjusting to fear, sadness, perplexity, and anger. If these issues are unaddressed, they may lead to serious psychiatric disorders, including depression, anxiety, and confusion (Lloyd-Williams, 2008). Lloyd-Williams lists psychosocial needs in palliative care as desires for understanding, acceptance, self-esteem, safety, belonging, love, spirituality, and hope. She explains that people in palliative care have needs in multiple contexts of their lives, including, social, emotional, psychological, cultural, sexual, and ethical areas.

The two following studies report the most important and common needs of patients in palliative care. In the first study, with patients diagnosed with advanced cancer or ALS, the most significant personal values were benevolence, self-direction, and universalism (Fegg, Wasner, Neudert, & Borasio, 2005). Osse, Vernooij-Dassen, Schade, and Grol (2005) found that among the multitude of issues that patients identified, the five that required further attention were: informational needs, coping with the unpredictability of the future, fear of metastases, fear of physical suffering, and difficulties remembering what was discussed during consultations. The needs of patients in palliative care are numerous and often require the assistance of professionals to alleviate suffering. Nevertheless, patients in palliative care have key personal characteristics and strengths that help them to cope with issues and even grow from the experience.

Spiritual Needs

Palliative care patients often have spiritual needs near the end of life, regardless of their religious or cultural background. Murray, Kendall, Boyd, Worth and Benton (2004) discovered that patients and caregivers expressed needs for love, meaning, purpose, and sometimes transcendence. Other spiritual needs include the need for positivity, hope, and gratitude; the need to give and receive love; the need to review beliefs; the need to have meaning; and needs related to religiosity and preparation for death (Johnston, 2003). In one study of advanced cancer patients, researchers found that many advanced cancer patients' spiritual needs were not supported by religious communities or the medical system; however, spiritual support was associated with better quality of life. They also discovered that religious individuals more frequently wanted aggressive measures to extend life (Balboni et al., 2007). Spiritual needs are an important area of care that may be neglected in certain settings or situations, and it is vital for medical staff and caregivers to recognize the importance of addressing these issues.

Patient Strengths

Strengths demonstrated by patients in palliative care embody creativity, dignity, honour, and sense of identity (Proulx & Jacelon, 2004). With respect to a patient`s hope, Hermsen and Henk (2004) describe the strength required to have hope in themselves and the future. Other research utilizing interviews focused on patients' hope in palliative care identified a subtheme of inner strength and energy and confidence in treatment (Benzein & Saveman, 1998). Additional strengths include preserving dignity in the face of adversity (Chochinov, 2002; Enes, 2003; Proulx & Jacelon, 2004; Street & Kissane, 2001).

Musical Characteristics

Terminal illnesses affect people of any age, race, ethnicity, and religious background. This makes it difficult to define musical characteristics of this population, as every person has different environmental influences that affect their relationship with music. One patient may have been a music performer before he/she was hospitalized, while a patient in the same room may have never played a musical instrument and only used music as a listening tool. Music may have religious meaning to some patients, while it may be a profession or lifestyle choice of others. Every patient is accompanied by diverse musical experiences, and a wide variety of musical characteristics may be present in different patients. Also, depending on the illness and the severity of symptoms, patients may be limited in their ability to use music in the same way they did before the illness occurred. For example, a singer who develops throat cancer may have used music as personal enjoyment and as a part of his/her career, but now is unable to sing. People's ability to play instruments may be affected by strength and pain, and cognitive issues such as delirium may affect a patient's receptive listening skills. The individual variance with this population makes it difficult to define specific musical characteristics, and there is a lack of research in this area. Most commonly, musical characteristics are identified in individual case studies in music therapy and therefore cannot be generalized to the general population of patients in palliative care. One example is brought forward by Aldridge (1996), who found that the patient in music therapy demonstrated music expressivity, originality, and musical intuition.

The variety of musical characteristics with palliative care patients informs practitioners that generalized music would not be as effective as client-specific preferred music. Hogan (1998) highlighted several benefits of preferred familiar music with terminally ill patients, including providing patients with a sense of achievement, greater control in their environment, and a physically and mentally stimulating experience, and heightening their awareness and exploration of emotional needs. Hogan also stated that familiar music can enhance purpose and self-worth by stimulating creative participation and that creating recordings of familiar music may provide comfort in times of fear and loneliness for the patient, while leaving behind a legacy gift for family members in the bereavement process. In one study investigating the effects of preferred music on pain perception, results showed that participants' own chosen music was found to increase tolerance and perceived control ratings in both male and female participants and that preferred music was both distracting and had a positive affective impact on the pain experience (Mitchell & MacDonald, 2006). When undergoing radiation therapy, patients who listened to self-selected music reported lower anxiety and treatment-related distress (Clark et al., 2006).

Referral and Assessment

As patient needs are vast and varying, referrals to music therapy are made for a combination of reasons, including physical, emotional, psychosocial, and spiritual issues. Referral trends show that nurses are the primary health care providers who refer patients, and the majority of patients are referred for symptom-based reasons, seconded by a need for additional support and coping (Horne-Thompson, Daveson, & Hogan, 2007). Referrals to music therapy by health care practitioners are largely based on their knowledge and experience with music therapy, and personal reasons and attitudes strongly influence the referral process (Hillmer, 2003). General reasons for referral include pain management, alteration in mental/neurological functioning, spiritual support, and coping (Houck, 2007).

Palliative care assessments can range from general medical-based assessments, disease-specific assessments, and symptoms-based assessments, to treatment-specific assessments. The following is an overview of popular assessment tools used in various palliative care settings.

Pain assessment is at the forefront of symptoms-based assessments. Typical assessment tools in this area include the following: McGill Pain Questionnaire, Brief Pain Inventory, Dartmouth Pain Questionnaire, West Haven–Yale Multidimensional Pain Inventory, Minnesota Multiphasic Personality Inventory, University of Alabama in Birmingham (UAB) Pain Behavior Scale, African Palliative Outcome Scale, Pain Assessment in Advanced Dementia (PAINAD) Scale, and pain intensity scales that include a visual analogue scale (VAS), numerical rating scale, and verbal descriptor scale (Powell, Downing, Ddungu, & Mwangi-Powell, 2010).

Using pain and symptom assessments helps guide clinical music therapy work in targeting specific symptoms to reduce pain and discomfort. Furthermore, allied health care professionals and nurses often administer these tools when working with the patients, and results are documented in the client chart.

Quality of life is a general goal in palliative care, and assessment forms that focus on quality of life also touch on other areas of need. Quality of life assessments often used in hospice and palliative care include: Edmonton Symptom Assessment Schedule (ESAS), European Organization for Research on Cancer Treatment (EORTC QLQ-C30), Hebrew Rehabilitation Centre for Aged Quality of Life (HRCA-QL), McGill Quality of Life Questionnaire (MQOL), McMaster Quality of Life Scale (MQLS), Palliative Care Assessment (PACA), Palliative Care Core Standards (PCCS), Rotterdam Symptom Checklist (RSCL), Support Team Assessment Schedule (STAS), Symptom Distress Scale (SDS), and Schedule for the Evaluation of Individual Quality of Life (SEIQoL) (Hearn & Higginson, 1997).

Using these standardized assessment scales is extremely valuable in music therapy practice, as they provide individualized information and guide specific interventions in clinical work.

Music Therapy Assessments

There is a small amount of research on music therapy assessments in palliative care, and the literature illuminates the need for standardized assessment materials in music therapy palliative/hospice care. Both the American Music Therapy Association and Canadian Association of Music Therapy provide general guidelines for practitioners to use in music therapy assessments. Hanser (1999) defines three types of assessments, including an initial assessment performed at the beginning of therapy to gather information about the client and develop treatment goals; comprehensive assessment, which allows the therapist to examine all aspects of a client's functioning and determine whether a client may benefit from music therapy; and ongoing assessment that continues throughout the treatment process and is reflected in session planning, treatment planning, and progress notes. Generally, music therapy practitioners use assessments that are standard tools implemented by medical staff at the facility to direct their interventions. This practice was highlighted by Groen (2007) in her study of current trends in pain assessment in end-of-life care for music therapy. She found that although there are a variety of popular assessment tools, 90% of hospice and palliative nursing professionals recommend the use of the FACES or picture scales by non-nursing health care professionals to assess patient pain; however, music therapists did not report using this scale as often as they did the Numerical Rating Scale (NRS) or a pain observation checklist. The main finding of Groen's study identified the majority of music therapists in the hospice setting incorporate formal pain assessment into their practice. The Numerical Rating Scale (NRS) and the Pain Behavior Observation Checklist were reported to be the most popular both among nursing and music therapy professionals.

Many assessments developed for music therapy involve utilizing assessments from the medical field to evaluate change in the client. Two of these tests include the Hospice Quality of Life Index–Revised (HQLI-R) and the Palliative Performance Scale (PPS) (Hilliard, 2003). Patients are frequently asked to complete a variety of self- assessments, including the European Organization for Research and Treatment of Cancer quality-of-life instrument (EORTC QLQ-C30), Edmonton Symptom Assessment System (ESAS), and the Hospital Anxiety and Depression Scale (HADS) (Strömgren et al., 2002).

Research is lacking in the area of music therapy assessment tools in palliative care. Maeu-Johnson and Tanguay (2006) created a hospice-based music therapy assessment tool based on clinical practice. The purpose of this assessment tool was to assist music therapists in achieving a clear and detailed portrayal of the current level of functioning of adult hospice patients, and also to help music therapists obtain relevant information to be used in forming a proper plan of care. Apart from this recent assessment tool, there are a limited amount of assessment tools available for the practicing music therapist. Clinicians should strive toward using assessment forms that are used by other health care professionals to provide unified patient treatment.

Overview of Methods and Procedures

The following methods and procedures are used most commonly with palliative care and hospice patients. These have not been sequenced to reflect relative significance, effectiveness, or complexity.

Receptive Music Therapy

- Music for Relaxation: using music, with or without additional relaxation techniques, to aid in achieving physical comfort.
- Guided Imagery: music and imagery techniques for in-depth exploration of emotional issues.
- Music for Reminiscence: music to retrieve memories and help bring them to life to recount in the therapy setting.
- Song Choice: encouraging the patient to choose and listen to preferred songs.
- Song (Lyric) Discussion: discussing song lyrics/themes to help client relate to or explore difficult emotions.
- Somatic Listening: using musical tones and vibrations to target specific physiological functioning.

Improvisational Music Therapy

- Empathic Improvisation: Therapist creates an improvisation that compassionately complements the client's current state of physical and mental being.
- Referential Improvisation: Therapist gives a verbal reference on which to base the improvisation, such as a story, a topic for fantasizing, or symbols.
- Active Improvisation: Client plays instruments, exploring their emotions freely with music.

Re-creative Music Therapy

- Vocal: vocalizations or singing, either individually or in a group setting.
- Instrumental: playing instruments freely or learning a new instrument, either individually or in a group setting.

Compositional Music Therapy

- Song Composition: writing instrumental parts or lyrics for a new song
- Song Stories: creation of a song telling the story of a client.
- Musical Autobiographies/Musical Life Reviews: client creating a list of songs that tells their story, either prearranged or composed by him/herself or the therapist.
- Music Collages: client creating a list of songs that depicts any story or theme not life-review specific, such as music that describes who he/she is, family, etc.

GUIDELINES FOR RECEPTIVE MUSIC THERAPY

Music for Relaxation

Overview. Music for relaxation is indicated if the client is experiencing tension, anxiety, difficulty sleeping, or pain (Bailey, 1986). Goals when using music for relaxation with palliative patients include: decreasing anxiety, improving physical comfort, increasing/initiating muscle relaxation, decreasing agitation/restlessness, and decreasing shortness of breath (Gallagher, Lagman, Walsh, Davis, & LeGrand, 2006). Grocke and Wigram (2007) state that music and relaxation may be used to reduce stress and tension as well as anxiety prior to medical procedures, alleviate pain and pain intensity, and regulate breathing. Schulberg (1981) affirms that relaxation training accompanied with music may be used to relieve high-level tension, eliminate insomnia, aid clients with tension-caused illnesses, and reduce tension to facilitate therapeutic conversation. Schulberg highlights that relaxation to music does not always intend to alter consciousness and put someone to sleep but can be used to facilitate a variety of goals (as listed above).

Music for relaxation should not be used if a client is struggling to remain conscious and wishes to remain conscious. If medication or aspects of the illness are making the client drowsy and he/she wishes to remain awake, music for relaxation is inadvisable because the music may affect their level of consciousness. Also, if the client is alert and wanting to participate in active music-making or discussion, music for relaxation might increase anxiety and restlessness. A proper assessment of the client's needs avoids this situation. Grocke and Wigram (2007) list contraindications for music and relaxation as patients who may be confused with abstract thought or scripts that involve embodied experiences, feel vulnerable being watched, have discomfort due to pain, have difficulty with deep breathing, and be embarrassed at paying attention to parts of the body in the presence of others. Depending on the client's discomfort level, relaxation sessions should be adapted or avoided. Clair (1996) notes that relaxation to music would not be appropriate if the client has no interest in relaxation or if orientation to reality is poor.

Music therapists with an undergraduate degree may be prepared to implement this technique with clients in palliative care, assuming that they had experience in doing so under supervision. If this is a new technique area, then a music therapist should research appropriate song choices related to goal areas and take steps to develop a listening protocol suitable to the client and their clinical needs.

Preparation. It is always beneficial to introduce the client to what the goals of music for relaxation are and then also to ask him/her if he/she has had any prior experience. Oftentimes, clients will have used music in their own lives to induce relaxation, and they may have certain genres, composers, or songs they know that help relax them and put them at ease. This can be very beneficial for clients, not only to help induce relaxation, but also to add a sense of personalization and comfort in a time when they may be away from home or in different schedules and circumstances than they are used to. It is also important to show the client your list of repertoire and explain that you have many valuable songs and techniques to use to help induce relaxation.

Grocke and Wigram (2007) present four major factors essential to an environment that fosters music relaxation. These include a comfortable position for the patient, light and dark, uninterrupted space, and monitoring the music reproduction (making sure equipment is properly placed and preparations are made in advance). Preparation of the session includes ensuring that all of these factors are suitable to the client; that the client is comfortable, the lighting is appropriate, medical staff and visitors know in advance that a relaxation session will take place, and all equipment is prepared.

Music selection should be individualized for the client. In general, if the client has not listed specific musical preferences, music should be predictable and steady, with a consistent tempo and minimal change in dynamics. Repetition is also important, and the harmony and melody are typically tonal and consonant. Wigram, Pederson, and Bonde (2002) listed important elements in music for relaxation as follows: stable tempo; stability or only gradual changes in volume, rhythm, timbre, pitch, and harmony; consistent texture; predictable harmonic modulation; appropriate cadences; predictable melodic lines; repetition of material, structure, and form; gentle timbre; and few accents.

What to observe. Both objective and subjective methods are used when assessing a client in a relaxation session. During the session, objective observation by a music therapist includes whether the client is breathing more deeply, if tension is being released from the body, a decrease in rigidity, and the client's level of consciousness. In some settings, it will be possible to monitor heart rate, respiratory rate, and extremity temperature via monitors in the patient's room. Clinicians should also pay attention to which musical selections contribute to the client's reaction and eliminate a song if it is causing tension or an adverse effect. If a song is effective and elicits positive effects in the client, it may be used again with that client, or perhaps with clients with similar musical preferences.

Clinicians can use patient self-rated questionnaires to determine if and how the relaxation session produced change. Self-rated questionnaires include: Spielberger's State–Trait Anxiety Inventory (STAI), Short-Form McGill Pain Questionnaire (SFMPQ), Linear Analog Self-Assessment Scale (LASA), and visual analogue scales (Calovini, 1993; Longfield, 1995).

Procedures. An important decision in using music for relaxation is whether to use live or recorded music. Recorded music captures a variety of musical elements and sounds, allows the therapists to focus on the vocal quality of the script, eliminates concerns regarding therapist performance fatigue, and allows for patient conditioning of the relaxation response. However, there is evidence that live music is more effective than recorded music. Bailey (1983) found that when hospitalized cancer patients listened to live music, they reported significantly less tension-anxiety and increased vigor compared to when listening to taped music. Also, when listening to live music, patients reported significantly less physical discomfort and an increase in positive mood and recommended music sessions for others.

Generally, the structure of a relaxation session is as follows:

Preparation:

- Find a comfortable position for client
- Keep light, noise, and distraction controlled to a minimum
- Prepare music selections and inductions

Induction (See Appendix A):

- Progressive muscle relaxation
- Structured/count down
- Autogenic-type
- Imagery such as color or light
- Tension and release to cues
- Meditative relaxation:

Music:

- Prerecorded Examples
  - Stephen Page, Steve Travis, Simon Cunliffe: The Therapy Collection: Meditation
  - Keith Hyett: Reflections
  - Various Artists: Healing music from around the world: Volume 1
  - Amy Clements-Cortés: Soothing Relaxation Journeys
  - David Bradstreet: Theracalm
- Live Music
  - Play a song repeatedly, gradually slowing down the tempo
    - Can choose a client's preferred song or song genre
    - Songs in 3/4 time are beneficial in relaxing a client (a traditional example is Brahms's "Lullaby")
  - Play within a simple chord progression, reducing the musical elements to soft, slow, and steady, or whatever variation seems appropriate at the time.

Return to alert state

- Structured
- Countdown

Verbal processing:

- How did the music make you feel?
- Do you notice any changes?
- How does your body feel?
- What words come to mind when you think of the music?
- What are you sensing or are aware of at present?

At times, music for relaxation can be a spontaneous and unplanned event. A music therapist may enter the room and the client may be experiencing physical or emotional stress/pain. Many times, music therapists go into a room to help a client fall asleep. In these situations, a planned induction or recorded music is not always possible. The music therapist can subsequently base the music he/she plays on the client's current state of being and attempt to relax the client and release tension.

Adaptations. Adaptations will almost always be made due to the variety of diagnoses and personal music preferences. Patient need and preferences may lead to variations in session length, abstract versus concrete thought, and changes in the order of the general procedure. Additionally, relaxation to music may also be carried out in group settings or with the client and their family members.

Guided Imagery

Overview. The Bonny Method of Guided Imagery and Music is an advanced practice method, which requires a therapist to complete three distinct levels of study in order to become a facilitator and to practice in the method. Goals of GIM for palliative patients include: improving mood, enhancing quality of life, decreasing emotional stress, reducing anxiety, decreasing sadness and depression, decreasing pain and nausea, facilitating emotional outlets, and providing an avenue for expressing grief and hope (Burns, 2001; Logan, 1998). An important goal of GIM is to reduce psychological distress, which can decrease a person's immune function through the positive effects that GIM has on immune and endocrine function in individuals with chronic illness (Short, 2002). If a client is experiencing psychological pain or suffering, guided imagery may be used to address emotional issues or provide emotional relief to aid in pain management and improve symptoms associated with the illness. If a client is experiencing difficulty feeling in control or is having feelings of hopelessness, music and imagery may be indicated as a way to visualize aspects of their disease to facilitate a gain in their sense of control and understanding. Clark (2000) states that in the medical setting, there are four ways to use guided imagery with clients: to decrease negative feelings, to promote healing, to improve problem-solving, and to prepare for upcoming situations.

Addressing psychological issues through music and imagery requires a certain amount of psychological strength on the part of the client before beginning an imagery session. If the client does not have the resilience to tackle difficult internal issues, their pain may be amplified (Dileo & Bradt, 1999). Wigram, Pederson, and Bonde (2002) list contraindications for traditional guided imagery and music as clients with reality (testing) problems, emotional instability, and intellectual impairment. Burns (2002) states the importance of clients receiving medical treatments when suffering from pain before using guided imagery and music, because acute pain can impede the imagery process. Marr (1998) maintains that if a patient has difficulty concentrating due to their illness, the patient will have trouble focusing and will not have sufficient energy to engage in a thorough imagery process. Other contraindications include clients suffering from hallucinations, personality disorders, and/or displaying suicidal ideations. Cohen (2002) highlights specific populations who should not receive guided imagery to music, which include clients who are mentally unstable, acutely psychotic, in acute phases of substance withdrawal, or without the necessary cognitive skills to interpret the abstract material from their unconscious.

Preparation. Preparation for music and imagery is similar to that for music and relaxation, in that the client should be as comfortable as possible before engaging in the activity. Bruscia (2002a) outlines the difference in guided imagery and music for relaxation, in that relaxation is used in guided imagery only to help the client achieve an open state of mind to explore expanded states of consciousness, and the goal of guided imagery is not focused solely on physical relaxation. Therefore, although there are similar types of inductions and techniques in guided imagery and relaxation, the preparation of the session and environment may be completely different. Similarities between imagery and relaxation include an uninterrupted space and a comfortable position for the client. Differences take account of the lighting used, as music and imagery can occur in a conscious state and therefore dim lights may not be necessary. A quality audio device is essential for the music to be played on, and items to assist the client in becoming comfortable. With this population, guided imagery and music is done with the client lying on his/her bed or sitting in a comfortable chair.

The Bonny Method of Guided Imagery and Music (BMGIM) requires a quiet space that will not be disturbed for approximately 70 to 120 minutes. This is not always practical in a hospital setting for palliative care patients, as there are often interruptions and potentially clients may also share their room. However, if a client is in a single room, or in care at home, a session can be executed provided the music therapist makes it clear to all medical staff that an interruption should not occur. The BMGIM involves the use of specifically sequenced classical music pieces, which last approximately 30 to 45 minutes and are known as "programs." There are over 18 music programs available in the BMGIM, each with different qualities and goals. The therapist must be very knowledgeable of all programs to be able to select the appropriate one for particular client issues (Grocke, 2002). Specific techniques for preparing the session and environment and executing the procedure are taught to clinicians in the BMGIM training program, and one cannot practice BMGIM techniques without official training. However, guided imagery to music is a universal technique belonging to the field of music therapy and can therefore be practiced by general music therapy clinicians.

What to observe. Grocke (2005) compiled a list of common types of experiences that clients may have in BMGIM. Collective experiences include visual experiences, memories, emotions and feelings, body sensations, body movements, somatic sensations, altered auditory perceptions, pure music transference (the client is fully engaged in the music), associations and transference to the music, abstract imagery, spiritual imagery/experiences, transpersonal experiences, archetypal figures, dialogue, aspects of the shadow part of the self, and symbolic shapes. Any of these experiences should be noted by the therapist, in order to be brought forth to the client postsession for client interpretation.

Grocke and Wigram (2007) list that the four essential items a therapist should observe are whether the client is able to listen to the relaxation induction and follow the instructions, concentrate on the therapist's voice when giving visualization, return from the relaxed state, and discuss the experience and gain benefit.

It is also highly important to observe if a client is having a traumatizing experience or physical discomfort. If clients imagine situations or feelings that are painful to them and they are not emotionally prepared to deal with those emotions, the imagery session should end and discussion should ensue. A large issue in guided imagery to music is transference and countertransference. In transference, the client reacts to the therapist as if the therapist is a significant person in the client's life, and in countertransference, the therapist reacts to the client's projections as though the therapist was a significant person in the client's life, or the therapist reacts to the client as though he/she was a significant person in the therapist's life (Bruscia, 1995). It is extremely important to be observant of the client's state of consciousness and the issues he/she might be projecting on the therapist, as a therapist must be cautious with his/her reactions to the client's transference. Bruscia (1995) also notes that the therapist's state of consciousness may also be altered, as he/she is experiencing the same stimuli as the client. It is important for a therapist to observe the client's level of consciousness and remain in control of awareness so that he/she can properly guide the client; however, Bruscia states that entering an altered state of consciousness for a brief period of time can be beneficial because it may loosen personal boundaries and free thinking to allow for more intuitive experiences.

Procedures. There are several methods for guided imagery to music, including regulative music therapy by Schwabe (1987), unguided music imaging, group music imaging, and guided music imaging. Grocke and Wigram (2007) list and describe different imagery methods. They describe directed music imaging as including a script for the imagery; unguided music imaging as occurring when the client generates imagery in response to the music solely; group music imaging as that in which each group member generates their own response to music; and guided music imaging as being where the client engages with the therapist in dialogue describing the imagery, and the therapist initiates questions and discussion. The variety in possible methods is valuable for music therapists working in palliative care due to vast client needs and the diversity of settings. The range presented in this setting requires a music therapist to have a large set of methods that are adaptable in any setting.

Clark (2000) provides guidelines for the session format when using guided imagery in a medical setting, which begins with achieving a relaxed state, imagining a safe and calming place, picturing the part that needs healing, reinforcing imagery ability, and returning to the present. Clark offers images to suggest in guided imaging, including picturing the client's white blood cells as animals eating the cancer cells, picturing radiant light, blood flow inside the body, giving cancer an image and voice, inner advisors, or images of health and wellness. Any of these images can be used for a variety of illnesses in palliative care. For pain, Clark suggests images of pain as a bird, colour, or time. This procedure or these images can be accompanied by music to achieve a deeper state of imagery.

The most popular technique for guided imagery in music therapy is the BMGIM. The Bonny Method involves five phases. Phase 1: An opening conversation serves as an introductory dialogue on issues of importance for the client. A focus or goal for the session is defined, and the therapist notes the energy level and mood of the client before choosing the music. Phase 2: A short relaxation induction procedure leading to a concentration on the client's inner world. This shift in focus is also called a transition to an altered state of consciousness. Phase 3: The music-listening period, where the client listens to one of the standard music programs or other sequences of music selection at the discretion of the therapist. At this point, the therapist dialogues with the client, supporting and encouraging the client's imagery. Phase 4: After the music ends, a return to normal state of consciousness as the therapist tries helps the client bring closure to the imagery. Phase 5: Closing conversation, which is time that allows the client and therapist to discuss and make sense of the client's music-imagery experience, and then apply the messages and meanings to the client (Bonny, 2002). Originally, there were four phases, but the final phase was split in to two phases: a return to consciousness and then evaluation.

Adaptations. Clark (2000) suggests one possible adaptation to guided imagery in medical settings that may occur if the clients are skeptical of the procedure or are having difficulty obtaining clear images. Here a clinician could add physical objects for the client to touch or begin with having the client look at visuals, close their eyes, and start with that image. Depending on the client's level of functioning and psychological need, music and imagery could be combined with other forms of therapy, including gestalt dream work therapy, Jung's analytical psychology, psychodynamic approaches, and incorporating spiritual growth (Bruscia, 2002b; Clarkson, 2002; Kasayka, 2002; Ward, 2002). BMGIM can also use metaphor and narrative solely as a means of self-transformation for the client (Bonde, 2000). Other guidelines for guided imagery and music in palliative settings include duration of the session; the client's music preferences; incorporating other sensory stimuli such as touch, sight, or smell; and using group music imaging to stimulate social support and unity. Every guided imagery session will be unique, and the therapist must be adaptable him-/herself to be adjustable for the client's needs.

Music for Reminiscence

Overview. Music for reminiscence is concerned with helping clients use music to retrieve memories and to help bring them to life to recount in the therapy setting. Music therapists require experience with choosing appropriate repertoire and require training in clinical counseling skills before using this technique with palliative patients. Music for reminiscence may bring numerous serious issues to the surface for clients dealing with a terminal illness, and music therapists need to be aware of all counseling issues associated with this level of therapy before implementing this technique without supervision.

There are several potential benefits of using music for reminiscence in palliative care. Jonas (2005) states that music for reminiscence can reinforce the patient's self-identity and promote communication between patient and family, and particular songs used for reminiscence may evoke memories of childhood, teenage, and adult years. Bailey (1984) maintains that when patients listen to important songs from their past, the patients as well as family members can remove their feelings and thoughts from the present situation, which may in turn reduce and/or alleviate pain. Therefore, music for reminiscence may be used to promote communication between the client and the therapist or their family, evoke positive memories, thereby increasing positive mood, and alleviate pain. O'Callaghan (2005) states that music for reminiscence in palliative care may improve communication between patients and friends and family, validate patients' lives, and enable self-esteem, sense of worth and identity, enhanced insight, and ethical and cultural affirmation.

Another major indicator for using music for reminiscence is if the client shows signs that he/she could benefit from life review. Berger (2006) states that creating a musical life review can bring different generations together in interactive, meaning-making ways, as well as aid in emotional connection, remembrance, and creating meaning for one's life. This is especially important if clients have received a terminal diagnosis and have a limited time to live. If the client is demonstrating signs of issues with self-concept and personal identity or is showing a decline in self-esteem, musical life review is a technique used to illustrate to the client their accomplishments and provide an avenue where they can reflect positively on their life. It is also a valuable way to help family members remember their loved one and potentially record some type of legacy gift to assist in the grieving process. Grocke and Wigram (2007) state that musical life review can outline and overview the uniqueness of one's life journey. This can increase positive emotions and add life completion. According to Clements-Cortés (2004), music is a reflection of our period of time, and when using music for reminiscence with dying clients, songs and significant music from various times in a person's life may facilitate a review of life's joys and disappointments and help clients look for meaning in their lives.

Music for reminiscence should not be used if the client has experienced a traumatic past (in particular, do not use music from that time period) and is not psychologically prepared to address issues of traumatic life events. O'Callaghan (1996) acknowledges that certain music can elicit negative memories from the past and that the therapist must be attentive and observant when playing certain song selections for clients. Further, certain instruments used by the therapist can remind clients of traumatic life events (e.g., low bass sounds reminding clients of bombs during war), indicating that proper assessment and questions should be asked to the client to prevent these situations. At times, music for reminiscence should not be used with clients who have difficulty with reality orientation or are challenged in differentiating their past from the present. In those situations, music for reminiscence may reinforce a client's belief that he/she is living in the past and should therefore not be used.

Preparation. When preparing a session for music for reminiscence, it is always important for the music therapist to learn about all phases of the person's life. A way to do this would be by interviewing the client or family members and asking about significant life events or periods in time about which the client may want to reminiscence. This can provide the music therapist with time periods and genres in which to search for music. The music therapist can also engage the client in a discussion about significant songs and stories from various points in his/her life. Many times, people can remember a significant song associated with a life event (e.g., a wedding song, graduation song, song they sang to their children, etc.). If the music therapist asks the client to list some songs, this can be extremely beneficial to personalizing the client's experience and provide meaning to the reminiscence experience. The music therapist should decide with the client about the reminiscence experience and determine jointly whether it should be one important event in their lives or music from all parts of life.

Edwards (2005) highlights the importance of the assessment process and explains that if a client had positive memories for a song once, it does not mean that he/she will have the same sentiments when listening to it in different life circumstances. Themes from songs of the person's past may once have seemed positive, but now that the person is in palliative care, he/she may feel bitter or resentful to certain themes in songs. Therefore, a therapist is cautioned to not solely use age as a factor when deciding what music a client listens to for reminiscence, but rather he/she should rely heavily on client-preferred music and details that the client gives during assessment.

If the client has given the therapist a list of songs, or the therapist and client have engaged in life review and chosen appropriate songs, the therapist can download the specific songs and place them in a usable format for the client and family. Equipment to prepare for a session may include audio or recording equipment and/or live music playing (Byrne, 1982). Visuals can also be added to stimulate reminiscence and complement the musical aspect (Forrest, 1990). Depending on what technology is available to the music therapist in a specific setting, several recording devices could be used to create a life review recording for the client or family. If the client wants live music recordings (the therapist playing the selected songs, the clients playing/singing the songs, or family member inclusion), the music therapist should choose reliable and appropriate sound recording devices.

What to observe. Grocke and Wigram (2007) affirm that when a client is listening to music, a therapist must scan the body language and facial expressions of the client and make periodic observations on how the client is relating to the song. This is important in ensuring that the client receives an optimal emotional experience, and is especially important if the therapist has chosen the songs for the client. As stated in the contraindications section for this technique, a client may respond negatively to certain song selections, and by monitoring the client's emotional and physical responses, the therapist can ensure that the client is benefiting from their song choice.

Procedures. Belgrave, Darrow, Walworth, and Wlodarczyk (2011) outline several clinical steps in putting a life story to music, beginning with the therapist asking the client to write their life story in five sentences, which assists the client in thinking about the most valuable aspects. Counseling techniques would be used to help the client process and discuss these events in a healthy manner. The therapist provides the client with song options and allows the client to choose the songs that best represent the emotional content of their life story, followed by discussion. If a client identifies important events and characteristics and wants to compose a song, the client can work with the therapist to create a living legacy project for family or friends. Belgrave and colleagues also discuss selecting certain songs for life review that have thematic content relating to life review, and engaging the client in lyric discussion.

The next step is to determine what type of discussion the therapist will have with the client about the song selections. The type of discussion could be open, in that the music therapist and client listen to the selection together and the client freely discusses any thoughts about the experience. The music therapist may also want to have prechosen questions associated with the musical selections to prompt the client in discussion. This will depend on the client's openness to discussion, the therapeutic relationship, and the stage or phase of music therapy sessions. The music therapist should be open to the client's comments and open to any suggestions that the client may have (e.g., wanting to learn how to play the song for a loved one).

Adaptations. Music for reminiscence in palliative care may also be used in a group setting. Koffman & O'Kelly (2007) maintain that group settings can help encourage individuals to support one another and may improve social interaction. In addition, music and poetry can serve as another medium to initiate life review or reminiscence (Wlodarczyk, 2009). Musical life review may include prerecorded music (from the original artists), music performed by the therapist or client, music recorded by the therapist and client, or music that includes family or friend participation.

Song Choice

Overview. Song choice is very important in music therapy and palliative care. When the therapist encourages the client to choose music to which to listen, it may lead to the attainment of other goals, including reminiscence, relaxation, or emotional expression. O'Callaghan (1996) states that patient choice is essential whenever possible and cautions therapists to be aware of projections by staff or family members regarding what they think the client would prefer. When clients are diagnosed with a terminal illness, a large amount of their autonomy is lost. Song choice can be a way to regain control and assist the client in expressing their emotions. Song choice may also be a way to introduce the client to music therapy and act as an avenue to other music therapy interventions, such as music for reminiscence, music for relaxation, musical life review, and active music-making.

O'Callaghan (1996) highlights adverse effects in music listening, which include lesions in the right temporal lobe in left hemispheric–dominant persons that can make listening to music painful, and musicogenic epilepsy, which is a condition that occurs when music directly triggers an epileptic seizure and unexplained negative emotional reactions. This suggests that music therapists should attend and consider the client's diagnosis and possible physical trauma. Depending on the situation and setting, music therapists should exude caution if clients choose music with negative lyrics or negative themes—although it may be their preferred music, it may be inappropriate in a hospital setting or may elicit negative emotions in the client he/she is not able to process at the time. The therapist needs to familiarize themselves with lyrics and themes in a client's song choice. This could be particularly important to be aware of if the client is cognitively unaware or delirious: Music from their past or songs that they suggest may be inappropriate or elicit a negative emotion in mentally unaware and unstable clients. Aldridge (1998) states that patients in hospice or palliative care may be hypersensitive to certain sounds, and when playing a client's preferred music either live or recorded, it is important to consider the tonality and range of the song, instrumentation used, and limitations of the client's auditory sensations. Apart from general contraindications to listening to music, if the client chooses the song, it is most likely a safe and appropriate choice.

Preparation. A music therapist requires a large repertoire including music in a variety of styles. If the client requests songs for the next session, the therapist should prepare those songs, either by playing them live or bringing in recordings to facilitate listening. The environment for song choice is similar to music for reminiscence (see above section for details).

What to observe. There are many similarities with music for reminiscence and relaxation when assessing a client's reaction to song choice. Juslin and Sloboda (2010) highlight emotional responses when listening to music and factors to consider such as other activities taking place during music listening that have their own complex sources of meaning and emotion. For example, if a client's roommate is receiving treatment, or a patient is crying or yelling in another room, this could adversely affect the listening experience, and therapists need to be aware of the surroundings and ascertain that negative associations are not attached to the client's preferred music. Grocke and Wigram (2007) note cautions in playing music as two levels: the client's tolerance of length, volume, and proximity of sound source, and the client's response to the style and characteristics of the music.

Procedures. Song choice can either be live or recorded. If the sessions are single-session interventions, the music will generally be live, but if the client requests music from the therapist for a future session, the therapist can bring recorded music for the client to use independently. Bruscia (1998) uses client song choice as song communication and outlines a session as follows: The therapist asks the client to select a song or bring in a recorded song (one that has relevance to the client), and then both the client and the therapist listen to the song, followed by an exploration of what the music communicates about the client, the client's life, or therapeutic issues.

To prepare for the session, a music therapist can interview the client, friends, or family members to ask about the client's preferred music. It is not always possible to have the client's preferred music, but as part of professional practice, music therapists should continually develop and expand their range of repertoire. Oftentimes, song choice or playing a client's favorite song/musical genre is an excellent way to get to know the client and introduce him/her to music therapy, as well as a good starting intervention to begin clinical work with a client. This technique adds personalization and choice to a situation in which both of those elements may be limited, and this can be extremely uplifting and positive for the client. This intervention can also lead to many different music activities (e.g., song (lyric) discussion, composition, etc.).

Adaptations. Adaptations for song choice include the client naming a genre and the therapist choosing a song within that category. Other adaptations include the client singing or playing instruments to music he/she has chosen. A client may also select music for their funeral when he/she is approaching the end of life (Aldridge, 1998; Cohen, Boston, Mount, & Porterfield, 2001).

Song (Lyric) Discussion

Overview. Song (lyric) discussion is an exceptional intervention in assisting clients who are having emotional difficulty relating to feelings that may be too difficult to express or who need help in defining feelings and emotions they are having difficulty understanding within themselves. Bruscia (1998) defines song (lyric) discussion as "the therapist brings in a song that serves as a springboard for discussion of issues that are therapeutically relevant to the client. After listening to the song, the client is asked to analyze the meaning of the lyrics and to examine (in dialogue with the therapist or other clients) the relevance of the lyrics to the client or the client's life" (p. 124). Clements-Cortés (2004) outlines goals for song (lyric) analysis in palliative care as encouraging a client to express feelings, stimulating cognitive function, facilitating the loss/grieving process, and regaining self-identity.

Similar to as with music for reminiscence, the music therapist must have advanced clinical counseling skills before introducing this type of activity with a client in palliative care. Song (lyric) discussion may help the client address serious issues he/she is facing, but if the therapist is not prepared to address those issues, it may cause harm or distress to the client instead of helping. Therefore, a music therapist would benefit from training or supervision during this type of session or activity and do research on possible techniques and methods of helping the client with spiritual, emotional, physical, or psychological needs.

Song (lyric) analysis should not be used if a client is mentally unstable or not at a point to explore difficult issues. If family members are also present and having emotional difficulty, the music therapist should not present a song for lyric analysis that might upset the family member or friend further. A music therapist should also never infer meaning onto a client, indicating that if the client is unable to communicate due to physical limitations, song (lyric) analysis should not be used. Also, if a client specifies a genre of music or artist that they do not like, the therapist should not use a song for lyric analysis that falls within that genre and instead search for another song with similar themes.

Preparation. If the client is choosing to bring in music for a session, the therapist should ensure that proper audio equipment is available. If the therapist is bringing the music, he/she must confirm that he/she has acceptable audio equipment and questions to ask the client about the music. If the music therapist is seeing the client for the first time but decides that song (lyric) analysis is an appropriate technique, the therapist needs to have a wide range of repertoire with appropriate themes and songs that will relate to the client. The therapist should come prepared with questions to ask the client about their chosen music and be adaptable to the client's comments and reactions to the music.

What to observe. A music therapist should observe the client's reactions to the lyrics or musicality of a song. If a client becomes upset, the therapist needs to decide whether or not to stop the song and discuss the emotional reaction, or to let the song continue and then discuss the emotions that arise after listening. The therapist needs to document all themes and emotions talked about, either during or after the session, as this record will be useful if the client has future sessions or if the client passes away and has left a thought or message for a family member or friend. Writing themes and topics that were discussed in song (lyric) analysis can be beneficial if the client grows spiritually or emotionally through the music therapy process, and the therapist and client can look back together, reflect, and chart progress.

Procedures. Grocke and Wigram (2007) outlined three stages in the song (lyric) analysis process. In stage one, the client chooses a song or piece of music. In stage two, the therapist and client listen to the song together, and in stage three, there is a discussion about the song, its meaning to the client and an analysis of the lyrics of the song. In palliative care, it may not always be feasible for the client to bring music, as they may be in the hospital and unable to leave. In that case, a family member could assist in bringing music to the session. In settings where visits are one session only (common in hospice and palliative care), the music therapist can either choose the song for the client or present the client with a list of songs from which to choose. The music therapist can have the client choose the song, or the music therapist can choose a song based on the clinical issues that the client brings forward during music therapy. For novice therapists, it may be beneficial to have a general list of repertoire that is appropriate for a variety of clinical issues. With this intervention, it is not always necessary to choose a song with which the client is familiar. Sometimes introducing a new song that addresses their issues can be inspiring, motivating, or interesting to the client, while learning new songs and lyrics may help him/her expand understanding of their issues or gain perspective.

Several themes commonly arise in discussions with palliative care patients. This facilitates development of a list of songs that might be beneficial in addressing these themes and, subsequently, discussion topics with appropriate songs that could be used in therapy settings, as a sort of reference guide. See Appendix B for a detailed list of themes, songs, and discussion points as an example of how music therapists can create a list of beneficial songs with subsequent discussion topics relevant to their clinical population.

Adaptations. Baumel (1973) outlined several uses of song (lyric) discussion in a group setting. These include: having clients select a song that reflects something about themselves, or a song that reflects the feelings of someone else in the group, or having the therapist select songs for the client or group. Other adaptations can include implementing lyric substitution after a song has been analyzed. The client may also want to create lyrics and attach a more personal meaning to the song. This can subsequently be a way to introduce songwriting to the client. A client's family members or friends can also present a music therapist with a song that they desire the client to listen to because of the significance of the lyrics.

Somatic Listening

Overview. Somatic listening refers to a medically centered approach of using musical tones and vibrations to target specific physiological functioning and is defined as vibrations, sounds, and music that directly influence the client's body (Wheeler, Shultis, & Polen, 2005). Somatic listening has the potential to influence the heart and brain on a physiological and psychological level simultaneously, reduce anxiety, and create a calming effect on the individual, as well as improve pain control (Freeman et al., 2006). If a client is presenting pain, anxiety, or difficulty sleeping/relaxing, somatic listening is indicated.

Music therapists may not have received in-depth training as to the effects of certain types of sound and the scientific principles supporting somatic listening. There are specific training courses focusing on somatic listening that may be beneficial for music therapists to learn about if they wish to include advanced somatic listening in their clinical work. Music therapists may also take vibroacoustic therapy training courses to further develop their somatic listening skills. Music therapists need to recognize their own limits and practice within the range of therapy appropriate to the amount of training that they have or have not received, especially when and if using vibroacoustic equipment such as vibroacoustic chairs.

Music used in the vibrational form (also known as vibroacoustic therapy) can help with pain management, anxiety relief, symptom reduction, physical therapy, and health improvement (Boyd-Brewer, 2003). Using music listening combined with vibroacoustic therapy significantly helps reduce pain and increase relaxation by engaging psychological processes through music listening combined with engaging physiological processes through applied musical vibration (Boyd-Brewer, 2004). It is important to note that there is some debate on whether vibroacoustic therapy is considered within the realm of music therapy. Cooper (2002) explains that because vibroacoustic therapy fulfills Bruscia's 1989 definition of music therapy in three criteria (three essential elements: a systematic intervention, a therapeutic relationship, and a musical experience), vibroacoustic therapy may be considered as music therapy.

The most commonly used instruments to facilitate somatic listening are harp and voice. Harp therapy provided in palliative care focuses on targeting pain with experimentally derived notes specific to the client. Harp therapy has been proven to relieve anxiety, fear, dyspnea, nausea, and pain, and also to provide awareness of the transcendent or spiritual dimension (Lewis, de Vedia, Reuer, Schwan, & Tourin, 2003). Harp therapists practice their discipline in the field known as music thanatology and not music therapy. Music thanatology unites music and medicine in end-of-life care by a music thanatologist using harp and voice at the bedside to address physical, emotional, and spiritual needs of a dying patient (Music Thanatology Association International, 2008). For the purpose of this chapter, the focus will remain on how clinical music therapists can use somatic listening in their clinical work, and not how clinical music thanatologists use harp therapy or somatic listening.

Somatic listening needs to be carefully and closely monitored in the medical setting with patients who are experiencing extreme pain and physical sensitivity. If clients present severe acute inflammations (excluding normal flu), major external or internal bleeding, or severe heart disease, their physician should be consulted before undergoing vibroacoustic therapy (Wigram, 1997). Vibroacoustic therapy in particular needs to be monitored and should be used only by a music therapist trained in this method, as damage or pain can be caused by improper implementation. For somatic listening using harp, voice, or other string instruments, the same carefulness and observation must be adhered to by music therapists when implementing the procedure to ensure that sounds or vibrations do not become painful or uncomfortable for the client. Vibroacoustic therapy that uses beds, tables, or chairs may be difficult to use in palliative or hospice care if the client is unable to be moved due to pain or is using the assistance of medical equipment such as a ventilator or IVs. Therefore, a music therapist should be cautious and consult medical staff before moving a client or bringing in extra equipment.

Preparation. The preparation of the session and environment depend on the type of somatic listening the music therapist is implementing. When using vibroacoustic music therapy, the preparation of the session requires arranging appropriate equipment and technology in the room. Boyd-Brewer (2004) outlines essential environmental elements during vibroacoustic music therapy as being quiet, lighting, isolation, comfort, and few distractions. In palliative/hospice care, many clients have roommates, and in that situation, the music therapist should arrange, if possible, to have the client moved to an area of less distraction or somehow block the activity from the other client if he/she does not want to participate.

What to observe. The therapist should pay attention to potential signs of pain or discomfort. If the music therapist is attempting to target specific notes or frequencies that affect the client's targeted pain, the therapist should have a systematic, precise method of evaluating the client's responses to specific tones, which include asking the clients about their sensations and subjectively evaluating their facial expressions or physical state and physiological responses via physiological measurement tools such as heart monitors.

Procedures. Begin by explaining to the client the procedures, intent, and goals of somatic listening. A vibroacoustic session is a process in which the patient reclines or sits on the vibroacoustic equipment and experiences vibrations of sound and/or music throughout the body; a relaxation intervention can be used at the beginning of the session to assist the patient in entering more deeply into relaxation (Patrick, 1999). Vibroacoustic therapy, not combined with musical instruments such as the harp or voice, uses sound to produce mechanical vibrations that are applied directly to the body. The technology used by trained vibroacoustic therapists involves speakers or transducers placed within mats, mattresses, chairs, recliners, tables, or soft furniture to provide a physiologic and auditory experience (Boyd-Brewer, 2003). Wigram (1995) describes a type of somatic listening experience that combined music as vibroacoustic therapy and employs the element of low frequency sound as a pulsed tone combined with underlying relaxing music.

Clinical music therapists may use the concepts and techniques behind vibroacoustic music therapy in their clinical work even if they are not trained in vibroacoustic therapy or do not have access to vibroacoustic therapy equipment. During prescriptive music-making, the clinician-musician observes physiological changes, cues, and breathing patterns of the patient. This is followed by synchronizing the music to reflect or support the patient's physiology and overall condition (Freeman et al., 2006). A music therapist could allow the client to play with various instruments to facilitate tactile vibratory stimulation and might also place the instrument against the client (e.g., guitar, small harps, etc.) if the patient is able to handle this type of tactile stimulation for an enhanced sensory experience. By placing the instrument on or near the client, he/she is able to experience the vibrations and resonance of the instrument, which would have positive effects on the client's physical and mental well-being. Even placing a client's hand on the music therapist's throat while they sing has helped in situations where a client has lost hearing and could feel the vibrations of the throat as a resonator. This helps connect the client to the music in a more meaningful way.

Adaptations. Adding guided imagery to the listening is a further extension to involve psychological processes along with the physical.

GUIDELINES FOR IMPROVISATIONAL MUSIC THERAPY

When engaging in improvisational music therapy with palliative care patients, the music therapist must ensure that their clinical music therapy skills are beyond the minimal level required for completing an undergraduate degree. Due to the serious emotional, spiritual, and psychological needs that patients may have, engaging in active improvisation can provide an open outlet for the patient to express, address, and tackle issues. The music therapist must be confident and knowledgeable about clinical issues concerning palliative care patients, and supervision is always essential if the music therapist does not have experience using this technique with palliative care patients.

Empathic and Referential Improvisation

Overview. Empathic improvisation involves the therapist creating an improvisation that compassionately complements the client's current state of physical and mental being (Wigram, 2004). Empathic improvisation is suitable for clients who are frustrated, feel misunderstood, or feel isolated or alone. Here improvisation may be used to reflect what the clients are feeling and subsequently allow them to feel understood by another person, and permit them to identify and experience their own emotions. With a music therapist portraying the client's physical, emotional, and mental state, the client can observe their own state of being performed, which may assist him/her in understanding their own emotions and provide feelings of relief and comfort.

Clients in palliative care often feel neglected, alone, isolated, and confused, and empathic improvisation may facilitate the client in feeling understood while further building an in-depth relationship between the client and therapist, which can be profound and meaningful for the client during the dying process (Lee, 1996). If a client feels a loss of relationship, friendship, or closeness, empathic improvisation can provide an outlet for the therapist and client to use to begin to build a therapeutic relationship and in turn be healing for the client. O'Kelly (2002) compares the support and reflection done by the music therapist in improvisation to the reflecting that a counselor does in verbal therapy. This support and reflection through the therapist's music can provide the client with emotional relief and comfort.

In referential improvisation, the therapist gives a verbal reference to base the improvisation on, such as a story, a topic for fantasizing, or symbols. Referential music therapy can be used to introduce clients to improvisation and help them think about and learn to express themselves with respect to difficult topics. Bruscia (1987) states that referential improvisation allows clients to project feelings through their improvisation based on the verbal reference. The music helps turn difficult or misunderstood emotions into live expressions and real experiences. Going through the process of expressing emotions may highlight what the feelings mean to the client and how those emotions arose. This can be enlightening for the client and assist in reducing psychological and emotional distress. If a client is demonstrating frustration, anxiety, denial, or a lack of motivation, referential improvisation can be used to symbolize and explore difficult emotions, in order to help the client transcend a lack of acceptance or emotional confusion.

Bunt (1994) summarizes general goals for musical improvisation with adults, including gaining awareness and insight about the self, physically, emotionally, intellectually, and socially. Some of the goals that Bunt mentions are applicable to adults in palliative care who are experiencing a deficit in physical, emotional, intellectual, or social awareness. Bunt (1994) states that during improvisation, clients can find release and resolution for a wide variety of hurtful and painful emotions. The concept of dying is difficult to grasp for some clients, and if death is approaching quickly, it may be challenging for them to express the emotions they are feeling. If clients are in denial of trying situations and emotions, they may be unwilling to discuss any emotions relating to their death and do not have the tools to express themselves, which would lead to emotional relief. Music improvisation is a way for clients to express themselves in a nonverbal modality that could lead to relief of tension and self-understanding.

A music therapist should not attempt empathic improvisation if the client is demonstrating behavior that indicates they are emotionally blocking the therapist or in a distant mood. The level of therapeutic intimacy that this requires may be unsuitable for a client who is not ready to open up to a new person and have their feelings portrayed back to them by the therapist. If the client is not prepared to address certain issues and the therapist chooses specific topics as a reference for referential improvisation, the client may become emotionally upset, agitated, frustrated, or confused. The music therapist needs to be precise and sensitive during the assessment process to ensure that the client is prepared to face specific issues through improvisation.

Preparation. The therapist must ensure that he/she has the proper instruments to accurately execute a reflection. Having a combination of rhythmic and melodic instruments will allow the music therapist to choose the exact sounds necessary to produce an accurate reflection of the client or allow the client to choose an instrument to properly express a reference chosen by the therapist or the client. Empathic improvisation is a suitable starting point to engage clients musically. For example, if the therapist begins the improvisation by playing for the client, this may spark an interest in the client to improvise, and the therapist should be prepared for this by having a wide selection of materials for the client to choose from to facilitate the client's active participation musically.

Referential improvisation is slightly more structured than free improvisation; therefore, the therapist might choose an instrument for the client on which to base their improvisation. For example, if the reference is a story, a melodic instrument such as xylophone or piano may be beneficial due to the tonal variety and melodic landscape that could be portrayed. However, a music therapist should not discount other instruments and should allow the client's interpretation of the reference to be the single most important factor in choosing an instrument for improvisation. Before the session begins, the therapist may have a reference in mind based on referrals from other health care professionals, family members, or friends. For example, a client may be referred to music therapy due to their difficult in accepting their illness. This information assists the music therapist in deciding on possible referents and advance preparation of the session. Nevertheless, if there is no referral, and the client presents issues on a single session visit, the music therapist could use a list of possible referents and themes to choose from, which will help guide their session planning and implementation of beneficial treatment.

The music therapist should strive for minimal disruptions and the creation of a safe, supportive environment.

What to observe. Careful observation of the client during empathic improvisation is essential to ensure that the therapist's musical reflections are not causing the client emotional stress or pain. For example, if the client is showing signs of sadness or depression, and the therapist decides to mirror those feelings, the music therapist needs to observe the client's reaction and assess that he/she is not putting the client into a further state of sadness. A music therapist should also observe whether the client is, through nonverbal communication, being understood by the therapist. If the client seems confused by the music being played during the improvisation, the therapist is not using proper improvisational techniques and needs to adapt their playing according to the client's reaction.

Procedures. The music therapist begins by observing the client's body posture, facial expression, and attitude. The therapist creates a musical interpretation of what mental, emotional, and physical state the client is in at that moment, matching what the client is feeling, and does not try to change or modify the client's state of being. The therapist is not matching the music of the client; rather, the therapist is matching the state of being that the client presents, and, therefore, the therapist's music may be quite different from what the client is playing.

Other techniques that demonstrate empathy toward the client's emotions are mirroring what the client is doing musically by copying exactly what the client is doing musically, verbally, and physically to show the client their own behaviors. A therapist can also imitate or copy what a client is doing musically as a reflection for the client of the client's own musical expression. These techniques not only show clients they are being listened to, but also that the therapist understands their emotions and can feel a deep emotional relation to the client's thoughts and feelings. In palliative care, patients often feel isolated, alone, and misunderstood by those who have not suffered a serious illness. By empathetically improvising with the client, the therapist can assist the client in feeling understood while also reflecting to the client their own emotions, which may facilitate the client understanding emotions that may have been confusing or strange. This self-awareness has the potential to be healing.

For referential improvisation, a music therapist or client can choose a referent, and the music therapist verbally defines what the referent is and explains that the client should attempt to illuminate, describe, or express the reference. Gardstrom (2007) lists three different types of referents: static, dynamic, and continuum. Static referents are topics or words that do not change over time. An example of a static referent used in palliative care could be emotions such as fear, strength, sadness, hope, or loss. Another type of static referent might be a place, such as hospital, home, or heaven. A static referent may also be an object, such as a needle, medicine, sunshine, or rain. Based on an assessment of the client's needs, the music therapist may suggest that the client attempt to portray a specific emotion, place, or object. A dynamic referent focuses on movement and change from beginning to end. In palliative care, possible dynamic referents include progression of illness, progression of a day, expressing emotions of a specific time period, etc. Continuum referents are lively in nature but refer to movement from one end of a continuum to another, such as birth to death and sickness to health. These referents would be helpful for clients who are having difficulty in expressing their emotions or understanding the progression of events of their life.

Wigram (2004) states that possible themes for improvisation consist of a guided fantasy or story, an object, a picture or image, the weather, an emotion, or the client's issues. By choosing a theme to improvise on, the client not only feels as though the therapist is choosing significant material for him/her and therefore empathized with, but also, for clients who are uneasy about free improvisation at first, choosing a theme helps to ease some of the uncertainty and provide structure to the improvisation. A theme can also help the client conceptualize an elusive topic such as "illness" or "healing." He/she can convey such feelings through their improvisation, and this may help relieve the stress of an inability to express such concepts. These themes are similar to static referents discussed by Gardstrom. Other themes that are suitable for palliative care are emotions and specific parts of the body, such as "sick" cells (e.g., cancer cells). A story improvisation can help the client in palliative care feel a sense of transcendence from their illness. The therapist would begin by asking the client to tell the story of their illness and finish the story by moving the client from being ill to being healed. Possible other stories could be the client's life story, which can serve as a tool for reminiscence and life review, or the story of a client's friendships or family. These stories are similar to dynamic referents explained by Gardstrom.

Adaptations. Empathic and referential improvisation could be used in a group setting in palliative care and would be extremely beneficial if there are a group of clients who have similar diagnoses (e.g., a group for clients with HIV/AIDS). This adaptation is an excellent method to foster social involvement and allow clients to connect with other people who are experiencing similar difficulties. Empathic improvisation may include verbal discussion of what the music therapist is attempting; however, verbal explanations should be used with caution. Often the music speaks for itself and verbal explanation may not be necessary. The client might also use empathic or referential improvisation to connect with their friends and family members and facilitate the friends and family members to feel understood by the client. By matching their companion's emotions or choosing a theme or referent that is important in the situation, a companion may feel more connected with the client, and this can improve their relationship, which may be important during the dying process.

Active Improvisation

Overview. Active improvisation involves the client playing instruments and exploring their emotions freely with music. The therapist can introduce a variety of techniques to support the client's exploration. If the client is feeling isolated and alone, misunderstood, or lacks direction, active client improvisation can help him/her explore their emotions and hopefully lead to improved understanding. Music improvisation provides an alternative, less threatening mechanism to explore the dying process (Hain, Wewinstein, Oleske, Orloff & Cohen, 2004). If a client has challenging emotions about dying or being ill, improvisation is a tool to facilitate exploring dying while releasing tension caused by emotional buildup. Music improvisation creates a means of expression and communication and can enhance mobility and motivation, while serving as a key to unconscious issues that are not easily addressed verbally, such as anger, jealousy, existential loneliness, and fear (Lee, 1996). When a client improvises on a musical instrument, he/she is able to express difficult emotions and demonstrate their personality and emotions to others.

A music therapist should not use active music improvisation if a client is emotionally unstable and not willing to explore their emotions. However, unlike empathic and referential improvisation, because the client is creating the music freely and without associations, the client is able to decide where the improvisation goes and what will be explored, decreasing the chance of the client bringing up difficult emotions until he/she is ready. If the client begins to become emotionally distressed or upset, the music therapist should use clinical judgment on whether to continue or end the improvisation. Becoming emotionally upset might be healing for the client, and it may be an expression of the emotions he/she needs to release in order to gain relief. If the client appears in extreme distress or anger, the music therapist needs to make an informed decision on whether or not to continue down the path the client is exploring or to redirect or end the improvisation.

Preparation. See Empathetic and Referential Improvisation.

What to observe. The music therapist should observe if the client is becoming extremely upset or distressed. Exploring deep psychological issues may be extremely difficult for the client, and he/she may need verbal counseling combined with the music improvisation to understand their emotions and feel that their emotions are accepted. A music therapist should pay careful attention to the musical characteristics of the client's improvisation to try to understand how the client is expressing him/herself and what musical parameters (structure, timbre, dynamic, harmonic and melodic form, level of intensity) the client is utilizing to explore their emotions. These observations are important in the therapist's understanding of the client's exploration, and can be verbalized to the client to allow him/her to gain understanding and reflection into their own improvisation. Recording sessions is always beneficial if the client is willing; however, it is not always possible to plan to record sessions in palliative care if the visits are single-session, and a music therapist should be mindful of not being intrusive on the client by asking to video or audio record their improvisation.

Procedures. A music therapist begins by allowing the client to explore a variety of instruments, both melodic and percussive, to determine what will fit their exploration most accurately. The client is encouraged to explore the sounds of the instrument and begin considering how to express their thoughts and feelings musically. The role of the music therapist is to support and guide the client's musical and emotional exploration. Bruscia (1987) listed 64 techniques for improvising with a client. For the purpose of this chapter, not all techniques will be listed or explained, because the improvisation will vary so immensely from client to client. Each technique relates to a specific function for the music therapist, whether it is supporting the client's improvisation in some way, redirecting their improvisation in a new way, or accompanying the client musically to allow for a completely individual improvisation. Depending on the needs the client presents emotionally and musically, a music therapist requires training in multiple techniques to provide the ultimate care for the client. Improvisation with a client requires a deep sense of empathy and strong clinical assessment skills.

If a client seems to be presenting questions or comments in their music, the music therapist can engage in musical dialogue with the client. Wigram (2004) discusses two types of musical dialogue with a client. The first is turn-taking dialogues, where the client and therapist take turns musically, allowing space for the other person to answer and respond to their improvisation. The second type is continuous "free-floating" dialogue, where the therapist and client play music at the same time, and musical ideas are heard and responded to with no pause in the improvisation and sound. Both of these techniques facilitate a client in feeling accepted and create understanding between the client and music therapist. If a client appears to require support in their improvisation, a music therapist can employ a number of techniques to provide a musical structure and base from which the client improvises. If a client needs their improvisation to be redirected due to emotional distress, or the music therapist feels as though it would be therapeutic to change the music to move to a new place, the music therapist should employ change and modulation to move the client emotionally and musically.

Adaptations. It is more difficult to use active improvisation in a group, as many different musical ideas and different types of explorations may ensue, and this may not allow the client to feel focused on or free to improvise what he/she needs to express. However, clients may begin to improvise off of each other and support one another musically, which may provide understanding and increase a feeling of social involvement. This should be monitored with caution, as clients who are untrained in improvisational techniques may overshadow or redirect another client's improvisation without realizing it, thus potentially leading to further frustration and anxiety from the clients.

Guidelines for Re-creative Music Therapy

A music therapist requires ear training, proficiency on a variety of instruments, and knowledge and skill in different styles and/or musical genres to implement these techniques. The music therapist should be prepared to give the client the opportunity to be creative and expressive in multiple ways, and this requires the music therapist to have exceptional music and clinical skills.

Vocal

Overview. Vocal re-creative music therapy involves the client producing vocalizations, sight-singing, chanting, taking voice lessons, and imitating/learning melodies (Bruscia 1998). Singing is a powerful tool for clients diagnosed with terminal illness as it holds the potential to increase confidence and mood, initiate reminiscence, improve interaction with family members, and release emotion (Aldridge, 1998). Singing also has physical benefits such as improving articulation, fluency, and breath control in speech, and can improve breathing by engaging the diaphragm and enhance physical relaxation and reduce discomfort (Clements-Cortés, 2004). The deep, regular breathing necessary to sustain vocalization during song increases vital capacity and maximizes oxygenation and relaxation and can also decrease the perception of pain (Rykov, 2001). Singing can contribute to self-awareness and create a sense of belonging (Clair, 1996). If clients have a low/anxious mood, are having breathing problems, or are having difficulty with family members and self-expression, singing is an extremely beneficial technique to implement in palliative care.

Singing is not indicated with clients who are having extreme difficulty speaking and would be frustrated by being asked to sing. The music therapist could begin with vocalizations, while being cautious with which vocalizations to use if the client is experiencing pain with certain sound production. Singing should not be used with clients who are having extreme difficulty breathing, as the breath required to sing may be strenuous to the client and cause further pain or frustration.

Preparation. Singing requires a small amount of preparation of the environment compared to other music therapy techniques. If the therapist has had previous sessions with a client, he/she can ask what types of songs the client likes to sing and bring the songs to the next session. The therapist assists the client in sitting up slightly or determines whether the client is comfortable singing lying down. If the client wants to record their singing, the music therapist would confirm that proper recording equipment is brought to the session. Also, microphones may prove effective in amplifying a client's singing and are an additional piece of equipment that a music therapist should consider bringing to the session.

What to observe. A music therapist observes the client's physical status and ensures the client is not becoming overtly weak or exhausted. Singing and vocalizing requires energy and physical stamina, and if a client is becoming physically stressed or tired, the music therapist should either slow down the singing or change activities. It is important to observe the client's mood while singing and to pay attention to reactions to different songs. A client may enjoy a song one day, and the next day dislike the song or have different attitudes toward the song. Even if the client states he/she has a favorite song, the therapist should carefully observe the emotional reaction of a client during singing to ensure the client does not have a negative emotional reaction to a piece.

Procedures. Vocalizations are a potential starting point if clients are wary about singing or having difficulty with sound production due to their illness. Vocalizing on a vowel sound is a helpful way to introduce the basic foundations of singing while possibly increasing the strength and range of a client's voice. Vocalizations (also called toning or chanting) often bring a sense of relief and emotional release for the client, if it is in a chant format and the music therapist is providing a musical background to chant sounds.

To introduce this technique to a client, the music therapist can give the client one tone and then one sound with which to begin. For example, the client could chant on "oh," "ah," "eh," "oo," or "ohm" to start and/or open vowel sounds. The therapist can follow this up by asking the client choose a sound and giving the client a note on which to vocalize. The therapist and client can also chant on one sound at the start and then suggest adding two, three, or four tones, or let the client experiment vocally while the therapist plays music or stays on a tonal center. Instruments that are beneficial to use during toning are flutes, or any variety of flutes, harps, or any instrument with resonance space and easily sustainable notes.

To introduce singing, the music therapist can ask the client what type of songs he/she likes to sing or inquire about the client's favorite songs. The music therapist may accompany the client or let the client sing on his/her own, or the therapist may sing along with the client. Lyrics should be provided for the client where possible and desired by the client. New songs may be introduced to the client by the therapist to increase client confidence and also help the client learn new vocal skills and increase their range and strength of voice. Subsequently, the music therapist can work with the client on preparing a piece for a family member as a song gift.

Adaptations. Singing and vocalizing in a group setting in palliative care is implemented to increase social interaction and provide feelings of connectedness and understanding between patients. The songs sung by the therapist and clients could also be recorded and given to family members or friends as a song gift and as a way of keeping a part of the client with the family beyond the death.

Instrumental

Overview. Playing instruments, whether percussive instruments (hand drums, shakers, ocean drums, etcetera) or melodic instruments (piano, guitar, xylophone, wind/brass instruments, other string instruments, etcetera,), can be very beneficial for clients in palliative care. General goals for playing instruments in palliative care are to promote participation, provide an alternate vehicle for self-expression, encourage choice making, and increase focus (Clements-Cortés, 2004). Playing instruments may increase expression of feelings, enhance mood, and improve quality of life (Halstead & Roscoe, 2007). Instrumental playing can open or maintain the field of communication between the client and family members, friends, and staff members (Gauthier & Dallaire, 1993). Instrumental playing can provide clients with a sense of competency by giving them a task to learn. Clients can use the new skills and hobby that they learned in music therapy outside of the therapy session and may gain a sense of confidence if they are unable to perform other tasks that they may once have before (Weber, 1998). If clients seem frustrated by their decreasing ability to perform tasks or hobbies they previously enjoyed, learning a new instrument could be a positive way for them to use their creativity and gain competency in a new skill, subsequently leading to improvements in self-esteem and self-efficacy.

Instrumental playing should not be attempted with clients who are too physically weak to lift an instrument or do not have the energy to actively play, as this may make the client feel frustrated and incompetent. Addressing other health care professionals and assessing the client's physical status are crucial in determining what should be attempted with the client. If the client is feeling negative emotions associated with incompetency due to deteriorating physical health, an activity that does not require a large amount of physical movement or strain is appropriate.

Preparation. It is important for the music therapist to have a wide variety of percussive instruments available to allow the client the freedom to choose the correct mode for expression, and also the right instrument based on their strength and physical ability. If the client has a history of playing an instrument, the music therapist should attempt to bring that instrument to the session but always ask the client what he/she would like to play. If the client wants to learn a new instrument, the music therapist must assess the client's previous musical background and take their prognosis into account; it might not be plausible for a client to learn standard musical notation or learn how to play an instrument in a short time period. If the client does present a desire to play an instrument that requires the ability to read notation (e.g., piano), the music therapist may adapt the song or adapt the method in which the client will learn to provide optimal playing time (e.g., learning tablature on guitar instead of standard notation, or learning one-note melodies on piano).

What to observe. A music therapist should observe whether the client is becoming fatigued or physically strained from instrumental playing. Playing instruments requires physical stamina and strength, and if the client is losing energy or experiences pain as a result of playing, the activity should be adapted immediately. If a client is learning a new instrument, the music therapist should carefully observe the client's progress and ensure the client is not becoming frustrated or disappointed in a lack of progress.

The learning process can subsequently be adapted to allow for more obtainable goals and help the client gain a sense of accomplishment.

Procedures. A good starting point is to allow the client to explore freely to become competent in the many different facets of the instrument. The music therapist or the client can choose a song. The client may create a song gift for family members and friends of a precomposed song with the client playing the instruments. The song can be recorded to leave as a gift for family members and friends or can be played at their funeral as well.

Adaptations. Instrumental playing is a great technique to use in group settings, as it fosters participation, creativity, and social interaction. Instrumental playing can be used to initiate musical activities such as call-and-response or conducting.

Guidelines for Compositional Music Therapy

The music therapist requires strong ear training skills and experience in composition to implement this technique. Experience in composition is not always extensive during an undergraduate degree, and music therapists may choose to further study composition and expand their knowledge of a variety of genres, instrumentation, and styles. Many continuing education workshops or presentations that discuss varied styles of composition are often available to pursue at music therapy conferences.

Song Composition (either with words or only instrumental)

Overview. Song composition is a highly important tool for music therapists to use when clients in palliative care are having difficulty expressing their emotions. Aldridge (1998) states that songwriting can help palliative care clients effectively deal with biopsychosocial issues affecting their experiences. If music therapists engage clients in the songwriting process, it can allow clients to externalize unexpressed feelings and stories, enable the collection and construction of shared experiences into song framework, and enable families and friends to speak the unspeakable (Blyth & Miles, 2012). O'Callaghan (1990) maintains that songwriting is a valuable medium that patients can use to ventilate pent-up feelings, gain support, send messages to special people, and help themselves feel that they are contributing something unique to this world, which can in turn help the client gain pleasure and self-esteem. Songs can also be composed for a client's children (O'Callaghan, O'Brien, Magill, & Ballinger, 2009). Bruscia (1998) lists several main goals of compositional music therapy, including developing the ability to document and communicate inner experiences, to promote exploration of therapeutic themes through lyrics, and to develop the ability to integrate and synthesize parts into wholes. If clients are having difficulty expressing their emotions, connecting with their family or friends, or feeling creative, or having difficulty understanding their own emotions, songwriting is a valuable tool for music therapists to implement.

Songwriting is contraindicated for emotional clients unprepared to express their feelings. For example, some clients may be unable to suppress certain emotions they are not ready to have surface in the presence of another person or the therapist. A music therapist should always ensure that a secure therapeutic relationship has been formed with the client before embarking on song composition, as it requires a level of expression and sharing with the therapist of which the client needs to be prepared.

Preparation. If a music therapist has asked the client in previous sessions if he/she would like to compose a song, the therapist should come prepared with all musical and compositional tools. For example, if a client described the type of song he/she wants to compose, the music therapist should be prepared with the correct instrumentation and musical styles. If the client does not know what direction he/she wants their composition to lead to, the music therapist may bring in examples of precomposed songs that fit the client's psychological needs. The client may want to record their song, and proper audio (and potentially visual) recording devices should be offered. Other materials include: paper and writing equipment for the client and staff paper for the music therapist and potentially the client if he/she is knowledgeable with standard musical notation.

What to observe. A music therapist should carefully note the lyrics chosen by the client and attend to recurring themes or ideas. It may be beneficial for the client to address these issues verbally and examine if there are any deep issues that need to be addressed. Negative emotional responses, reactions of sadness to the music or signs of frustration or limited creativity are indications for the music therapist to be aware of and verbally discuss with the client. A music therapist should pay attention to a client's reaction to the compositional process. If lyrics or instrumentation was created early on and the client begins to dislike or react in a negative way to their composition, the music therapist may perhaps offer to rewrite or change aspects of the composition.

Procedures. Song composition can be either instrumental or with lyrics. The music therapist asks the client what type of medium he/she wants to use for expression and offers a variety of musical choices. Song composition may be introduced by asking the client what ideas or thoughts he/she wants to express. If the client has lyrics he/she wants to create, the music therapist can work with the client to write down specific words, themes, or ideas that can be later set to music. If the client needs direction in writing lyrics, the music therapist can help summarize the feelings expressed by the client and offer to set a few lines to music or set their lyrics to an existing melody.

A music therapist can suggest topics to the client that have come up in conversations in previous sessions or specific issues that the client has brought up (e.g., anxiety about the future, finding strength, etc.). A music therapist can also choose precomposed songs that share similar themes that may be used by the client to act as a starting point for ideas, and the music therapist and client can listen together and brainstorm. The music therapist should also ask the client what their goal for songwriting is. This may help determine themes or ideas (e.g., giving a song gift to someone or to leave a legacy). If music therapists have examples from previous songwriting sessions with other palliative clients they have permission to disclose, they may share these songs with new clients to help inspire ideas.

The music therapist can also engage the client in lyric substitution, beginning with substituting one or two words into phrases that have significance to the client, and then moving to full sentences. O'Callaghan (1990) lists steps in conducting a compositional activity with a client in palliative care. The music therapist offers a choice of bright/happy major or mellow/sad minor keys, and improvises examples. Next, the music therapist presents various rhythmic styles and choices of melodies for each line in the verse. A choice of supportive harmonies, dynamics, tempo, and instrumentation and voicing is also important. The client is encouraged to make all decisions regarding the composition, and the music therapist brings their musical skills to assist this process.

Steps and Decisions for Assisting Clients in Song Creation

1) Brainstorming with Client

   - Music therapist brings notes from previous sessions to explore
   - Music therapist engages client in free association

2) Use of Precomposed Songs

    - Music therapist brings precomposed songs to assess lyrics with the client and uses the lyrics to act as a springboard for discussion and song creation

3) Suggestions of Melodies to Accompany Lyrics

    - Music therapist plays several melodies in varying keys as suggestions for lyrics and asks the client to select
    - Music therapist helps the client narrow down possible choices

4) Suggestions of Song Structure/Genre

    - Music therapist and client decide how many verses/choruses there will be in the song/what genre of music is preferred

5) Create Harmonies and Progressions for the Client to Listen To

    - Music therapist uses suggestions from client to create a phrase, starting with playing through possible harmonic progressions
    - Client chooses harmonic progression

6) Create Melodies within Harmonic Structure

    - Music therapist suggests melodies and word placement in phrase
    - Client creates phrases to add into song structure

7) Choose Themes or Ideas for Each Verse/Chorus

    - It is beneficial to have a theme for each verse as this can help the client decide the direction of the song

8) Create Song Together

    - In some cases, clients will want the music therapist to create the song based on the client's lyrics or suggestions
    - The music therapist can create the song and bring it in for the client to hear
    - The music therapist and client can then work together to edit the song and create as much client input as possible

Adaptations. Song composition is a unique tool to use in group music therapy. Creating lyrics together and contributing ideas to stories or themes provides opportunities for socialization for clients who may feel isolated due to their illness. Family members or friends may also be included in the music composition process, and it can be an excellent way for clients and family members/friends to relate to one another, share feelings, and engage in a creative activity. The client may choose to perform a self-composed piece or may ask the music therapist to perform the piece for others or to the client as well.

Song Stories, Musical Autobiographies, Musical Life Review, Music Collages

Overview. Song stories, musical autobiographies/musical life review, and music collages are unique ways for clients to leave legacies and memories for important people in their lives. A song story is a song telling the story of a client. Musical autobiographies/musical life reviews involve the client creating a list of songs that tells their story, either prearranged or composed by him/herself or the therapist. A music collage could depict any story or theme not life-review specific, such as music that describes who he/she is, family, etc.

A client may not be ready to compose songs or projects based on their life if he/she is feeling extreme remorse and not prepared to deal with difficult emotions. Through the assessment process, the music therapist can determine whether creating a musical life review would be appropriate.

Preparation. Most of the preparation occurs after an initial conversation about the intervention with the client. A music therapist can prepare for a session by introducing the client to the idea of creating a musical life review and determining whether the client wants to compose their own songs or compile songs from other music mediums. Depending on either case, the music therapist can come prepared for the next session with the appropriate music and compositional instruments and materials.

What to observe. The music therapist must pay special attention to adverse emotional reactions. If the client becomes more distressed or frustrated by life review and seems to be put in to a negative mood by reviewing their life, the music therapist uses their clinical verbal and musical skills to address the issues and adapt the activity.

Procedures. To create a musical life review, or musical chronology, Duffey (2008) lists several suggested steps to follow.

1) The therapist explains the purpose of musical life review and sets goals with the client.
2) The client compiles a list of significant songs that trigger associations to important life events.
3) The therapist and/or client play the music, and the client discusses and considers significant memories and meaning behind each song to discuss further. In this activity, the client can either pick prerecorded songs or compose songs about significant life events and accomplishments.
4) The therapist and client decide if and how they want to share the song (e.g., recording the song, playing it for family and friends together, writing down the songs/lyrics and giving the lyrics to family/friends).
5) The client and/or music therapist perform/record the song and share it with the desired audience (or record it for the client's use).
6) The therapist and client discuss the outcome of the life review and go back to the goals and purpose of creating the life review to review the successes of the activity.
7) The music therapist and client can work on another project or edit their first project together. The music therapist can suggest other types of compositional activities, such as composing songs or writing music together.

For any compositional activity involving life review or review of the self, the client should always be the main motivator in decision-making. Even if the client has no musical background, the therapist should use their clinical and musical skills as tools for the client to use for their creation.

The music therapist can use a wide variety of methods to choose songs and significant life events. A music therapist can interview the client, staff, friends, and family members to address significant life events and important music for the client. These songs provide a good starting point for the client, and the client can then choose to add prerecorded music, or even to compose new music to describe any important life events.

Adaptations. Musical life review/autobiographies may be used as a technique for clients to participate in with family and friends. If clients are having difficulty remembering positive aspects of their lives or difficulty seeing accomplishments, family members and friends often can help the client see and feel that he/she has achieved things in their life. Musical autobiographies and musical life reviews can be recorded and given to family members and friends as meaningful gifts before or after the client has died. A client's composition could also be played at their funeral or memorial service to provide family and friends with an overview of the client's life and to ensure that the client's voice is heard.

Working with Caregivers

Working with caregivers is a central component of music therapy work in palliative/hospice care. Facing the serious illness of a loved one can be traumatic and lead to numerous life changes for family members and friends of the dying patient. During the dying process and after a loved one dies, many family members and friends will suffer from grief. Grief is defined by the Webster's New World Medical Dictionary, 3rd edition (Shiel & Stoppler, 2008a), as "the normal process of reacting to a loss. Emotional reactions of grief can include anger, guilt, anxiety, sadness, and despair. Physical reactions of grief can include sleeping problems, changes in appetite, physical problems, or illness" (para. 1). Family members who are watching their loved one's health deteriorate may experience anticipatory grief. Webster's New World Medical Dictionary, 3rd edition (Shiel & Stoppler, 2008b), defines anticipatory grief as "The normal mourning that occurs when a patient or family is expecting a death. Anticipatory grief includes depression, extreme concern for the dying person, preparing for the death, and adjusting to changes caused by the death" (para. 1). Aldrich (1974) defines anticipatory grief as "any grief occurring prior to a loss, as distinguished from the grief which occurs at or after a loss" (p. 4).

Music therapists may work with clients who have complicated or unresolved grief. Horowitz, Siegel, Holen, Bonanno, Milbrath, and Stinson (1997) state that "[c]omplicated grief disorders may include symptoms such as intrusive images, severe pangs of emotion, denial of implications of the loss to the self, and neglect of necessary adaptive activities at work and at home" (p. 290). Webster's New World Medical Dictionary (Shiel & Stoppler, 2008c) defines complicated/unresolved grief as "[g]rief that is complicated by adjustment disorders (especially depressed and anxious mood or disturbed emotions and behavior), major depression, substance abuse, and posttraumatic stress disorder. Complicated grief is identified by the extended length of time of the symptoms, the interference in normal function caused by the symptoms, or by the intensity of the symptoms (e.g., intense suicidal thoughts or acts)" (para. 1). Rando (1984) lists factors that can inhibit children from moving through the mourning process, including the surviving parent denying his or her feelings and their expression, fear about the vulnerability of the surviving parent and the security of the self, a lack of the security of a caring environment, the lack of a caring adult who can stimulate and support the mourning process, confusion about the death and his/her part in it, ambivalence toward the deceased parent, cognitive inability to accept the finality and irreversibility of the death, and instability of family life after the loss. These issues can affect a child's ability to process the death of a loved one, and they may need extra guidance and support through the grieving process.

Music therapy holds the potential to assist caregivers in multiple ways, including during the dying process of their loved one, and in bereavement and grief work after the death. The majority of music therapy literature concentrating on grief and bereavement has been conducted with children and adolescents, and the research with adult caregivers is focused on family members/friends diagnosed with Alzheimer's/dementia, although some research has been conducted with adult caregivers in hospice/palliative care. Both types of clients will be discussed below together with techniques that can be implemented in music therapy.

Children and Adolescents

Although children are not necessarily caregivers for their loved ones, they are directly affected emotionally and psychologically by a death, and music therapy is an effective intervention to ease suffering. Some symptoms of grief and difficulties with grief that children and adolescents demonstrate include sudden personality changes, withdrawal, extensive depression, psychosomatic headaches and stomachaches on a recurring basis, losing friends through aggressiveness or withdrawal, lack of energy and enthusiasm, and extreme denial such as fantasies of reunion or refusal to admit that the person is dead (Hamilton & Masecar, 1997). Other symptoms of grief that children or adolescents may demonstrate are mood swings, feelings of hopelessness and helplessness, risk-taking, self-harming, anger, withdrawal from adults, and problems focusing (Jacobs, 2011). Hilliard's (2007) study of bereaved children using Orff-based cognitive behavioral music therapy techniques, found that the intervention allowed for emotional healing, building positive social relationships, and cognitive reframing, and helped decrease behavioral problems.

Adults

Adults who lose a parent in their lives may be having difficulty coping or grieving with losses. Becvar (2001) states that symptoms of grief for young adults include pulling back to their family of origin, which may threaten the newly defined sense of self; guilt over unresolved conflicts; loss of a parent who may have been a primary source of emotional support; feeling abandoned and not knowing how to move forward in their lives; and resurgence of grief with each milestone, graduation, wedding, birth of a child, and birthday. Adults who experience grief may feel a loss of the longest of life's relationships, security, and unconditional love (especially for those that saw the parent as a caretaker, provider of praise); feelings of abandonment; anger toward others or over things that did or did not happen in the relationship with the deceased parents; guilt, denial, and/or depression symptoms; and physical feelings such as such as tightness in the throat or a heaviness in the chest, loss of appetite, restlessness, having difficulty sleeping, and dreaming of the deceased parent frequently (Dane, 1991).

Music therapy may facilitate coping with grief and loss, pain and anxiety, disorientation and dementia, lack of meaning, and hopelessness (Hilliard, 2001a). Music therapy with caregivers can support clients and caregivers in finding resolution and relationship completion through singing, selecting songs, and participating in the lyrical and musical interactions; music itself plays a vital role in helping motivate and inspire love in caregivers during the course of music therapy and during bereavement (Magill, 2009). Caregivers may find it difficult to express feelings, thoughts, and last wishes to their loved one who is dying; music therapy can aid communication between the family and the patient who is actively dying and also provide a comforting presence (Krout, 2003). Music therapy with adults can be used in the dying process of their loved one, as well as after the death, while dealing with the loss and change that comes with losing a significant person in their lives.

Music therapy can be a valuable tool in assisting caregivers of clients who are in palliative or hospice care. By fostering communication with loved ones during the dying process, completing relationships, and providing care through the grief process, caregivers can receive emotional and psychological support though the entire process.

Bereavement Groups

Bereavement groups offer a supportive opportunity for caregivers to cope with the loss of a loved one. General guidelines for running a bereavement group include recognizing differences between complicated and uncomplicated bereavement reactions, identifying risk factors that may make certain individuals more vulnerable to bereavement (and related complications), appreciating and monitoring for potential adverse outcomes associated with bereavement, and taking actions to prevent or minimize maladjustment to the loss (Zhang, El-Jawahri, & Prigerson, 2006). These guidelines are important for music therapists to consider when designing a bereavement group. Other factors to consider are the psychological model that the therapist follows. For example, is the group going to be run under a cognitive behavioral, humanistic, or psychodynamic model? The type of psychological model the therapist practices under affects assessment, interventions, and evaluation of progress with the group.

Music therapy bereavement groups are extremely important for children who have lost a parent to prevent psychological issues from arising later in their life. One study that focused on a cognitive behavioral model of music therapy (involving behavior modification, identifying and expressing emotions, and challenging/reshaping cognitive distortions) was conducted with children in a bereavement group who had lost a loved one within two years of the study (Hilliard, 2001b). Music therapy techniques used in this study included singing, songwriting, rap writing, rhythmic improvisation, structured drumming, lyric analysis, and music listening. Children receiving group music therapy from these techniques demonstrated significant reductions in grief symptoms and a reduction in behavioral problems. Implementing the techniques used in this study could be extremely beneficial for children who are experiencing grief.

Music therapy bereavement groups are a valuable intervention for clients who are suffering from complicated or unresolved grief. Dalton and Krout (2005) studied adolescent grief and found that participants who engaged in songwriting in groups were better able to process their grief than those without music therapy treatment. Skewes (2001) also provided group music therapy to six bereaved adolescents, using improvisation and group music sharing/discussion. The six adolescents who participated were better able to express feelings and share memories of their loved ones while maintaining developmental needs such as freedom, control, fun, and group cohesion. Amir (1998) found that using folk songs and singing folk songs from one's culture helped adult women in a music therapy bereavement group create and strengthen identity and facilitated the expression of feelings and implications of a death.

Music therapy bereavement groups offer a constructive way to create group cohesion and understanding and assist clients in feeling connected while creating relationships.

Suggested bereavement group outline. A music therapist should prepare a variety of assessment activities to determine the varying needs of clients when designing a bereavement group. Some clients may be more adjusted or secure, while others may be having a more difficult time. To prevent certain clients from receiving inadequate treatment, a music therapist should always conduct proper assessments to gauge the client's position in the grief process. There are a multitude of possible assessment activities that could be used with bereavement groups. Free improvisation on instruments could be used to assess the client's willingness to express their emotions and help reveal the emotional position of the client. Lyric substitution and songwriting can also reveal a client's current state of being. Assessing a client's reaction to a song chosen by the therapist can also help the therapist assess the client's level of emotional preparedness and their needs. Family members and other health care professionals alongside the client may be interviewed to further assess client needs.

Once the therapist has determined the group dynamic and the needs of the group, treatment may begin. A session should include a wide variety of music therapy activities to engage the clients in different ways and ensure that each client is benefiting from participating. Possible interventions include songwriting, music and art, lyric analysis/discussion, lyric substitution, music listening, music improvisation, and music and imagery. Within those broad areas, a music therapist can structure the session according to the clients' needs. A conceivable session outline could include a greeting song or activity, music for lyric analysis (either brought by the therapist or brought by the clients), instrumental/vocal improvisation, songwriting, music for imagery/relaxation, and a closing song or activity. By using different musical modalities, clients will be able to explore their own emotions and find the venue of expression that works best for them.

Krout (1999) composed a series of songs to help clients through the grieving process and to explore and validate their feelings. Certain themes from his songs based on sessions with clients were rearranging, celebrating life, taking care of oneself, sending messages to loved ones, taking journeys, and changes. These are all themes that he experienced with clients, and these themes, songs, and activities are excellent tools to use with those who are bereaved.

Needs of the Music Therapist

Working with clients in palliative care can be physically, emotionally, and spiritually challenging. If a music therapist is dealing with his/her own issues surrounding death and dying, it may be extremely difficult to provide appropriate care for someone who is dying. It is important for a music therapist to have a support system in place so that if issues do arise, he/she is able to deal with concerns effectively and continue to provide exceptional care. Factors that may lead to burnout among music therapists who work in palliative care include a lack of understanding by health care professionals of the role of the music therapist, ongoing loss, differing palliative care philosophies among members of the interdisciplinary team, difficult referrals, and overidentifying with clients, (Clements-Cortés, 2006). Other stressors included feelings of helplessness, juggling multiple roles, advocating for music therapy, not feeling valued or appreciated, and relationships with other interdisciplinary team members.

Boston and Mount (2006) found that transference and countertransference, cumulative grief, a lack of time to process loss, and differences in religious/cultural views are issues that may arise for health care providers working in palliative care. Although it is acknowledged more openly that nursing staff and medical staff may require support in working with persons who are actively dying and/or in poor health, music therapists also feel the effect of loss and sadness when clients die, and they see death on a regular basis with people whom they have developed a therapeutic relationship (Rykov, 2001).

A music therapist benefits from the support of coworkers and allied health care professionals in their immediate work environments. Feeling unsupported can make the music therapist's work extremely difficult if he/she is constantly trying to advocate and provide care at the same time. A music therapist also may benefit from the emotional support, guidance, and creative programming ideas of fellow music therapists. This is not always feasible in the day-to-day work setting, but may be fostered through classmates, professional colleagues, and social networks such as LinkedIn or local music therapy organizations. A music therapist also needs support from family, friends, or other members who might be in a personal/social network. If a music therapist is isolated in his/her personal life, it may be difficult to tackle tough situations and/or feel supported.

Research Evidence

Although there is an abundance of research on the efficacy of music therapy in palliative care, there is a need for more meta-analyses across research and further summaries of the expansive literature. Hilliard (2005) focused on research studies that followed a quantitative model of measurement, where most studies in music therapy in palliative care had taken a qualitative approach. In Hilliard's study, he found that of the 11 studies analyzed, all studies' results showed promise for the use of music therapy in palliative care, yet limitations prevented generalized applicability to the broad population of palliative care. Hilliard acknowledges a serious lack of controlled studies with large sample sizes and maintains the need for studies with higher levels of control and randomization of subjects. In the following section, research is highlighted on each technique; additional specific research about each technique has been provided above within the previous section outlining the indications, goals, and level of therapy.

Bradt, Dileo, Grocke, and Magill (2011) completed a Cochrane Review of the literature using a wide variety of medical and professional databases to compare the effects of music therapy or music medicine interventions and standard care with standard care alone, or standard care and other interventions in patients with cancer. Their review included 30 trials with a total of 1,891 participants and found that music therapy may have a beneficial effect on anxiety, pain, mood, quality of life, heart rate, respiratory rate, and blood pressure in cancer patients, but that most trials were at high risk of bias and, therefore, these results need to be interpreted with caution. They also concluded that music therapy in cancer care may lead to small reductions in heart rate, respiratory rate, and blood pressure. The areas of need that did not have conclusive positive results were regarding the effect of music interventions on distress, body image, oxygen saturation level, immunologic functioning, spirituality, and communication outcomes. This study shows the positive effect of music therapy as an intervention in cancer care and also highlights the areas of need for further research in the world of music therapy.

Receptive Methods

There are a number of efficacy studies concerning receptive music therapy in palliative care. A graphical analysis of nine terminally ill patients' perceived pain relief, physical comfort, relaxation, and contentment scores after their listening to recorded music showed that music has the power to positively affect each of those areas (Curtis, 1986). Several case studies demonstrate that pain is reduced and relaxation increases when listening to recorded music (Magill-Levreault, 1993; Mandel, 1991; Munro & Mount, 1978; Munro, 1984). Kemper and Danhauer (2005) found that when patients listened to classical music, they showed decreased tension, and when they listened to prescribed music (music designed to enhance a sense of well-being), patients reported significantly more relaxation, mental clarity, vigor, and compassion and significantly decreased hostility, sadness, fatigue, and tension. Troesch, Rodehaver, Delaney, and Yanes (1993) found that patients who participated in guided imagery while receiving chemotherapy treatments experienced more delayed symptoms of chemotherapy than did those in the control group. They also reported feeling significantly more prepared, relaxed, and in control prior to chemotherapy than subjects in the control group. Jonas (2005) states that music for reminiscence can reinforce the patient's self-identity and promote communication between patient and family, and particular songs used for reminiscence may evoke memories of childhood, teenage, and adult years. In one study of patients in palliative care comparing live vs. taped music, the results indicated that both taped and live music conditions resulted in significant reductions in pain measures, but that live music was relatively more effective in terms of the magnitude of the pain reduction and enhancement of physical comfort (Clements-Cortés, 2011).

Song choice is also proven to be beneficial in music therapy with palliative patients. In Gallagher, Lagman, Walsh, Davis, and LeGrand's (2006) study, song choice was the fifth most common technique out of 14 interventions and was implemented to facilitate goals in several areas: providing enjoyment, decreasing anxiety and depression, decreasing perception of pain, providing coping skills/support, improving mood, and providing distraction. Any of these goals could be an area of focus or importance depending on client need at the referral or assessment stage. Standley (1992) found that patients who were exposed to their own choice of music experienced either a reduced or delayed incidence of nausea after chemotherapy treatment. Clements-Cortés (2004) states that song choice provides clients with choice and a voice, and song choice can help clients express feelings that are too difficult to verbalize, increase self-esteem, help patients regain self-identity, encourage choice-making, and promote social interaction.

Improvisational Methods

In a study on the effects of vocal improvisation with in-patient hospice clients, Batzner (2003) documented a decrease in discomfort behaviors of clients receiving music therapy. Lee (1996) found that empathic improvisation can allow the client to feel understood and further build an in-depth relationship between the client and therapist, which can be profound and meaningful during the dying process for the client. Bunt (1994) states that during improvisation, clients in palliative care were able to find a release and resolution for a wide variety of hurtful and painful emotions. Further, during free improvisation, Lee (1996) found that improvisation can enhance mobility and motivation, while serving as a key to unconscious issues that are not easily addressed verbally, such as anger, jealousy, existential loneliness, and fear.

Re-creative Methods

Singing proved to increase confidence and mood, initiate reminiscence, improve interaction with family members, and release emotions with clients in palliative care (Aldridge, 1998). Singing can contribute to self-awareness and can create a sense of belonging (Clair, 1996). Dileo (1999) notes that toning and chanting can help to reduce stress and provide physical and emotional relief for clients. Playing instruments was found to increase expression of feelings, enhance mood, and improve quality of life with clients in palliative care (Halstead & Roscoe, 2007) and helped maintain the field of communication between the client and family members, friends, and staff members (Gauthier & Dallaire, 1993).

Compositional Methods

O'Callaghan (1994) analyzed the themes of 64 songs written by 39 palliative care patients in music therapy sessions. The expression of these themes through songwriting indicates that songwriting can offer patients an opportunity to find refuge and diversion from their current situation, and that this place of safety may aid in symptom control. O'Callaghan (1990) states that songwriting is a valuable medium that patients can use to express buried feelings, gain support, send messages to special people, and feel that they are contributing something unique to this world, which can in turn help the client gain pleasure and contribute to positive self-efficacy. Blyth and Miles (2012) found that songwriting allowed clients to externalize unexpressed feelings and stories, enable the collection and construction of shared experiences into song framework, and enable families and friends to speak about challenging situations.

Musical life review is another form of compositional music therapy that can improve the quality of life for palliative patients. O'Callaghan (1984) discusses how musical life review enables clients to overview the uniqueness of their life and affirms significant life events. This can be very crucial with clients who fear death or have regret in their lives and are having existential concerns about life and death. Halstead and Roscoe (2007) state that musical life review can be used to alleviate spiritual distress, and Duffey (2008) maintains that musical life review can also facilitate clients' access to their emotional responses to life, help clarify negative aspects and relationships of a client's life that he/she may regret, and help the client address and re-author those life events. A client who is dying young may have feelings of guilt, regret, and remorse about their lack of life experience. Song stories and musical autobiographies are excellent tools to highlight achievements and positive memories and the impact the client has had in their life.

SUMMARY AND CONCLUSIONS

Music therapy is a recognized treatment in palliative and hospice care that offers an innovative approach benefiting clients throughout the dying process. Music therapy interventions can range on a continuum of passive to active techniques and include music listening, lyric discussion and analysis, GIM, improvisation, songwriting, musical life review, production of legacy gifts, relaxation, and singing/playing instruments. There is an abundance of literature on the efficacy of music therapy interventions in palliative care, although there is a need for greater sample size and meta-analyses of the existing studies. Music therapy can help clients going through the dying process to improve communication with family and friends and gain a sense of legacy and finality near the end of life. Music therapy has proven effects on anxiety, pain, mood, quality of life, heart rate, respiratory rate, and blood pressure in palliative care clients. Music therapy is strongly recommended as an intervention to be used in palliative/hospice care.

REFERENCES

Aldrich, C. K. (1974). Some dynamics of anticipatory grief. In B. Schoenberg, A. C. Carr, A.H. Kutscher, D. Peretz, & I.K. Goldberg (Eds.), *Anticipatory grief* (pp.3-9). New York: Columbia University Press.

Aldridge, D. (1999). *Music therapy in palliative care: New voices*. Philadelphia, PA: Jessica Kingsley.

Aldridge, G. (1996). A walk through Paris: The development of melodic expression in music therapy with a breast-cancer patient. *The Arts in Psychotherapy*, 23, 207–223.

ALS Society of Canada. (2011). Glossary. Retrieved from http://184.107.204.92/en/research/glossary

Alternative Medicine Foundation Inc. (2010). *Relaxation and meditation practices*. Retrieved from http://www.amfoundation.org/relaxation.htm

Alzheimer Society of Canada. (2009). Diagnosis. Retrieved from http://www.alzheimer.ca/english/disease/diagnosis.htm

American Heritage. (2008). The American heritage medical dictionary. Houghton Mifflin Harcourt Publishing Company.

Amir, D. (1998). The use of Israeli folk songs in dealing with women's bereavement and loss in music therapy. In D. Dotker (Ed.), *Arts therapists, refugees, and migrants: Reaching across borders* (pp. 217–235). Philadelphia, PA: Jessica Kingsley.

Bailey, L. M. (1983). The effects of live music versus tape-recorded music on hospitalized cancer patients. *Music Therapy, 3*(1), 17–28.

Bailey, L. M. (1984). The use of songs in music therapy with cancer patients and their families. Music *Therapy, 4*(1), 5-17.

Bailey, L. M. (1986). Music therapy in pain management. *Journal of Pain and Symptom Management, 1*(1), 25–28.

Balboni, T. A., Vanderwerker, L. C., Block, S. D., Paulk, M. E., Lathan, C. S., Peteet, J. R., & Prigerson, H. G. (2007). Religiousness and spiritual support among advanced cancer patients and associations with end-of-life treatment preferences and quality of life. *Journal of Clinical Oncology, 25*(5), 555–560.

Batzner, K. W. (2003). The effects of therapist vocal improvisation on discomfort behaviors of in-patient hospice clients (Unpublished master's thesis). University of Kansas, Lawrence, KS.

Baumel, L. (1973). Psychiatrist as music therapist. *Journal of Music Therapy, 10,* 83–85.

Becvar, D. S. (2001). *In the presence of grief: Helping family members resolve death, dying, and bereavement issues.* New York: The Guilford Press.

Belgrave, M., Darrow, A. A., Walworth, D., & Wlodarczyk, N. (2011). *Music therapy and geriatric populations: Handbook for practicing music therapists and other healthcare professionals.* Silver Spring, MD: American Music Therapy Association, Inc.

Benzein, E., & Saveman, B. I. (1998). Nurses' perception of hope in patients with cancer: A palliative care perspective. *Cancer Nursing, 21*(1), 10–16.

Berger, J. S. (2006). *Music of the soul: Composing life out of loss.* New York: Taylor & Francis Group.

Bernstein, D. A., & Borkovec, D. (1973*). Progressive relaxation training: A manual for the helping professions.* Champaign, IL: Research Press.

Blyth, L., & Miles, L. (2012). We're all in this together: Inpatient and community based music therapy for children and families experiencing terminal illness. *Palliative Care Australia.* Online PDF retrieved from http://www.palliativecare.org.au/Portals/46/Together%20conference/C4%20Louise%20Miles.pdf

Bonde, L. O. (2000). Metaphor and narrative in guided imagery and music. *Journal of the Association for Music and Imagery, 7,* 59–76.

Bonny, H. (2002). *Music & consciousness: The evolution of guided imagery and music.* Gilsum, NH: Barcelona Publishers.

Borysenko, J., & Rothstein, L. (1987). *Minding the body, mending the mind.* Reading, MA: Addison-Wesley Pub. Co.

Boston, P. H., & Mount, B. M. (2006). The caregiver's perspective on existential and spiritual distress in palliative care. *Journal of Pain and Symptom Management, 32*(1), 13–26.

Boyd-Brewer, C. (2003). Vibroacoustic therapy: Sound vibrations in medicine. *Alternative and Complementary Therapies, 9*(5), 257–263.

Boyd-Brewer, C. (2004). Vibroacoustic sound therapy improves pain management and more. *Holistic Nursing Practice, 18*(3), 111–118.

Bradt, J., Dileo, C., Grocke, D., & Magill, L. (2011). Music interventions for improving psychological and physical outcomes in cancer patients. *Cochrane Database of Systematic Reviews, 2011(8),* Article. CD006911, doi: 10.1002/14651858.CD006911.pub2.

Bruscia, K. E. (1987*). Improvisational models of music therapy.* Springfield, IL: Charles C. Thomas Publications.

Bruscia, K. E. (1995). Modes of consciousness in guided imagery and music (GIM): A therapist's experience of the guiding process. In C. B. Kenny (Ed.), *Listening, playing, creating: Essays on the power of sound,* pp. 165–198. Albany, NY: State University of New York Press.

Bruscia, K. E. (1998*). Defining music therapy (2nd ed.).* Gilsum, NH: Barcelona Publishers.

Bruscia, K. E. (2002a). The boundaries of guided imagery and music (GIM) and the Bonny method. In K. E. Bruscia & D. Grocke (Eds.), *Guided imagery and music: The Bonny method and beyond. Gilsum,* pp. 37–62, NH: Barcelona Publishers.

Bruscia, K. E. (2002b). A psychodynamic orientation to the Bonny method. In K. E. Bruscia & D. Grocke (Eds.), *Guided imagery and music: The Bonny method and beyond*, pp. 225–244. Gilsum, NH: Barcelona Publishers.

Bunt, L. (1994). *Music therapy: An art beyond words.* London: Routledge.

Burns, D. (2001). The effect of the Bonny method of guided imagery and music on the mood and life quality of cancer patients. *Journal of Music Therapy, 38*(1), 51–65.

Burns, D. (2002). Guided imagery and music (GIM) in the treatment of individuals with chronic illness. In K. E. Bruscia & D. Grocke (Eds.), *Guided imagery and music: The Bonny method and beyond,* pp. 171–186. Gilsum, NH: Barcelona Publishers.

Byrne, L. A. (1982). Music therapy and reminiscence: A case study. *Clinical Gerontologist, 1,* 76-77.

Calovini, B. S. (1993). The effect of participation in one music therapy session on state anxiety in hospice patients(Unpublished master's thesis). Case Western Reserve University, Cleveland, OH.

Canadian Hospice Palliative Care Association. (2011). Hospice palliative care fact sheet. Retrieved from http://www.chpca.net/family-caregivers/faqs.aspx

Canadian Hospice Palliative Care Association. (2011). What is hospice palliative care? Retrieved from http://www.chpca.net/Homev

Canadian Liver Foundation. (2011). Liver disease. Retrieved from http://www.liver.ca/liver-disease/

Chochinov, H. M. (2002). Dignity-conserving care—a new model for palliative care: Helping the patient feel valued. *Journal of the American Medical Association, 287*(17), 2253–2260.

Clair, A. A. (1996). *Therapeutic uses of music with older adults.* Baltimore, MD: Health Professions Press, Inc.

Clark, C. C. (2000). *Integrating complementary health procedures into practice.* New York: Springer Publishing Company, Inc.

Clark, M., Isaacks-Downton, G., Wells, N., Redlin-Frazier, S., Eck, C., Hepworth, J. T., & Chakravarthy, B. (2006). Use of preferred music to reduce emotional distress and symptom activity during radiation therapy. *Journal of Music Therapy, 43*(3), 247–265.

Clarkson, G. (2002). Combining gestalt dreamwork and the Bonny method. In K. E. Bruscia & D. Grocke (Eds.), *Guided imagery and music: The Bonny method and beyond,* pp. 245–256. Gilsum, NH: Barcelona Publishers.

Clements-Cortés, A. (2004). The use of music in facilitating emotional expression in the terminally ill. *American Journal of Hospice and Palliative Medicine, 21*(4), 255– 260.

Clements-Cortés, A. (2006). Occupational stressors among music therapists working in palliative care. *Canadian Journal of Music Therapy, 12*(1), 30–60.

Clements-Cortés, A. (2011). The effect of live music vs. taped music on pain and comfort in palliative care. *Korean Journal of Music Therapy, 13*(1), 105-121.

Cohen, N.S. (2002). Ethical considerations in guided imagery and music (GIM). In K. E. Bruscia & D. Grocke (Eds.), *Guided imagery and music: The Bonny method and beyond.* Gilsum, NH: Barcelona Publishers.

Cohen, S. R., Boston, P., Mount, B. M., & Porterfield, P. (2001). Changes in quality of life following admission to palliative care units. *Palliative Medicine, 15*(5), 363– 371.

Cooper, J. (2002). Is VA therapy, music therapy? Music Therapy Today (online). Retrieved from http://musictherapyworld.net

Curtis, S. L. (1986). The effect of music on pain relief and relaxation of the terminally ill. *Journal of Music Therapy, 23,* 10–24.

Dalton, T. A., & Krout, R. E. (2005). Development of the grief process scale through music therapy songwriting with bereaved adolescents. *The Arts in Psychotherapy, 32*(2), 131–143.

Dane, B. O. (1991). Counseling bereaved middle-aged children: Parental suicide survivors. *Clinical Social Work Journal, 19*(1), 35–48.

Davis, M., Eshelman, E. R., & McKay, M. (2008). *The relaxation & stress reduction workbook (6th ed.).* Oakland, CA: New Harbinger Publications, Inc.

Dileo, C., & Bradt, J. (1999). Entrainment, resonance, and pain-related suffering. In C. Dileo (Ed.), *Music therapy and medicine: Theoretical and clinical applications* (pp. 181-188). Silver Spring, MD: American Music Therapy Association.

Duffey, T. (2008). Using music and a musical chronology as a life review with the aging. In L. C. Rubin (Ed.), *Popular culture in counseling, psychotherapy, and play- based interventions* (pp. 81–92). New York: Springer Publishing Company, LLC.

Edwards, J. (2005). The contribution of music therapy to the process of therapeutic change for people receiving hospital care. In C. Le Navenec & L. Bridges (Eds.), *Creating connections between nursing care and the creative arts therapies: Expanding the concept of holistic care* (pp. 149–155). Springfield, IL: Charles C. Thomas Publisher, Ltd.

Enes, S. P. D. (2003). An exploration of dignity in palliative care. *Palliative Medicine, 17*(3), 263–269.

Fegg, M. J., Wasner, M., Neudert, C., & Borasio, G. D. (2005). Personal values and individual quality of life in palliative care patients. *Journal of Pain and Symptom Management, 30*(2), 154–159.

Field, T. (2009). *Complementary and alternative therapies research.* Washington, DC: American Psychological Association.

Forrest, M. (1990). Reminiscence therapy in a Scottish hospital. Health Libraries Review, 7(2), 69–72.

Freeman, L., Caserta, M., Lund, D., Rossa, S., Dowdy, A., & Partenheimer, A. (2006). Music thanatology: Prescriptive harp music as palliative care for the dying patient. *American Journal of Hospice and Palliative Medicine, 23*(2), 100–104.

Gallagher, L. M., Lagman, R., Walsh, D., Davis, M. P., & LeGrand, S. B. (2006). The clinical effects of music therapy in palliative medicine. *Support Care Cancer, 14,* 859–866.

Gardstrom, S. C. (2007*). Music therapy improvisation for groups: Essential leadership competencies.* Gilsum, NH: Barcelona Publishers.

Gauthier, P. A., & Dallaire, C. (1993). Music therapy. *Canadian Nurse, 89*(2), 46–48.

Grocke, D. E. (2002). The Bonny music programs. In K. E. Bruscia & D. Grocke (Eds.), *Guided imagery and music: The Bonny method and beyond.* Pp. 99–136.Gilsum, NH: Barcelona Publishers.

Grocke, D. E. (2005). The role of the therapist in the Bonny method of guided imagery and music. *Music Therapy Perspectives, 23*(1), 45–52.

Grocke, D., & Wigram, T. (2007). *Receptive methods in music therapy: Techniques and clinical applications for music therapy clinicians, educators, and students.* Philadelphia, PA: Jessica Kingsley.

Groen, K. M. (2007). Pain assessment and management in end-of-life care: A survey of assessment and treatment practices of hospice music therapy and nursing professionals. *Journal of Music Therapy, 44*(2), 90–112.

Hain, R., Weinstein, S., Oleske, J., Orloff, S.F., & Cohen, S. (2004). Holistic management of symptoms. In B. S. Carter, M. Levetown, & S. E. Friebert (Eds.), Palliative care for infants, children, and adolescents: A practical handbook (pp. 163-195). Baltimore, MD: The Johns Hopkins University Press.

Halpin, D. M. G., Seamark, D. A., & Seamark, C. J. (2009). Palliative and end-of-life care for patients with respiratory disease. *European Respiratory Society Monograph, 43,* 327–353.

Halstead, M. T., & Roscoe, S. T. (2007). Restoring the spirit at the end-of-life: Music as an intervention for oncology nurses. *Clinical Journal of Oncology Nursing, 6*(6), 332–336.

Hamilton, L., & Masecar, D. (1999*). Counselling the bereaved: Caregiver handbook.* Suicide prevention training programs, Calgary, Alberta.

Hanser, S. M. (1999). *The new music therapist's handbook* (pp. 75–97). Boston, MA: Berklee Press Publications.

Hearn, J., & Higginson, I. J. (1997). Outcome measures in palliative care for advanced cancer patients: A review. *Journal of Public Health, 19*(2), 193–199.

Hermsen, M. A., & Henk, A. M. J. (2004). Pastoral care, spirituality, and religion in palliative care journals. *American Journal of Hospice and Palliative Care, 21*(5), 353–356.

Higginson, I., Wade, A., & McCarthy, M. (1990). Palliative care: Views of patients and their families. *British Medical Journal, 301*(6746), 277–281.

Hilliard, R. E. (2001a). The use of music therapy in meeting the multidimensional needs of hospice patients and families. *Journal of Palliative Care, 17*(3), 161–166.

Hilliard, R. E. (2001b). The effects of music-therapy based bereavement groups on mood and behaviour of grieving children: A pilot study. *Journal of Music Therapy, 38*(4), 291–306.

Hilliard, R. E. (2003). The effects of music therapy on the quality and length of life of people diagnosed with terminal cancer. *Journal of Music Therapy, 40*(2), 113– 137.

Hilliard, R. E. (2005). Music therapy in hospice and palliative care: A review of the empirical data. *Evidence-based Complementary and Alternative Medicine, 2*(2), 173–178.

Hilliard, R. E. (2007). The effects of Orff-based music therapy and social work groups on childhood grief symptoms and behaviors. *Journal of Music Therapy, 44*(2), 123– 138.

Hillmer, M. G. (2003). Survey of nurses' attitudes and perceptions toward music therapy in the hospital setting (Master's dissertation). University of Kansas, KS.

Hogan, B. (1998). Music therapy at the end-of-life: Searching for the rite of passage. In D. Aldridge (Ed.), *Music therapy in palliative care: New voices*. Philadelphia, PA: Jessica Kingsley.

Horne-Thompson, A., Daveson, B., & Hogan, B. (2007). A project investigating music therapy referral trends within palliative care: An Australian perspective. *Journal of Music Therapy, 44*(2), 139–155.

Horowitz, M. J., Siegel, B., Holen, A.,, Bonanno, G. A., Milbrath, C., & Stinson, C. H. (1997). Diagnostic criteria for complicated grief disorder. *American Journal of Psychiatry, 154*, 904-910.

Houck, A. J. W. (2007). The development of a music therapy protocol for determining the spiritual needs of hospice patients (Doctoral dissertation). Ann Arbor, MI: ProQuest Information and Learning Company.

Ikezoe, J., Godwin, J. D., Hunt, K. J., & Marglin, S. I. (1995). Pulmonary lymphangitic carcinomatosis: Chronicity of radiographic findings in long-term survivors. *American Journal of Roentgenology, 165*(1), 49–52.

Jacobs, B. (2011). Grief in children and teens. Retrieved from http://www.bill-jacobs-lpcc.com/grief-in-children-and-teens.html

Jacobson, E. (1938). *Progressive relaxation*. Chicago: University of Chicago Press.

Johnston, E. T. (2003). Spiritual needs of patients with cancer and family caregivers. *Cancer Nursing, 26*(4), 260–266.

Jonas, J. (2005). Reflections: Music therapy in palliative care. *Humane Medicine Health Care, 13*(3).

Juslin, P. N., & Sloboda, J. A. (2010). *Handbook of music and emotion: Theory, research, applications*. New York: Oxford University Press.

Kasayka, R. (2002). A spiritual orientation to the Bonny method: To walk the mystical path on practical feet. In K. E. Bruscia & D. Grocke (Eds.), *Guided Imagery and Music: The Bonny method and beyond*. Gilsum, NH: Barcelona Publishers.

Kemper, K. J., & Danhauer, S. C. (2005). Music as therapy. *Southern Medical Journal, 98*(3), 282–288.

Kidney Foundation of Canada. (2011). What is kidney disease? Retrieved from http://www.kidney.ca/page.aspx?pid=320

Koffman, J., & O'Kelly, J. (2007). Multidisciplinary perspectives of music therapy in adult palliative care. *Palliative Medicine, 21*(3), 235–241.

Krout, R. E. (1999). *Songs from sorrow, songs from joy: Contemporary songs from grief to healing*. St. Louis, MO: MMB Music Inc.

Krout, R. E. (2003). Music therapy with imminently dying hospice patients and their families: Facilitating release near the time of death. *American Journal of Hospice and Palliative Medicine, 20*(2), 129–134.

Lawton, J. (2000). *The dying process: Patients' experiences of palliative care.* New York, NY: Routledge.

Lee, C. (1996). *Music at the edge: The music therapy experiences of a musician with AIDS.* London: Routledge.

Lewis, C. R., de Vedia, A., Reuer, B., Schwan, R., & Tourin, C. (2003). Integrating complementary and alternative medicine (CAM) into standard hospice and palliative care. *American Journal of Hospice and Palliative Medicine, 20,* 221– 228.

Lloyd-Williams, M. (Ed.). (2008). *Psychosocial issues in palliative care.* New York: Oxford University Press, Inc.

Logan, H. (1998). Applied music-evoked-imagery for the oncology patient: Results and case studies of a three month music therapy pilot project. Unpublished manuscript.

Longfield, V. (1995). The effects of music therapy on pain and mood in hospice patients (Unpublished master's thesis). St. Louis University, St Louis, MO.

Magill- Levrault, L. (2009). The meaning of the music: The role of music in palliative care music therapy as perceived by bereaved caregivers of advanced cancer patients. *American Journal of Hospice and Palliative Medicine, 26*(1), 33–39.

Magill-Levrault, L. (1993). Music therapy in pain and symptom management. *Journal of Palliative Care, 9(4),* 42–48.

Maluso-Bolton, T., & Schlecter, B. (2002). Neurological symptoms. In B. M. Kinzbrunner, N. J. Weinreb, & J. S. Policzer (Eds.), *Twenty common problems in end-of-life care* (pp. 187–207). New York: McGraw-Hill, Inc.

Mandel, S. E. (1991). Music therapy in the hospice: "Musicalive." *Palliative Medicine, 5*(2), 155-160.

Marr, J. (1998). GIM at the end-of-life: Case studies in palliative care. *Journal of the Association for Mental Imagery, 6,* 37–54.

Maue-Johnson, E. L., & Tanguay, C. L. (2006). Assessing the unique needs of hospice patients: A tool for music therapists. *Music Therapy Perspectives, 24*(1),13-20.

McKinnis, E. A. (2002). Dyspnea and other respiratory symptoms. In B. M. Kinzbrunner, N. J. Weinreb & J. S. Policzer (Eds.), *Twenty common problems in end-of-life care* (pp. 147–162). New York: McGraw-Hill, Inc.

McKinnon, S. E., & Miller, B. (2002). Psychosocial and spiritual concerns. In B. M. Kinzbrunner, N. J. Weinreb, & J. S. Policzer (Eds.). *Twenty common problems in end-of-life care* (pp. 257–274). New York: McGraw-Hill, Inc.

Merriam-Webster. (2012a). Dyspnea. Retrieved from http://www.merriam-webster.com/dictionary/dyspnea

Merriam-Webster. (2012b). Ascites. Retrieved from http://www.merriam-webster.com/dictionary/ascites

Mitchell, L. A., & MacDonald, R. A. (2006). An experimental investigation of the effects of preferred and relaxing music listening on pain perception. *Journal of Music Therapy, 43*(4), 295–216.

Mount, B., Hanks, G., & McGoldrick, L. (2005). The principles of palliative care. In M. Fallon & G. Hanks (Eds.), *ABC of Palliative Care (2nd ed.)*(pp. 1–3). Malden, MA: Blackwell Publishing Inc.

The Multiple Sclerosis Society of Canada. (2011). What is MS? Retrieved from http://mssociety.ca/en/information/ms_what.htm

Munro, S., & Mount, B. M. (1978). Music therapy in palliative care. *Canadian Medical Association Journal, 119*(9), 1029–1034.

Munro, S. (1984). *Music therapy in palliative/hospice care.* St. Louis, MO: MMB Music, Inc.

Murray, S. A., Kendall, M., Boyd, K., Worth, A., & Benton, T.F. (2004). Exploring the spiritual needs of people dying of lung cancer or heart failure: A prospective qualitative interview study of patients and their carers. *Palliative Medicine, 18*(1), 39–45.

Music-Thanatology Association International. (2008). What is music-thanatology? Retrieved from http://www.mtai.org/index.php/what_is

National Consensus Project for Quality Palliative Care. (2009). What is palliative care? Clinical Practice *Guidelines for Quality Palliative Care (2nd ed.).* Retrieved from http://www.nationalconsensusproject.org

National Hospice and Palliative Care Association. (2009). An explanation of palliative care. Retrieved from http://www.nhpco.org/i4a/pages/index.cfm? pageid=4646&openpage=4646

National Hospice and Palliative Care Organization (NHPCO). (2012*). NHPCO facts and figures: Hospice care in America.* Alexandria, VA: National Hospice and Palliative Care Organization.

National Institute of Neurological Disorders and Stroke. (2011). NINDS spinal cord injury information page. Retrieved from http://www.ninds.nih.gov/disorders/

O'Callaghan, C. (1984). Musical profiles of dying patients. *Australian Music Therapy Association Bulletin, 7*(2), 5-11.

O'Callaghan, C. (1990). Music therapy skills used in song-writing within a palliative care setting. The *Australian Journal of Music Therapy, 1,* 15–22.

O'Callaghan, C. (1994). Songwriting in palliative care(Master's thesis). University of Melbourne, Australia.

O'Callaghan, C. (1996). Pain, music creativity, and music therapy in palliative care. *American Journal of Hospice and Palliative Medicine, 13*(2), 43–49.

O'Callaghan, C. (2004). The contribution of music therapy to palliative medicine. In D. Doyle, G. Hanks, N. J. Cherny, & K. Calman (Eds.), *Oxford textbook of palliative medicine* (pp. 1041–1046). New York: Oxford University Press.

O'Callaghan, C., O'Brien, E., Magill, L., & Ballinger, E. (2009). Resounding attachment: Cancer inpatients' song lyrics for their children in music therapy. *Supportive Care Cancer, 17*(9), 1149–1157.

O'Kelly, J. (2002). Music therapy in palliative care: Current perspectives. *International Journal of Palliative Nursing, 8*(3), 130–136.

Osse, B. H., Vernooij-Dassen, M. J., Schad é, E., & Grol, R. P. (2005). The problems experienced by patients with cancer and their needs for palliative care. *Supportive Care Cancer, 13*(9), 722–732.

Palliative Care Australia. (2008). Palliative and end-of-life care glossary of terms (1st ed.). *Palliative Care Australia.* ISBN: 978-0-9758254-8-8.

Patrick, G. (1999). The effects of vibroacoustic music on symptom reduction: Inducing the relaxation response through good vibrations. *IEEE Engineering in Medicine and Biology, 18*(2), 97–100.

Powell, R. A., Downing, J., Ddungu, H., & Mwangi-Powell, F. N. (2010). Pain history and pain assessment. In A. Kopf & N. B. Patel (Eds.), *Guide to pain management in low-resource settings* (pp. 67–78). Seattle, WA: International Association for the Study of Pain.

Proulx, K., & Jacelon, C. (2004). Dying with dignity: The good patient versus the good death. *American Journal of Hospice and Palliative Care, 21*(2), 116–120.

Rachlis, M. (2006). Presentation to the Local Health Integration Networks (LHIN). Education Session, Toronto, Ontario, April 6, 2006.

Rando, T. (1984). *Grief, dying and death: Clinical interventions for caregivers.* Champaign, IL: Research Press.

Rykov, M. H. (2001). Facing the music: Speculations on the dark side of our moon. *Journal of Palliative Care, 17*(3), 188–192.

Schulberg, C. H. (1981*). The music therapy sourcebook: A collection of activities categorized and analyzed.* New York: Human Sciences Press, Inc.

Schwabe, C. (1987). *Regulative musiktherapie.* Leipzig: VEB Gustav Fischer

Shiel, W. C., & Stoppler, M. C. (2008a). Definition of grief. *Webster's New World Medical Dictionary* (3rd ed.; online). Retrieved from http://www.medterms.com/script/main/art.asp?articlekey=24274

Shiel, W. C., & Stoppler, M. C. (2008b). Definition of anticipatory grief. *Webster's New World Medical Dictionary* (3rd ed.; online). Retrieved from http://www.medterms.com/script/main/art.asp?articlekey=26258

Shiel, W. C., & Stoppler, M. C. (2008c). Definition of unresolved grief. Webster's New World Medical Dictionary (3rd ed.; online). Retrieved from http://www.medterms.com/script/main/art.asp?articlekey=26263

Short, A. (2002). Guided imagery and music (GIM) in medical care. In K. E. Bruscia & D. Grocke (Eds.), *Guided imagery and music: The Bonny method and beyond.* pp. 51–170. Gilsum, NH: Barcelona Publishers.

Skewes, K. (2001). The experience of group music therapy for six bereaved adolescents(Unpublished dissertation). University of Melbourne, Australia.

Smith, J. (2005). *Relaxation, meditation, & mindfulness: A mental health practitioner's guide to new and traditional approaches.* New York, NY: Springer Publishing Company, Inc.

Smith, L., & Stephen, J (n.d.). *Circlework: A Manual for relaxation and support group facilitators.* British Columbia Cancer Agency: PDF retrieved from http://www.cw.bc.ca/library/pdf/CircleWorksManual.pdf.

Standley, J. M. (1992). Clinical applications of music and chemotherapy: The effects of nausea and emesis'. *Music Therapy Perspectives, 10*(1), 27–35.

Statistics Canada. (2004). Population projections for Canada, provinces and territories—2000–2026. Statistics Canada, Catalogue #91-520, p. 124.

Street, A. F., & Kissane, D. W. (2001). Constructions of dignity in end-of-life care. *Journal of Palliative Care, 17*(2), 93–101.

Strömgren, A. S., Goldschmidt, D., Groenvold, M., Petersen, M. A., Jensen, P. T., Pedersen, L., ... Sjogren, P. (2002). Self-assessment in cancer patients referred to palliative care: A study of feasibility and symptom epidemiology. *Cancer, 94*(2), 512–520.

Troesch, L. M., Rodehaver, C. B., Delaney E. A., & Yanes, B. (1993). The influence of guided imagery on chemotherapy-related nausea and vomiting. *Oncology Nurse Forum, 20*(8), 1179–1185.

Ward, K. (2002). A Jungian orientation to the Bonny method. In K. E. Bruscia & D. Grocke (Eds.*), Guided imagery and music: The Bonny method and beyond*, pp. 207–244. Gilsum, NH: Barcelona Publishers.

Watson, M., Lucas, C., Hoy, A., & Back, I. (2005). *Oxford handbook of palliative care.* New York: Oxford University Press.

Weber, S. (1998). Music: A means of comfort. In D. Aldridge (Ed.), *Music therapy in palliative care: New voices* (pp. 95–105). Philadelphia, PA: Jessica Kingsley.

Wedro, B. (2012). Superior vena cava syndrome. Retrieved from http://www.medicinenet.com/superior_vena_cava_syndrome/article.htm

Wheeler, B. L., Shultis, C. L., & Polen, D. W. (2005). *Clinical training guide for the student music therapist.* Gilsum, NH: Barcelona Publishers.

Wigram, T. (1995). The psychological and physiological effects of low frequency sound and music. *Music Therapy Perspectives, 13*(1), 16–23.

Wigram, T. (1997). The effect of VA therapy on multiple handicapped adults with high muscle tone and spasticity. In T. Wigram & C. Dileo (Eds.), *Music vibration and health* (pp. 143–148). Cherry Hill, NJ: Jeffrey Books.

Wigram, T. (2004). *Improvisation: Methods and techniques for music therapy clinicians, educators, and students.* Philadelphia, PA: Jessica Kingsley.

Wigram, T., Pedersen, I. N., & Bonde, L. O. (2002). *A comprehensive guide to music therapy: Theory, clinical practice, research and training.* London: Jessica Kingsley Publishers.

Wlodarczyk, N. (2009). The use of music and poetry in life review with hospice patients. *Journal of Poetry Therapy, 22*(3), 133–139.

World Health Organization. (2011a). WHO definition of palliative care. Retrieved from http://www.who.int/cancer/palliative/definition/en/

World Health Organization. (2011b). Cancer. Retrieved from http://www.who.int/topics/cancer/en/

World Health Organization. (2011c). Cardiovascular diseases. Retrieved from http://www.who.int/topics/cardiovascular_diseases/en/

World Health Organization. (2011d). Chronic respiratory diseases. Retrieved from http://www.who.int/respiratory/en/index.html

World Health Organization. (2011e). HIV/AIDS. Retrieved from http://www.who.int/topics/hiv_aids/en/

Wright, R., & Culverhouse, O. (2011). Palliative care: Themes & songs (Unpublished internship project). University of Windsor, Windsor, Ontario.

Zhang, B., El-Jawahri, A., & Prigerson, H. (2006). Update on bereavement research: Evidence-based guidelines for the diagnosis and treatment of complicated bereavement. *Journal of Palliative Medicine, 9*(5), 1188–1203.

APPENDIX A

Relaxation Techniques

Progressive Relaxation

Bernstein and Borkovec (1973) devised basic procedures of progressive relaxation, which include an introduction, tensing instructions, and additional instruction. The introduction includes explaining the procedures that will occur and recognizing the feelings a patient has at the beginning of the session. Tensing instructions encompass direction on tensing different muscle groups, and additional instructions include the release of tension on cue and light changes. The progressive relaxation method can be accompanied with music to further initiate relaxation.

Progressive muscle relaxation was developed by Jacobson in 1934, and the protocol involved tensing and relaxing 16 muscle groups (Field, 2009). Jacobson's Progressive Muscle Relaxation has been adapted for group and individual use by many psychologists and therapeutic health care workers, but the basic outline remains consistent throughout adaptations. Below is a summary of a standard progressive muscle relaxation session created by Jacobson (1938).

The recommended sequence for the tensing of muscles is as follows: right foot, right lower leg and foot, entire right leg, left foot, left lower leg and foot, entire left leg, right hand, right forearm and hand, entire right arm, left hand, left forearm and hand, entire left arm, abdomen, chest, neck and shoulders, face.

There are two steps: Step 1: Tension, Step 2: Release. Follow the list of muscle groups in the sequence given and work through your entire body, completing Step 1 and Step 2 for each muscle group before moving on the next part of the body.

Step One: Tension.

First, focus your mind on the muscle group. Then inhale and squeeze the muscles as hard as you can for approximately 8 seconds.

Step Two: Releasing the Tension.

After the 8 seconds, quickly and suddenly let go and release the tension. Let all the tightness and pain flow out of the muscles as you simultaneously exhale. Feel the muscles relax and become loose and limp. Focus on and notice the difference between tension and relaxation. Stay relaxed for about 15 seconds, and then repeat the tension-relaxation cycle with the next muscle group.

Structured/Countdown

Structured/countdown is a simple tool to use that can effectively help a client move into a deeper sense of relaxation. Smith (2005) provides an example of a 5-point countdown, although a 10-point can also be used. "5: Let yourself become more relaxed. 4: Let feelings of tension flow away. 3: Notice how you feel as you become increasingly calm. 2: Your entire body becomes relaxed and calm. 1: Enjoy the feelings of relaxation you have created" (p. 255).

In this example, Smith (2005) uses a script combined with counting. A clinician can also use inhalation and exhalation with a countdown, by pairing inhalation and exhalation with each number and increasing the amount of breath inhaled and time spent exhaling. For example:

5: Inhale, exhale; 4: Inhale, exhale; 3: Inhale, exhale; 2: Inhale, exhale; 1: Inhale, exhale, with the clinician increasing the time spent in between each number.

Autogenic-type

Autogenic training involves mentally repeating phrases or images that are associated with somatic relaxation, and specifically reductions in autonomic arousal (Smith, 2005). Smith (2005) outlines a protocol for administering autogenic-type relaxation session:

> Step 1: Select format, provide overall orientation, conduct assessment.
> Step 2: Exercise Rationale. This involves explaining the key idea of the connection between body and mind. There are four main categories of sensation: heaviness, warmth in the extremities, evenly beating heart, and warmth in the abdomen.
> Step 3: Demonstration/Warm-up.
> Step 4: Practice. This involves going through the four main categories of sensations and suggesting to the client key phrases or images that he/she will repeat internally. For example, for heaviness, the client could think the words "Arms and legs, very heavy."
> Steps 5 and 6: Review, Revision, and Special Problems. (pp. 134–136)

Imagery

Imagery relaxation is effective in helping clients release thoughts and stresses that are preventing them from achieving relaxation. Although imagery and relaxation can be used as an entire session, imagery can subsequently be implemented as an induction tool to help clients achieve a deeper level of relaxation. Smith and Steven (n.d.) provide a guide for using imagery with palliative care patients and suggest using images from the client to enhance the client's interests in inducing relaxation. If the client has no images chosen, the authors suggest several possible examples, including sanctuaries, a desert image of peace and expansiveness, the ocean, a calm lake, the tranquil light of the forest, an alpine meadow, tree, cactus, rainbow, stream, eagle, clouds, deer, a storm, wind, a container to hold all of one's worries, balloons set free, leaves drifting on a stream, and debris washed away by waves (pp. 54–55).

I have found light images highly effective in enhancing relaxation techniques. Smith (2005) describes that using a moving spot of light can help the client imagine that tension is melting away. The therapist can also use an image of light to bring energy and health. Moving light can be focused on a client's specific needs, to include sending a light to areas that are more tense or in pain, to help the client feel as though they can stop focusing on the pain and move into a deeper sense of relaxation.

Tension and Release to Cues

Davis, Eshelman, and McKay (2008) state that cue-controlled relaxation involves building an association between a cue (e.g., the command "relax") and muscle relaxation. They list a protocol for cue-controlled relaxation, which is adapted and expanded below:

1) Find a comfortable position. Take a deep breath in and hold it for a moment. Exhale and let your stomach and chest relax.
2) Relax yourself from your forehead all the way to your toes.
3) Continue to breathe deeply and regularly.
4) Repeat these words over and over until all tension is released (pp. 78–80).

The client and/or the therapist can choose cues, such as "breathe in, relax" or "breathe in, breathe out." The words serve as the cues for tension and release. Depending on the time available, the therapist may go through every muscle group (as practiced in progressive muscle relaxation), or the focus may be on the entire body. Cue words allow the client to focus and follow a rhythmic procedure to gain a deeper sense of relaxation.

Meditative Relaxation

The Alternative Medicine Foundation Inc. (2010) maintains that meditation practices are specific to the cultural and/or religious contexts in which they were created. It would be beneficial for the therapist to ask the client whether or not he/she has any cultural or religious meditation practices that he/she would like to use. If not, a general format for meditative relaxation is listed below:

1) Choose a quite spot
2) Sit in a comfortable position
3) Close your eyes
4) Relax your muscles sequentially from head to foot
5) Become aware of your breathing, noticing how the breath goes in and out, without trying to control it in any way.
6) Repeat your focus word silently in time to your breathing
7) Don't worry about how you're doing. Each time you notice that you've drifted into thought, try labeling where you were, for instance, "thinking, thinking" or "anger, anger" or "judging, judging," and then let it go, getting back to the anchor.
8) Practice at least once a day for 10 to 20 minutes. (Borysenko & Rothstein, 1987, pp. 42–45)

For Step 6, the focus word could be a secular or nonsecular word or phrase. Examples could be "one," "om," "peace," or any word that the client feels represents stress release or relaxation.

APPENDIX B

Discussion Points for Songs

Adapted from Palliative Care: Themes and Songs by R. Wright & O. Culverhouse, 2011, Internship Project, pp. 1–5. Adapted and reprinted with permission.

Theme: Change

"Que Sera, Sera"—Doris Day
- What are your thoughts about taking it one day at a time and letting things be, so to speak?
- As a child, did you have dreams of a certain job that you might like or things you wanted to accomplish?
- Do you want to talk about the future today?

"She Will Be Loved"—Maroon 5
- What feels like compromise?
- Which part of you has stayed the same, and which has changed?
- How open are you to change in life?

"Turn, Turn, Turn"—Pete Seeger
- What do you think about the seasons changing?
- What storms have you weathered in your life and how did you get through them?

"Uprising Down Under"—Sam Roberts
- What will live on from you?
- How can you turn stress and sadness into relief and happiness?
- Do you have spiritual sources of strength?

Theme: Christianity

"Amazing Grace"
"Blessed Assurance"
"Blessed Be Your Name"
"Come, Thou Fount
"Go Now in Peace"
"How Great Thou Art"
"Little Light of Mine"
"Lord, I Lift Your Name on High"
"Old Rugged Cross"
- What has your faith meant to you before and during this time?
- What is waiting for you after death?
- Who supports your faith in your life?
- How does your faith help you?
- How can you use your faith during this time?
- Who will you meet after death?

Theme: Family

"Daddy Sang Bass"—Johnny Cash
- What was an activity that brought the family together?
- Did your family all sing together?

- What kinds of songs did you sing and at what occasions?
- What were times like when you were young?

"Family"—Dar Williams

- What does your family mean to you?
- Have they been there during times of celebrations, trouble, or sadness?
- Who are important people in your life?

"I'll Be"—Reba McEntire

- Do you have children, nieces, nephews, or younger siblings?
- How are you a supportive person in your family?
- Who has been there for you in your life?

"Mama"—Spice Girls

- What is your relationship like with your mother?
- Are you a mother/father? If so, what were some moments of joy or sorrow in that role?
- How has your mother/father been there for you in the past, present, and future?

"My Yiddish Mamme"

- What roles did your parents play in raising your family?
- What are some moments that you remember in particular (perhaps family meals or trips)?

"Wind Beneath My Wings"—Bette Midler

- Who is your hero?
- Who has lifted you up and supported you in life?
- When was a troubled time in your life when your family was there for you?
- Have you been a hero to others?

"You Needed Me"—Anne Murray

- Who have you supported in your life?
- How are you a strong friend and family member?
- How do families support one another?

Theme: Home

"Home"—Michael Bublé

- How do you feel
- being far from home?
- Is it difficult meeting so many new people?
- Why do you want to go home?
- Have you done a lot of travel for work or pleasure?

"Homeward Bound"—Simon and Garfunkel

- What makes home special to you?
- Do you get homesick when you travel?
- Who is special at home?

"This Is Home"—Switchfoot

- What are some good memories from home?
- Is home where the heart is?
- What about home makes you feel like you belong and are safe?
- What makes a house a home?

Theme: Hope

"Here Comes the Sun"—Beatles

- Has your illness ever felt like a long winter?
- What do thoughts of spring make you feel like?
- What brings sunshine to your life?

"I Can See Clearly Now"—Johnny Nash

- What have been some obstacles in your life?
- What are some sad days or memories that you can let go of?
- What makes your days bright?

"If We Hold On Together"—Diana Ross

- Who gives you hope?
- What helps our dreams stay alive?
- Is faith, hope, or glory a part of your life story?

"Keep Holding On"—Avril Lavigne

- What do you fight for?
- What do you hold on to?
- Who is always by your side?

"You'll Never Walk Alone"—Carousel

- What storms are you facing in your life?
- What helps you tackle fear?
- What keeps you going forward?
- Who has walked beside you in your life?

Theme: Individuality

"Blowin' in the Wind"—Peter, Paul, and Mary

- What are your views on life?
- What questions do you ask about the world around you?
- What makes you an individual in the world?

"My Way"—Frank Sinatra

- How were you unique in the world?
- What roles, jobs, or tasks did you take on in life?
- What makes your life special?

Theme: Love

"A Moment Like This"—Kelly Clarkson
"Can't Help Fallin' in Love"—Elvis Presley
"Happy Together"—Turtles
"I Got You"—Leona Lewis
"I'll Cover You"—RENT
"I'll Stand By You"—The Pretenders
"I Love You"—Sarah McLaughlin
"I Love You Truly"—Perry Como
"I Will Always Love You"—Dolly Parton
"Let Me Call You Sweetheart"—Bing Crosby
"LOVE"—Frank Sinatra
"Love Me Truly"—Carrie Bond
"Maybe I'm Amazed"—Paul McCartney
"Sentimental Reasons"—Nat King Cole
"Your Song"—Elton John

- Who is the love of your life?

- What have been some important relationships in your life?
- How has the support of loved ones helped you throughout your life?
- What is special about your significant other?
- How have you formed your lives together?
- What is a way to keep your relationship strong through this time?
- How have you changed each other for the better?

Theme: Reminiscence

"In My Life"—Beatles

- What are the most significant places you remember?
- Who has made the most impact in your life?
- What are some affectionate memories?

"It Was a Very Good Year"—Frank Sinatra

- What were the best years of your life?
- How is your life like "vintage wine"?
- What was changing through the years like?

"I Will Remember You"—Sarah McLaughlin

- What will you be remembered for?
- Are there special people or places you remember?
- What were some of the good times in your life?

"Remember When"—Alan Jackson

- What was being young like?
- What were some of the special small moments in your life?
- What goals and dreams did you have when you were younger?

Theme: Strength

"Believe"—Josh Groban

- What are you capable of achieving?
- What helps you believe in your goals?
- What do you believe in?

"Dream On"—Aerosmith

- What are your hopes and dreams?
- What is strong about you?
- Is there anything negative that happened in your life that has made you a stronger person?

"I'm Not Afraid"—Eminem

- What storms have you been facing?
- Who is beside you for help and support?
- Have you ever felt alone in your journey?

"Lean on Me"—Bill Withers

- Who have you leaned on in life?
- Is it hard for you to ask for help?
- Who do you support in life?
- Who has leaned on you?

Chapter 13

Caring for Caregivers

Barbara A. Daveson

Despite the valuable contribution of caregivers, their effort often goes unrecognised. We have yet to establish a clear evidence base regarding how best to support carers. In this chapter, the role of the caregiver is defined and the needs and resources of this group are identified. Clinical applications of the four music therapy methods for this group are examined, and research that has examined the capacity for music therapy interventions to result in change is identified. Future challenges and recommendations are shared in order to help advance the potentiality of music therapy with this important group.

Diagnostic Information

By 2030, approximately three-quarters of all global deaths will be from noncommunicable conditions (World Health Organisation, 2008). Diseases that impact the patient's ability to make decisions for themselves, such as dementia, will result in caregivers becoming more involved in the care of medical patients (Silveira, Kim, & Langa, 2010). The need for surrogate decision-making for the elderly was demonstrated by nationally representative US cohort data from 2000—2006 that showed that 42·5% of individuals aged ≥60 years (N = 3,746) required treatment-related decisions before death; however, the large majority (70%) lacked capacity to make these decisions (Silveira, Kim, & Langa, 2010). One-third of surrogate decision-makers experience often substantial negative emotional consequences that typically last months (or sometimes years) due to making treatment-related decisions (Wendler & Rid, 2011). Research has shown that in the context of serious illness, many patients want family, other relatives, and friends to be involved in making decisions about their medical care (Daveson et al., 2013).

Increased aging populations around the world will place a strain on the financial resources of health care systems nationally and globally. Financial imperatives are expected to continue to drive the need for shorter stays in hospital. This means that caregivers may need to provide more care for patients in their own homes. For example, previously the majority of deaths in England occurred in hospitals (58%) (Department of Health, 2008); however, these trends are beginning to reverse with a recent increase in the proportion and numbers of cancer patients dying in their own home.

People are also living longer and longer with chronic disease, and this means a future strain on long-term care systems around the world. Long-term care systems rely on the contribution of family and friends who provide unpaid care for those with ongoing care needs. It is widely recognised that unpaid caregivers contribute substantially to long-term care. In fact, in many countries the contribution of long-term care from caregivers surpasses the formal contribution of paid workers (Organisation for Economic Cooperation and Development [OECD], 2011b). Altogether, this means that the role of music therapy with caregivers may expand in the future.

Defining caregiver

While many different definitions of caregivers exist, the definition of caregivers used in this chapter is as follows. Carers, who may or may not be family members, are lay people in a close supportive role who share in the illness experience of the patient and who undertake vital care work and emotion management (National Institute for Clinical Excellence [NICE], 2004). Family is defined broadly and includes relationships formed in many different ways due to various reasons. Family may include, for example, same- or different-sex relationships, and relationships formed through biology, adoption, or cohabitation. Friends, neighbours, and relatives may be caregivers, and older couples often may be codependent carers.

Caregivers usually provide assistance to individuals who experience difficulties with activities of their daily living due to physical, cognitive, psychological, or emotional impairments. Caregivers usually go unpaid for the work they contribute, although family caregivers and/or the patient sometimes institute informal payment arrangements.

In the literature, caregivers are referred to in many different ways. For example, the following terms have been used: informal carers, unpaid carers, and caregivers. It is good practice to ask each individual how they wish to be referred to, as individuals have particular preferences. For example, some may not like the term "informal carer," as they may feel it detracts from their contribution.

Identifying caregivers

Identifying the demographic characteristics of caregivers is difficult. Demographic data that helps us to identify caregivers within the different fields of medicine, for example, palliative care or rehabilitation, are not widely available. Local service-provider and population-based data may be useful sources of data for therapists working with caregivers. For example, in the first instance, identifying the number of primary carers of patients in any one service will help. An assessment of the patient's social support network may also be useful to help with identifying caregivers at an individual level. Sociograms may help depict and identify the relationships that patients have with their caregivers and the relationships that caregivers have with others in their broader support network.

Many carers may not define themselves as a caregiver even though they are providing unpaid care to the patient. The assumption of a caregiver role may be influenced by various factors, including culture, the availability or lack of another caregiver in the patient's support network, gender roles, and the availability of financial resources to support the taking on of this role. For example, the Fair Work Act in Australia indicates that employees are entitled to 10 days of paid personal/carer leave each year in order to take care of a person in their immediate family or household (Office of Legislative Drafting and Publishing, 2011). This entitlement may help individuals with taking on the role of caregiver. However, for others, taking on the role on the role of a caregiver may be more of a natural phase within their own life (Payne et al., 2010).

Diversity acknowledged, we do know that on average women spend more time providing care than men (OECD, 2012). Also, caregivers are older in age in many developed countries (Payne et al., 2010). Research has shown that long-term care is associated with age. In many countries, one in five long-term care users is greater than 65 years, while around half of all users are over 80 years old (OECD, 2011a).

How much time do we spend caring?

Data from time-use surveys help us to understand the profile of different caregivers. Time-use surveys require people to record information on how they spend their time on different activities. This is usually done through the use of a diary for a defined time period (e.g., for a number of consecutive days). Even though useful, time-use surveys generally do not separate the time spent caring for children and time spent caring for an adult, for example, an elderly mother or father, or an unwell partner. An exception to this is in Korea, where data regarding time spent caring for a parent, spouse, or other family member is available. It is best to ask the caregiver to estimate the amount of time they spend providing care. Estimations from individual caregivers will help understand the impact that caring has on their own opportunities, for example, on their leisure and employment opportunities. A study in music therapy reported that the caregivers involved in the study spent an average of two to nine hours per day or two to five hours per day providing care (Choi, 2010). This report is notably higher than population-based data. It may provide a useful example of the realities involved in providing care for someone in the hospital.

Three more reasons for providing care

Providing care to caregivers is important due to at least three reasons. First, caregiver health is important, as without caregivers, the care of the person they are caring for may become compromised. Second, caregivers' health is important in and of its own right. Everyone is entitled to good health and well-being. Third, caregivers have increased health risks due to their caring role. A meta-analysis (analysis of findings from many studies combined) showed that caregivers may be at increased risk of psychiatric difficulties and financial hardship (OECD, 2011a). In essence, caregivers have a unique role, as they both provide and require care (Northouse & Peters-Golden, 1993).

The pros and cons of caring

Over the last 30 years, research into caregivers has been underpinned by the assumption that taking on the role of a caregiver has a detrimental effect on the caregiver's health. Although there are many reports of negative consequences of taking on this role, the impact of providing care isn't always negative. Positive benefits of providing care are beginning to emerge, including reports of feelings of competence, kinship, and importance (Cohen, Colantonio, & Vernich, 2002; Kramer, 2012). Also, research is beginning to examine the complexities involved in caring. For example, data show that caregivers who report higher levels of benefit are more likely to report more depression and grief (Boerner, Schulz, & Horowitz, 2004; Kramer, 2012).

Music therapists will encounter caregivers in every field of medicine in which they work. Cross-cutting themes of caregiver experience may be evidenced across fields of medicine. This may include caregiver burden. Burden includes feelings of embarrassment, feeling overloaded, and feeling trapped, isolated, or resentful (Zarit, Reever, & Bach-Peterson, 1980). Burden associated with caregiving may also include feelings of being out of control or losing control, experiences of poor communication (Morris, Morris, & Britton, 1998), and increased work pressures (Stephens, Kinney, & Ogrocki, 1991). Keeping in mind the pros and cons involved with caregiving may help assess the needs and resources of caregivers.

Needs and Resources

Three factors should be considered when assessing the needs and resources of caregivers. First, identify the symptomatology and disease/illness trajectory of the person receiving care from the caregiver. Identifying symptoms and trajectories helps us to understand caregivers' experiences and the duration of these experiences. For example, the majority of caregivers of persons with dementia will be subjected to physical and psychosocial demands for three to 15 years, including anger, paranoia, and agitation from the person receiving their care. Caregivers will most probably compensate for the loss of function of the person in their care over this period of time. They will also be mindful of the cognitive deterioration of the person they care for (Vitaliano & Zhang, 2003).

Second, consider the impact of chronic stressors associated with illness. Third, investigate the personal qualities and resources that may buffer caregivers from any potential negative consequences of providing care, such as marital (partner) status, financial hardship, and social support.

In summary, the needs and resources of caregivers are complex, and these needs are best understood through an assessment of the individual's response and their circumstance alongside an understanding of caregiver research findings in general and also in relation to the therapist's field of practice. An appreciation of chronic stress literature and pathways to illness will help. Early identification of needs and strengths is critical to good quality and timely care.

Guidelines for Music Therapy

There is wide acknowledgement within the literature that caregivers have their own needs. These needs are diverse and are related to informal support, financial challenges, anxiety, information, and isolation. The application of music therapy with caregivers is a neglected area of clinical work and research (Brown, Götell, & Ekman, 2001); nonetheless, good examples of music therapy practice and research are available, and it is widely accepted by music therapists that music therapy can help caregivers.

The recommendations provided in this section are based on the author's clinical experience from work with carers in medical settings and findings from a systematic review of the literature that identified 11 articles regarding music therapy for carers. The review was conducted in June 2012. The databases searched were the International Index for Music Periodical (IIMP) (full text), the Nordic Journal of Music Therapy (NJMT) website, and the ScienceDirect database for articles published within *The Arts in Psychotherapy* journal. This transparent method of identifying the research identified a number of resources relevant to the topic of caregivers and music therapy.

Overview of Music Therapy Methods

The following methods and procedures have not been sequenced to reflect relative significance, effectiveness, or complexity.

Receptive Music Therapy

- Music Listening for Relaxation and Other Tasks: Carers listen to music to relax or to evoke images, and discuss the experience.
- Music Listening, Verbal Processing, and Intimate Sharing: Carers listen to (and/or accompany) songs sung by the therapist and discuss their thoughts and feelings.
- Music Legacies: Carers create music videos or other music collages for later listening, usually after the death of the patient.

Improvisational Music Therapy

- Carers improvise music, either based on something other than the music itself, for example, a story, a picture, or an event, or without referring to anything except the improvisation itself.

Re-creative Music Therapy

- Carers engage in musical tasks that require them to reproduce music in some way. This may include participating in a sing-along, rehearsing music, music lessons, and music performance.

Compositional Music Therapy

- Carers write their own music with the therapist's assistance, with the idea of repeating that music at another point in time.

Guidelines for Receptive Methods

When receptive methods are used, the caregiver is engaged primarily in music listening experiences. In the literature, there are many examples of receptive methods being used with caregivers. This includes music listening by itself or listening coupled with one or several elements. Music therapists have coupled music listening with: (1) progressive muscle relaxation (PMR) (Choi, 2010) and PMR with positive visual imagery, gentle exercise, discussion, images, or artistic media (Hanser, Butterfield-Whitcomb, Kawata, & Collins, 2011); (2) verbal processing and intimate sharing (Hinman, 2010); (3) reminiscence (Zabin, 2005); and (4) the creation of music legacy videos (Cadrin, 2006) or other types of outputs or products (Baxter & O'Callaghan, 2010) that are listened to at a later point in time by the caregiver, usually after the death of the patient.

The review procedure used to inform the writing of this chapter didn't identify much information about guided imagery and music (GIM) with caregivers, except for Cadrin's work focused on the creation of legacies with those at the end of life. This may be because literature about GIM is mostly published elsewhere (for example, in books on guided imagery and music-specific journals), or it may have been that there were no GIM articles that focused specifically on caregivers within the parameters of the search that was completed. Regardless, GIM is another method that could be used with caregivers, but it is not extensively addressed here. Nevertheless, there are many methods described in this chapter that are similar to Bonny's guided imagery and music method. The caregivers identified in the search as being involved in receptive music therapy sessions included spouses/partners, mothers of adult patients, siblings of adult patients, and adult children of adult patients (Chaput & Silverman, 2012; Choi, 2010; Thorgrimsen, Schweitzer, & Orrell, 2002).

Length of session and programmes

The literature shows that music therapy sessions that involve receptive methods vary in length and programme duration. The briefest description of a music therapy intervention for a research study to date is one single dose of 20 minutes of music listening. A second study involved comparatively similar session lengths of 30-minute sessions. However, four sessions were administered over a two-week period in this program (Choi, 2010). An example of a longer programme involved listening to an individualised CD three days a week after an initial two-hour training session (facilitated by the therapist with the caregiver). After the training, the caregiver determined the number of sessions to implement. This ranged from a target of eight to 20 sessions (Hanser, Butterfield-Whitcomb, Kawata, & Collins, 2011).

As with most fields of music therapy, in medicine the length of the session and programme duration is mostly based on what's feasible (e.g., only one session may be able to be conducted before the patient is discharged) and the goals to be addressed by the intervention. The literature mostly shows that music therapy programmes with caregivers are short-term in nature. However, there are exceptions to this. For example, within rehabilitation contexts, carers may participate in music therapy sessions over a much longer period of time. This may especially be the case when a long period of patient rehabilitation is required. In these scenarios, the duration of the programme with carers may continue over a span of months and sometimes years. In contrast, a predefined number of sessions may be offered when working with bereaved carers, and the program that is offered may be agreed upon in advance. For example, one session may focus on the use of music and imagery for relaxation, while another session may rely on music listening and PMR for tension release. In essence, the needs of the carer should determine the length of the program.

Music Listening for Relaxation and Other Tasks

Overview. The literature contains two good examples of using music listening with caregivers. The intervention described by Choi (2010) involved music listening combined with progressive music relaxation (PMR). Hanser et al., (2011) described the use of music listening, including at times PMR, with positive visual imagery, gentle exercise, discussion, images, or artistic media Choi used prerecorded music. Hanser and colleagues burned the music and instructions onto a CD for use with patients diagnosed with dementia and their caregiver/s.

Preparation. Choi highlighted some of the items that need to be prepared or organised before a music listening and PMR session. These included:

- Find a quiet room that is free from distractions so that the session can be conducted without distraction/s. If a quiet room isn't available, then a quiet area may need to be used.
- Select the music to be used with the participant. To this end, before the session, meet with the caregiver (and patient, if relevant) in order to determine their musical preferences. Based on this information, compile a music programme.
- When compiling the programme, assess the different musical components in the recordings that will be used, including the music's timbre, rhythm, tempo, melody, and instrumentation. Pelletier's meta-analysis showed that instrumental music, music with slower tempo and low pitch, and music that is predictable help with relieving stress. Music without lyrics was shown to be more useful in reducing stress (Pelletier, 2004).
- An audio-player also needs to be organized for the session. For example, you may arrange for a CD player to be used, or you may stream your music from another source.
- If you are unfamiliar with facilitating a relaxation induction, it may also be useful to prepare a relaxation script beforehand.

In addition, when working in a hospital environment, it is sometimes helpful to prepare a "do not disturb" sign to put on the door of the room where the session will take place. If you are facilitating the session in a shared cubicle in a hospital room, you can also draw the curtains around the patient's bedside so that the caregiver and patient can participate in the session in a private manner. The "do not disturb" sign can be placed on the drawn curtains, just like you would place it on a closed door.

Preparation. Both Choi and Hanser and colleagues provided information about the procedures involved in the sessions. Choi (2010) helpfully outlined the following procedures:

1) Explain the purpose of the method to the participant(s) and invite them (the caregiver and the patient) to participate in the music listening experience.

2) Invite them to make themselves comfortable. They may wish to lie down on a mat or sit in a comfortable chair or sofa.
3) Begin going through the relaxation induction with the participant(s).
4) Introduce the music after or at the same time as the PMR induction.
5) Close the session and reorient the participant(s) back to their surroundings.
6) Explore the participant's feelings, responses, and thoughts and support them in sharing their responses.

Hanser (2011) and colleagues also published a protocol for use with patients and caregivers living with dementia. She developed eight different music listening protocols to be used in different sessions. For example, you may use protocol number two in one session and protocol number three in another session. These protocols may be used with many different types of caregivers and patients. Admittedly, some of these protocols don't rely solely on music listening.

1) The caregiver and patient to listen to the caregiver's musical selection. This is followed by discussion of associated memories and feelings.
2) The caregiver and patient listen to either the patient's musical selection or the caregiver's piece that has been chosen for the patient. This is to be followed by discussion about the piece.
3) The caregiver and patient do some gentle exercise and gentle movement to music.
4) The caregiver and patient complete a PMR induction. This is then followed by the use of imagery.
5) The caregiver and the patient draw while listening to music. They then discuss the images that have been drawn. A variation on this is for the caregiver and patient to share and discuss the images that are evoked by the music listening.
6) The caregiver and patient listen to music that is not familiar to them or music that is not well-known to them. They freely share the words that enter their mind while listening to the music.
7) The caregiver and patient use the music they are listening to as an accompaniment. They sing, improvise, or play instruments while listening to the music.
8) The caregiver and patient use music listening to achieve certain outcomes. For example, they use music listening to help them sleep or relax, or they use music listening to distract them.

What to observe. Throughout the session, observe for changes in the person's bodily tension, observe for changes in their respiratory rate, and observe any changes in their presentation that may suggest they are relaxing. The researchers who have investigated interventions used a number of measurement scales to help determine the effect of the intervention. Evaluating the outcome of your session may be of benefit to the caregiver and patient.

Both Choi and Hanser and colleagues used visual analogue scales (VASs) along with a number of other measures. A VAS is usually a straight line of 100 millimetres in length. On each end of the line, the extreme response is located. For example, at one end, a response of relaxation may be identified. At the opposite end, a response of not relaxed may be placed. The participant(s) are usually asked by the therapist to rate their response on the VAS. Alternatively, the participants use these scales independent of a therapist.

When determining what to observe within a session, it is also useful to consider what outcome measure you will use to help work out whether your intervention had the desired outcome. When selecting which outcome measure to use, it's important to look at both the psychometric properties of the scale and the clinimetric properties. The psychometric properties help work out whether the measure is valid and reliable. The clinimetric properties help work out whether the tool is suitable for use with the participants with whom you are working (Bausewein, Daveson, Benalia, Simon, & Higginson, 2012).

Adaptations. These protocols can be adapted in many different ways. The work by Hanser and colleagues illustrates some of the different variations that are possible. In essence, the adaptations should be based around the needs of the caregiver and their patient and the aims of the session. Some of the possible variations include using live music instead of recorded music. The ways that imagery is combined with the PMR induction could also be varied, and there is scope to vary the amount of time you may devote to the induction as compared to the reflection component of the session.

Music Listening, Verbal Processing, and Intimate Sharing

Overview. Hinman's work (2010) provides a good illustrative example of verbal processing and intimate sharing facilitated through music listening (and sometimes active music participation). Hinman (2010) described her intervention as primarily influenced by music psychotherapeutic, psychodynamic, and humanist approaches. It involves sessions that enable openness, intimacy, connections, and interactions between couples, despite being located within a medical environment.

Preparation. Within the sessions, Hinman (2010) used both prepared music and improvisation. This means that preparation for the session may involve learning songs and instrumental pieces in order to reproduce them within the sessions. It might also involve working out with the couple when the best time to visit might be. This will ensure participation of all partners. In some medical settings, a referral may also be required before the patient (and or couple can be seen).

What to observe. Observations for the therapist to attend to within the sessions include attending to the couples' behaviours (including within the music) and their physical responses, such as observing gestures of intimacy and warmth between the couple. This might involve, for example, one or both partners moving closer toward each other, hand-holding, and other gestures of intimacy. The level of emotionality may also be observed, the content that is shared, and the ways in which the couples are able to attend to both of their needs and their needs as a couple. Changes over time should be noted. For example, as the programme continues, the therapist might assess whether the partners are able to share their feelings and gestures of intimacy more frequently within the hospital environment.

Procedures. The procedures outlined by Hinman illustrate how to facilitate the session:

1) Start the session with a welcome, including a verbal and musical greeting.
2) Offer a variety of instruments for the couple to choose from to use in the session.
3) Explore their musical preferences. Ask them what their favorite songs and types of music are.
4) Start engaging the couple in active music-making or alternatively sing a song for them to listen to.
5) Invite the sharing of thoughts and feelings in response to the music. Explore the significance of the music to them.
6) Invite the couple to select music to play and/or listen to. Consider inviting them to improvise together.
7) Continue to work with the couple in an iterative manner.

Adaptations. Hinman (2010) described her intervention as primarily influenced by music psychotherapeutic, psychodynamic, and humanist approaches. This procedure can therefore be adapted in line with other models. Also, the use of alternating musical offerings could be incorporated into the session in order to increase awareness and expression of the needs of each individual within the partnership. For example, one partner may choose a piece of music for both partners to listen to. This may be followed by the second partner selecting the next piece of music for both of them to listen to. Admittedly, in some cultures, more than two partners may be present with the session. Hinman illustrated primarily the use of live music within sessions. Prerecorded music could also be integrated into the session. Also, the couple could be invited to use imagery together, they could draw while listening to the music to help externalize and portray their feelings, and they could collage together to help explore their feelings of intimacy and connectedness.

Music Listening and Reminiscence

Overview. Zabin (2005) described her intervention as making a connection through music with the patient through using the therapist's capabilities such as their own heart, their mind, and their physicality in order to help with loss and frustration.

Preparation. As the intervention relies on both improvisation and reproducing familiar songs, the therapist must have well-developed improvisatory skills and a large repertoire of music from which to draw during the session.

What to observe. Zabin (2005) described that she would very carefully observe the patient's expression during the session. Even though caregivers may be present in the room, her observations would mainly be focused on the patient. Zabin would also observe her own internal responses throughout the session. Zabin would access the ways that she was connecting with the patient in order to help shape the music and interactions.

Procedures. Zabin highlighted the following procedures involved with facilitating music listening and reminiscence sessions:

1) Ask if the patient would like to have some music. If the patient doesn't respond, ask the caregiver whether they think the patient would like to have some music.
2) Ask what instrument they would like the music to be played on.
3) Explore the patient's musical biography. Explore their musical history, their musical preferences, their feelings toward and about music, the memories that they have with certain pieces of music, and their associations with certain pieces.
4) Assess the patient's cognitive, psychological, and emotional state.
5) Convey this state back to the patient and caregiver through the music that is played.
6) Ask for them to immediately share any negative responses that they may have in response to the music.
7) Observe the patient for their expressions to the music and invite the patients and, if the patient is unable to communicate, invite their caregivers to share their responses verbally.
8) Promote the expression of their thoughts and feelings. This might be aided through sharing your own reflections about the music.
9) Bring the music to a close.
10) Ask whether the patient or their caregivers require anything else and attend to these needs where possible.

Adaptations. This intervention can be adapted in many different ways. Indeed, Zabin provides many examples of how she varies this protocol. Zabin shared a case study where only one piece of music was administered during the session. For example, the piece of music was sung quietly and the melody was hummed over and over throughout the session. Alternatively, the music in the session may be themed. For example, the music that is played might be Christian music only. Many different Christian songs may be played in the session to enhance someone's Christian identity. Zabin also highlighted that the intervention might involve more discussion about feelings and responses in the now, and not as much focus on reminiscence. Also, Zabin highlighted that rather than administering a live session, a tape may be made by the therapist for the patient to use by themselves. The structure used on the tape may follow the outline of a session.

Music Legacies

Overview. A music legacy involves the creation of music videos (Cadrin, 2006) or other types of outputs or products (Baxter & O'Callaghan, 2010) that are listened to at a later point in time by the caregiver, usually after the death of the patient. A modified version of Guided Imagery and Music (GIM) was administered by Cadrin in order to produce a music legacy for the patient. After the death of the patient, the partner listened to (or experienced) the patient-created legacy; in this respect, the method was a receptive one for the caregiver. Cadrin defined legacy work as a creative process that involves documenting the patient's life with the purpose of leaving the legacy behind for others after they have died.

Preparation. For Cadrin, the preparation for the caregiver's listening experience involved the facilitation of a GIM session (or modified version of GIM). The session varied from a traditional GIM session, as the idea of a legacy was also introduced to the patient.

What to observe. Currently, there is limited work regarding the observations of caregivers' responses to legacy work. There are some reports of increased emotional expression during the use of legacy material at patients' funerals.

Procedures. The procedures used in Cadrin's example were:

1) Introduce the concept of legacy to the patient.
2) With the patient, combine the transcripts of the GIM sessions, including other relevant components. This may include combining the transcripts with life affirmations, life stories, and special insights.
3) The patient provides permission for the sharing of this legacy.
4) The therapist shares the legacy with the caregiver upon the death of the patient.

Adaptations. In addition to Cadrin's work, the work shared by Baxter and O'Callaghan (2010) highlights the complexities involved in facilitating the steps of legacy creation with the patient. They provide an extensive discussion of some of the considerations that require attention, along with some of the preparation that is required before the session. These include, for example, considering the organisational procedures involved in gaining informed consent for the use of the materials after the death of the patient and understanding the legal requirements for the management of the legacy after the patient's death. Baxter and O'Callaghan also highlight the varied ways that legacy materials can be used with caregivers. For example, in their article, one patient did not want the legacy shared with a family member while they were alive but they were happy for the material to be shared with them after their death. Another patient was willing for the legacy to be shared with others while they were still alive.

GUIDELINES FOR IMPROVISATIONAL MUSIC THERAPY

The improvisatory method can be used in hospital, hospice, and specialist inpatient/outpatient environments, ideally within a private room to ensure confidentiality.

Improvisation

Overview. Referential improvisation is improvisation that is based on something other than the music itself, for example, a story, a picture, or an event. Nonreferential improvisation is improvisation that refers to nothing else except for the improvisation itself. Four examples, based on my clinical and research experience, are suggested here. This information is shared from my own clinical experience as the search that was used to inform this chapter did not reveal any research that investigated the use of music therapy with caregivers. Nevertheless, it is acknowledged that many therapists most probably use referential and nonreferential improvisation with caregivers in order to help them cope with the hospitalisation of the patient; express feelings around the patient's illness and to aid their coping; enhance their relationship with the patient; release tension; improve relaxation; and decrease frustration associated with the patient's illness and their care.

Preparation. The preparation for this method involves the consideration of the needs of the caregiver in order to determine what the caregiver may wish to improvise about. For example, are they engaging in risky behaviours due to the stress associated with providing long-term care to the patient? Are they emotionally depleted due to neglecting their own needs due to the high-care needs of the patient? An assessment of their needs may provide clues as to what themes might be useful during the session. The selection and preparation of instruments is also required before the session. Plus, if the session is to be audio-recorded, then equipment for this task needs to be prepared. Some therapists prepare different themes to be used with the caregiver. This can be presented to caregivers in a number of different ways. For example, the themes can be written down on pieces of paper and presented as options to the caregiver. They can all be laid out on a table in front of the caregiver, and they can choose the theme that stands out to them. There are many different creative options that the therapist may consider in order to prepare for improvisatory sessions. Several procedures will be presented below for various situations.

Procedures for exploring caregiver's experiences during hospitalization are:

1) Ask the caregiver to improvise music about some aspect relating to their experiences of hospitalisation. For example, they may wish to improvise on the pressures of balancing their own personal needs while continuing to provide support to the patient in hospital. They may wish to improvise on the theme of lost opportunities that result from prolonged periods of hospitalization.
2) After the improvisation, invite the caregiver to verbally describe their improvisatory experience.
3) Invite the caregiver to share how their improvisation expresses some of their feelings related to hospitalisation.
4) Invite the caregiver to identify the coping strategies that they use to cope with the hospitalisation of the person they care for.
5) During the discussion, assist the caregiver in identifying useful coping strategies and help them to identify what might need to change and what can be improved upon in order to cope with the patient's hospitalisation.

Procedures for expression of feelings concerning illness and to aid with coping are:

1) Ask the caregiver to bring in an object that symbolises their current experience of the patient's illness and or their experience of the patient's illness.
2) Ask the caregiver to illustrate this symbol/experience through improvisation.
3) After the improvisation has finished, invite the carer to express how the improvisation felt to them.
4) Invite them to describe their experience of the improvisation and/or their feelings and thoughts about the illness that they had before, during, or after the improvisation.
5) Use this discussion and improvisation to allow for self-expression about the illness and help them to identify strategies and resources to cope.

Procedures for enhancing relationships are:

1) Introduce the idea of improvisation to the carer and patient.
2) Outline the potential benefits of music therapy improvisation.
3) Invite the caregiver to improvise a musical message to the patient and then explore the interpretation/intent of this message with the caregiver and patient.
4) Invite the carer and patient to reflect on other shared and enjoyable experiences that have taken place outside of the hospital environment that also involved music. Use these offerings to facilitate additional improvisations.

Procedures for tension and frustration release and relaxation are:

1) Share information about the potential effects of improvisation to allow for increased relaxation and reduction of tension and frustration.
2) Provide the caregiver with a selection of instruments on which to improvise, including vocal improvisation.
3) Engage the carer in improvisation for a specified amount of time or an unspecified amount of time.
4) Encourage the caregiver to use this experience to help release their tension, relax, and lessen feelings of frustration.

Guidelines for Re-creative Music Therapy

Overview. The re-creative method involves engaging the caregiver in musical tasks that require the caregiver to reproduce music in some way. This may include participating in a sing-along, rehearsing music, music lessons, and music performance. Within the literature reviewed for this chapter, there were fewer examples of the re-creative method being used with carers as compared to the other three methods. Nevertheless, re-creative methods can be used with carers to address items related to coping and mood. For example, uncertainty is often experienced by both patients and carers. Uncertainty may be experienced in relation to the prognosis of the patient, the course of treatment involved, options for care that may or may not be involved, and financial uncertainty due to medical bills. These concerns in turn may challenge pre-existing repertoires of coping strategies and may impact negatively on mood. Music-based assisted counseling can be used to discuss these items in order to equip carers with adaptive coping strategies and explore mood-based items. These sessions can be run with other members of the multidisciplinary team, such as pastoral care workers, psychologists, counselors, and social workers. This work can be facilitated via group or individual sessions.

Procedures. The procedures used for re-creative methods with caregivers are similar those already specified in this chapter. In particular, see the procedures outlined by Hinman and protocol seven identified by Hanser and colleagues. In addition, Zabin's procedures can be used with patients for re-creative purposes. This would involve modifying step five outlined in the Zabin example to include active music-making by the caregiver.

Adaptations. Adaptations of this method are plentiful. Different instruments can be used in the sessions. Different themes can be used in the sessions. For example, songs from a certain period of the caregiver's life can be re-created. Alternatively, the songs that symbolize a certain aspect of their relationship with the patient can be re-created.

Guidelines for Compositional Music Therapy

Overview. The compositional music therapy method involves engaging the caregiver in the writing of new music with the idea of repeating that music at another point in time. The process of composition may last for the duration of one session. Alternatively, the caregiver may be engaged in composing music over an entire music therapy programme that spans several sessions. Three examples of the creative or compositional method are available within the music therapy literature (Baxter & O'Callaghan, 2010; Cadrin, 2006; Hinman, 2010). These examples involved spousal/partner caregivers and/or the involvement of extended family, occasionally involving many generations. One of the papers demonstrated the role of the compositional method to assist with self-expression and processing of information related to an acute event. In this paper, the blues form was provided by the therapist to allow the patient and wife to engage in a songwriting process about a sudden admission to hospital that resulted from a ruptured gall bladder. The songwriting process allowed for different views about the event to be shared (Hinman, 2010).

Procedures. The procedures used in the Hinman example were as follows:

1) Engage the patient and the caregiver in the re-creative method (e.g., playing familiar songs). The suggestion of writing a song is then introduced into the session. This suggestion may be volunteered by the patient, for example. If it is volunteered by the caregiver or patient, then affirm their suggestion and begin to engage them in the process of songwriting.
2) Ask them what type of song they would like to write. Establish a theme for the song if appropriate.
3) Explore what role the patient and the caregiver might take in the songwriting process or allow these roles to emerge organically.
4) Provide musical expertise to assist the patient and caregiver in the compositional process.
5) Provide structure for the compositional process.
6) Record the composition and provide assistance for this to happen.

Adaptations. Other authors have written about the use of songwriting by patients and/or carers and the subsequent audio- and video-recording of these products. The benefits of songs being used by caregivers after a patient's death have been identified, including aiding with bereavement and the maintenance and sustenance of bonds with the deceased (Baxter & O'Callaghan, 2010). Songwriting (Hinman, 2010), the creation of journals emerging from Guided Imagery and Music sessions, and legacy videos have also been used with caregivers (Cadrin, 2006). This work is facilitated before the patient's death, both before and after their death, or after their death only. The sessions can be conducted with the patient and spouse/partner alone, with many family members (or caregivers) with the patient, or with the caregiver alone.

Selecting the Music for Use with Caregivers and Patients

A special consideration when working with both caregivers and patients at the same time is: Who will direct the session and who will choose the music? Within some of these examples, the patients selected the music. In other examples, the music was selected based on the caregiver's musical preferences and biography. The process of selecting music for use with caregivers is similar to selecting music with other types of participants, such as patients. However, as caregivers are sometimes seen with the patient, the music used is occasionally patient-preferred music, rather than based on the caregivers' preferences. This is illustrated in one study that involved the use of patient-preferred live music administered to both patients and caregivers in one joint session (Chaput & Silverman, 2012). This means that there is an additional level of complexity involved when selecting which music to use when both carers and patients are involved in the same session. Music selection should be approached carefully. Even though the caregiver and patient may have shared some significant moment in their life that involved a certain piece of music, the caregiver and patient may have different associations and emotional responses to that same piece of music. Therefore, if the caregiver is involved in the sessions, then the therapist may need to establish the needs of the caregiver and ensure their access to care to enable their support alongside supporting the patient.

Research Evidence

A systematic review conducted by the author before writing this chapter identified 11 articles regarding music therapy research with carers. Systematic reviews aim to identify, evaluate, and summarise the findings of all existing evidence in order to inform clinical practice, research, and the commissioning of services. The 11 articles that were identified included five research studies and six articles that detailed aspects of music therapy clinical work shared here in this chapter. All of these articles have been referred to within the methods section. There is scope to further the research into music therapy for carers through both quantitative and qualitative research. Qualitative research could be used to further our understanding of music therapy for carers. For example, what experiences are perceived as helpful for caregivers when supporting an adult receiving medical care? In terms of quantitative research, a study to evaluate the use of improvisation to increase energy levels among carers caring for people with advanced cancer could be completed. Plus, a sufficiently powered trial to examine the effectiveness of interventions with caregivers may help to refine how we work with caregivers and the interventions that we use.

Contraindications

At the time of the writing of this chapter, only one contraindication written about music therapy for caregivers was found. This involved the scenario of conflicting needs between the patient and caregiver. The example identified involved the clinical scenario where the patient wanted to express their feelings about the seriousness of their condition but the caregiver preferred this not to be spoken about (Hinman, 2010). As the role of music therapy for caregivers grows, the balance between attending to patients' and caregivers' needs may benefit from further discussion and attention.

ADDITIONAL CONSIDERATIONS

Based on my clinical experience, seven additional considerations are worthy of attention in relation to music therapy for caregivers. They are:

1) Consider the musical preferences of both the patient and their caregiver/s. Caregivers are sometimes seen with patients in sessions, and sometimes they are seen without the patient present. If the caregiver and patient are seen at the same time, then the integration of the caregivers' musical preferences needs to be considered alongside the patient's preferences.
2) Negotiate the duty of care with the patient and their caregiver/s. When commencing a music therapy programme, the patient may have an expectation that the therapist will work with them and help to address their need/s. However, caregivers may not hold this expectation. They may hold the expectation that the therapist will prioritize and address the patient's needs. It is helpful for the therapist to discuss the role, application, and benefit of music therapy with both the patient and caregiver/s. These discussions will help the therapist determine whether or not to open a duty of care for the caregiver. Discussion about this also provides the caregiver with the opportunity to say whether or not they wish to be a recipient of music therapy.
3) Establish a separate clinical record for the caregiver/s. Within hospital settings, patient records often include information about encounters with carers; however, detailed notes of interventions with caregivers are not typically kept within the patient's record. If a duty of care is opened for a caregiver, then a separate clinical record may need to be developed and maintained.
4) Negotiate boundaries between patient and caregiver sessions early on—respect the wishes of both the patient and the caregiver and plan for different scenarios. When working with caregivers, it is not uncommon for them to inquire about the work that the therapist is completing with the patient. A discussion early-on regarding what information can be shared between the patient and carer will assist with responding to questions that may emerge during treatment. Discussing this will ensure that both the patient's and caregiver's wishes are respected. It may be useful to discuss different scenarios with the patient, as they may hold different preferences for what can be shared before their death and after their death, or in scenarios where they have lost mental capacity or competence.
5) Schedule caregiver sessions around their availability and the patient's schedule of care. Caring for patients is potentially time-consuming and labor-intensive. Caregivers are committed to providing care for patients, and they sometimes prioritize the needs of the patient over their own needs. Scheduling clinical sessions and research activity around the patient's priorities and schedules may therefore help caregivers with attending sessions.
6) Measure the outcomes of your interventions. The use of measures that are able to detect the minimal clinically important difference is needed in our field. Using good measures will help us to improve our practice and establish data to clarify the role of music therapy in medicine. The challenge of evaluating music therapy with patients is clear. We have a similar challenge in identifying fit-for-purpose measures for our work with caregivers.

7) Remember to acknowledge the benefits of caregiving. Caregivers don't often view the role of providing care to a loved one as burdensome. Providing care to a loved one is sometimes viewed as a way of acknowledging their special relationship with the patient. The consequences of providing care to a patient are not always negative. Literature is starting to show that caregivers may experience increased feelings of altruism and kinship as a result of providing care. Therapists should acknowledge these benefits alongside acknowledging the negatives.

THE FUTURE ROLE OF MUSIC THERAPY WITH CAREGIVERS

In the future, the need to provide care for caregivers will probably increase. There is a growing body of music therapy research and clinical literature regarding the role of music therapy with adult caregivers. This information is valuable and should be used to inform our clinical interventions. Future challenges include the delivery of research that is adequately powered to detect the difference that music therapy may (or may not) make to caregivers (i.e., studies with sufficient sample sizes are required), and the selection of outcome measures is vitally important. Selecting the right measures will help us detect clinically meaningful changes. Also, the inclusion of sufficient detail in case studies will help us identify the profile of caregivers who access music therapy and the interventions that are useful to them. Addressing these factors will help us realise the potential of music therapy for caregivers and help us form strong, credible partnerships with this group.

REFERENCES

Bausewein, C., Daveson, B. A., Benalia, H., Simon, S. T., & Higginson, I. J. (2012). *Outcome measurement in palliative care: The essentials.* PRISMA and King's College, London.

Baxter, C., & O'Callaghan, C. (2010). Decisions about the future use of music therapy: Products created by palliative care patients. *The Australian Journal of Music Therapy, 21,* 20–25.

Boerner, K., Schulz, R., & Horowitz, A. (2004). Positive aspects of caregiving and adaptation to bereavement. *Psychological and Aging, 19,* 668–675.

Brown, S., Götell, E., & Ekman, S. L. (2001). "Music-therapeutic caregiving": The necessity of active music-making in clinical care. *The Arts in Psychotherapy, 28,* 125–135.

Cadrin, M. L. (2006). Music therapy legacy work in palliative care: Creating meaning at end of life. *Canadian Journal of Music Therapy, 12,* 190–237.

Chaput, J., & Silverman, M. J. (2012). Effects of music therapy with patients on a post-surgical oncology unit: A pilot study determining maintenance of immediate gains. *The Arts in Psychotherapy, 39* (5), 1–27.

Choi, Y. K. (2010). The effect of music and progressive muscle relaxation on anxiety, fatigue, and quality of life in family caregivers of hospice patients. *Journal of Music Therapy, 47,* 53–69.

Cohen, C. A., Colantonio, A., & Vernich, L. (2002). Positive aspects of caregiving: Rounding out the caregiver experience. *International Journal of Geriatric Psychiatry, 17,* 188.

Daveson, B. A., Bausewein, C., Murtagh, F., Calanzani, N., Higginson, I. J., Harding, R., et al. (2013). To be involved or not to be involved: A survey of public preferences for self-involvement in decision making involving mental capacity (competency) within Europe. *Palliative Medicine.* (Electronic version). Available at http://pmj.sagepub.com/content/early/recent

Department of Health. (2008). *End of life care strategy: Promoting high quality care for all adults at the end of life.* (Rep. no. 9840). Washington DC: U. S. Department of Health.

Hanser, S. B., Butterfield-Whitcomb, J., Kawata, M., & Collins, B. E. (2011). Home-based music strategies with individuals who have dementia and their family caregivers. *Journal of Music Therapy, 48,* 2–27.

Hinman, M. L. (2010). Our song: Music therapy with couples when one partner is medically hospitalized. *Music Therapy Perspectives, 28,* 29–36.

Kramer, B. J. (2012). Gain in the caregiving experience: Where are we? What next? *The Gerontologist, 37,* 218–232.

Morris, L. W., Morris, R. G., & Britton, P. G. (1998). The relationship between marital intimacy, perceived strain, and depression in spouse caregivers of dementia sufferers. *British Journal of Medical Psychology, 13,* 231–236.

National Institute for Clinical Excellence (NICE). (2004). *Guidance on cancer services improving supportive and palliative care for adults with cancer.* Oxford: Author.

Northouse, L. L., & Peters-Golden, H. (1993). Cancer and the family: Strategies to assist spouses. *Seminar in Oncology Nursing, 9,* 74–82.

Organisation for Economic Cooperation and Development (OECD) (2011a). Help wanted? Providing and paying for long-term care. In *Long-term care: growing sector, multifaceted systems* (pp. 37–59).

Organisation for Economic Cooperation and Development (OECD) (2011b). Policies to support family carers. In *Help wanted? Providing and paying for long-term care* (pp. 121–158). OECD.

Organisation for Economic Cooperation and Development (OECD) (2012). *Society at a glance 2011: OECD social indicators.* OECD publishing.

Office of Legislative Drafting and Publishing, A.-G. D. (9-7-2011). Fair Work Act. Terms and conditions of employment, 95–96.

Payne, S., Hudson, P., Grande, G., Oliviere, D., Tishelman, C., Pleschberger, S., et al. (2010). White Paper on improving support for family carers in palliative care: Part 1. *European Journal of Palliative Care, 17,* 238–245.

Pelletier, C. L. (2004). The effect of music on decreasing arousal due to stress: A meta-analysis. *Journal of Music Therapy, 41,* 192–214.

Silveira, M. J., Kim, S. Y., & Langa, K. M. (2010). Advance directives and outcomes of surrogate decision making before death. *New England Journal of Medicine, 362,* 1211–1218.

Stephens, M. A. P., Kinney, J. M., & Ogrocki, P. K. (1991). Stressors and well-being among caregivers to older adults with dementia: The in-home versus nursing home experience. *Gerontologist, 31,* 217–223.

Thorgrimsen, L., Schweitzer, P., & Orrell, M. (2002). Evaluating reminiscence for people with dementia: A pilot study. *The Arts in Psychotherapy, 29,* 93–97.

Vitaliano, P. P., & Zhang, J. (2003). Is caregiving hazardous to one's physical health? A meta-analysis. *Psychological Bulletin, 129,* 946–972.

Wendler, D., & Rid, A. (2011). Systematic review: The effect on surrogates of making treatment decisions for others. *Annals of Internal Medicine, 154,* 336–346.

World Health Organisation. (2008). *The global burden of disease: 2004 update.* Switzerland: The World Health Organisation.

Zabin, A. H. (2005). Preview lessons learned from the dying: Stories from a music therapist. *Music Therapy Perspectives, 23,* 70–75.

Zarit, S. H., Reever, K. E., & Bach-Peterson, J. (1980). Relatives of the impaired elderly: Correlates of feelings of burden. *Gerontologist, 20,* 649–655.

A

B

C

R

Guidelines for Music Therapy Practice
A Four Volume Series

GUIDELINES FOR MUSIC THERAPY PRACTICE IN DEVELOPMENTAL HEALTH
Edited by Michelle R. Hintz

1) Introduction: *Michelle R. Hintz*
2) Early Intervention: *Elizabeth K. Schwartz*
3) Autism: *Michelle R. Hintz*
4) Rett Syndrome: *Jennifer M. Sokira*
5) Developmental Speech and Language Disorders: *Kathleen M. Howland*
6) Attentional Deficits in School Children: *Michelle R. Hintz*
7) Learning Disabilities in School Children: *Michelle R. Hintz*
8) Behavioral and Interpersonal Problems in School Children: *Patricia McCarrick*
9) Children with Hearing Loss: *Christine Barton*
10) Visually Impaired School Children: *Paige A. Robbins Elwafi*
11) Mild to Moderate Intellectual Disability: *Douglas R. Keith*
12) Severe to Profound Intellectual and Developmental Disabilities: *Donna W. Polen*
13) Physical Disabilities in School Children: *Jennifer M. Sokira*
14) Individuals with Severe and Multiple Disabilities: *Barbara Wheeler*

GUIDELINES FOR MUSIC THERAPY PRACTICE IN MENTAL HEALTH
Edited by Lillian Eyre

1) Introduction: *Lillian Eyre*
2) Adults with Schizophrenia and Psychotic Disorders: *Andrea McGraw Hunt*
3) Adult Groups in the Inpatient Setting: *Lillian Eyre*
4) Adults in a Recovery Model Setting: *Lillian Eyre*
5) Children and Adolescents in an Inpatient Psychiatric Setting: *Bridget Doak*
6) Foster Care Youth: *Michael L. Zanders*
7) Survivors of Catastrophic Event Trauma: *Ronald M. Borczon*
8) Women Survivors of Abuse and Developmental Trauma: *Sandra Lynn Curtis*
9) Adult Male Survivors of Abuse and Developmental Trauma: *Jeffrey H. Hatcher*
10) Children and Adolescents with PTSD and Survivors of Abuse and Neglect: *Penny Rogers*
11) Adults with Depression and/or Anxiety: *Nancy A. Jackson*
12) Adults and Adolescents with Borderline Personality Disorder: *J. M. Dvorkin*
13) Adults and Adolescents with Eating Disorders: *Peggy Tileston*
14) Adults with Substance Use Disorders: *Kathleen M. Murphy*
15) Adolescents with Substance Use Disorders: *Katrina Skewes McFerran*
16) Adult Males in Forensic Settings: *Vaughn Kaser*
17) Adult Females in Correctional Facilities: *Karen Anne Litecky Melendez*
18) Adjudicated Adolescents: *Susan Gardstrom*
19) Juvenile Male Sexl Offenders: *Lori L. De Rea-Kolb*
20) Elderly Residents in Nursing Facilities: *Elaine A. Abbott*

21) Persons with Alzheimer's and Other Dementias: *Laurel Young*
22) Professional Burnout: *Darlene M. Brooks*
23) Stress Reduction and Wellness: *Seung-A Kim*
24) Musicians: *Gro Trondalen*
25) Spiritual Practices: *Annie Heiderscheit*

GUIDELINES FOR MUSIC THERAPY PRACTICE IN PEDIATRIC CARE
Edited by Joke Bradt

1) Introduction: *Joke Bradt*
2) Pain Management with Children: *Joke Bradt*
3) Premature Infants: *Monika Nöcker-Ribaupierre*
4) Full-Term Hospitalized Newborns: *Helen Shoemark*
5) Pediatric Intensive Care: *Claire Ghetti*
6) Surgical and Procedural Support for Children: *John Mondanaro*
7) Burn Care for Children: *Annette Whitehead-Pleaux*
8) Children with Cancer: *Beth Dun*
9) Palliative and End-of-Life Care for Children: *Kathryn Lindenfelser*
10) Brain Injuries and Rehabilitation in Children: *Jeanette Kennelly*
11) Respiratory Care for Children: *Joanne Loewy*
12) Medically Fragile Children in Low Awareness States: *Jennifer Townsend*
13) Children in General Inpatient Care: *Christine Neugebauer*

GUIDELINES FOR MUSIC THERAPY PRACTICE IN ADULT MEDICAL CARE
Edited by Joy Allen

1) Introduction: *Joy Allen*
2) Surgical and Procedural support: *Annie Heiderscheit*
3) Pain Management with Adults: *Joy Allen*
4) Adults in Critical Care: *Jeanette Tamplin*
5) Adults in Cardiac Care: *Christine Pollard Leist*
6) Adults with Stroke: *Simon Gilbertson*
7) Adults with Traumatic Brain Injury: *Victoria Policastro Vega*
8) Adults with Neurogenic Communication Disorders: *Nicki Cohen*
9) Adults with Neurogenerative Diseases: *Wendy Magee*
10) Adults with HIV/AIDS: *Douglas Keith*
11) Adults with Cancer: *Joy Allen*
12) Adults in Palliative/Hospice Care: *Amy Clement-Cortes*
13) Caring for Caregivers: *Barbara Daveson*

THE BARCELONA COLLECTION OF PRINT AND E-BOOKS 2013

ANALYTIC MUSIC THERAPY

- Essays on Analytical Music Therapy (Priestley)
- Music Therapy in Action (2nd Edition) (Priestley)
- The Dynamics of Music Psychotherapy (Bruscia)
- Group Analytic Music Therapy (Ahonen-Eerikäinen)

CASE STUDIES

- Case Examples of Guided Imagery and Music (Bruscia)
- Case Examples of Improvisational Music Therapy (Bruscia)
- Case Examples of Music Therapy for___ (Bruscia):
    - Alzheimer's Disease
    - Autism and Rett Syndrome
    - Children and Adolescents with Emotional or Behavioral Problems
    - Developmental Problems in Learning and Communication
    - End of Life
    - Event Trauma
    - Medical Conditions
    - Mood Disorders
    - Multiple Disabilities
    - Musicians
    - Personality Disorders
    - Schizophrenia and other Psychoses
    - Self-Development
    - Substance Use Disorders
    - Survivors of Abuse
- Case Examples of the Use of Songs in Psychotherapy (Bruscia)
- Studies in Music Therapy (Bruscia)
- Inside Music Therapy: Client Experiences (Hibben)
- Psychodynamic Music Therapy: Case Studies (Hadley)

CHILDREN WITH SPECIAL NEEDS

- Alike and Different: The Clinical and Educational Uses of Orff-Schulwerk – Second Edition (Bitcon)
- The Miracle of Music Therapy (Boxill)
- Music for Fun, Music for Learning (Birkenshaw-Fleming)
- Music: Motion and Emotion: The Developmental-Integrative Model in Music Therapy (Sekeles)
- Music, Therapy, and Early Childhood (Schwartz)
- Music Therapy in Special Education (Nordoff & Robbins)

- Therapy in Music for Handicapped Children (Nordoff & Robbins)

COMMUNITY MUSIC THERAPY
- Elaborations Toward a Notion of Community Music Therapy (Stige)
- Culture-Centered Music Therapy (Stige)

INFANCY AND EARLY CHILDHOOD
- Music, Therapy, and Early Childhood (Schwartz)
- Music Therapy for Premature and Newborn Infants (Nöcker-Ribaupierre)

END OF LIFE
- Music Therapy: Death and Grief (Sekeles)

FEMINISM
- Feminist Perspectives in Music Therapy (Hadley)

FIELDWORK AND INTERNSHIP TRAINING
- Clinical Training Guide for the Student Music Therapist (Wheeler, Shultis & Polen)
- Music Therapy: A Fieldwork Primer (Borczon)
- Music Therapy Supervision (Forinash)

GROUP WORK
- Music Therapy: Group Vignettes (Borczon)
- Music Therapy Improvisation for Groups: Essential Leadership Competencies (Gardstrom)

GUIDED IMAGERY AND MUSIC (BONNY METHOD)
- Guided Imagery and Music: The Bonny Method and Beyond (Bruscia & Grocke)
- Music and Consciousness: The Evolution of Guided Imagery and Music (Bonny)
- Music and Your Mind: Listening with a New Consciousness (Bonny & Savary)
- Music for the Imagination (Bruscia)

GUITAR
- Guitar Skills for Music Therapists and Music Educators (Meyer, De Villers, Ebnet)
- Use of the Guitar in Music Therapy (Oden)

IMPROVISATIONAL MUSIC THERAPY
- The Architecture of Aesthetic Music Therapy (Lee)
- Essays on Analytical Music Therapy (Priestley)
- Creative Music Therapy: A Guide to Fostering Clinical Musicianship – Second Edition with Four CDs (Nordoff & Robbins)
- Group Analytic Music Therapy (Ahonen-Eerikäinen)
- Healing Heritage: Paul Nordoff Exploring the Tonal Language of Music (Robbins & Robbins)
- Improvising in Styles: A Workbook for Music Therapists, Educators, and Musicians (Lee & Houde)
- Music as Therapy: A Dialogal Perspective (Garred)
- Music-Centered Music Therapy (Aigen)
- Music Therapy: Improvisation, Communication, and Culture (Ruud)
- Music Therapy Improvisation for Groups: Essential Leadership Competencies (Gardstrom)
- Paths of Development in Nordoff-Robbins Music Therapy (Aigen)

- Playin' in the Band: A Qualitative study of Popular Music Styles as Clinical Improvisation (Aigen)
- Sounding the Self: Analogy in Improvisational Music Therapy (Smeijsters)

MUSIC FOR CHILDREN TO SING AND PLAY

- Distant Bells (Levin & Levin)
- Learning Songs (Levin & Levin)
- Learning Through Music (Levin & Levin)
- Learning Through Songs (Levin & Levin)
- Let's Make Music (Levin & Levin)
- Music for Fun, Music for Learning (Birkenshaw-Fleming)
- Snow White: A Guide to Child-Centered Musical Theatre (Lauri, Groeschel, Robbins, Ritholz & Turry)
- Symphonics R Us (Levin & Levin)

NORDOFF-ROBBINS MUSIC THERAPY (CREATIVE MUSIC THERAPY)

- The Architecture of Aesthetic Music Therapy (Lee)
- Being in Music: Foundations of Nordoff-Robbins Music Therapy (Aigen)
- Conversations on Nordoff-Robbins Music Therapy (Verney & Ansdell)
- Creative Music Therapy: A Guide to Fostering Clinical Musicianship – Second Edition with Four CDs (Nordoff & Robbins)
- Healing Heritage: Paul Nordoff Exploring the Tonal Language of Music (Robbins & Robbins)
- Here We Are in Music: One Year with an Adolescent Creative Music Therapy Group (Aigen)
- A Journey into Creative Music Therapy (Robbins)
- Music Therapy in Special Education (Nordoff & Robbins)
- Paths of Development in Nordoff-Robbins Music Therapy (Aigen)
- Playin' in the Band: A Qualitative study of Popular Music Styles as Clinical Improvisation (Aigen)
- Therapy in Music for Handicapped Children (Nordoff & Robbins)

MUSIC THERAPY PRACTICE

- Guidelines for Music Therapy Practice in Mental Health (Eyre)
- Guidelines for Music Therapy Practice in Developmental Health (Hintz)
- Guidelines for Music Therapy Practice in Pediatric Care (Bradt)
- Guidelines for Music Therapy Practice in Adult Medical Care (Allen)

MUSIC PSYCHOTHERAPY

- The Dynamics of Music Psychotherapy (Bruscia)
- Essays on Analytical Music Therapy (Priestley)
- Emotional Processes in Music Therapy (Pellitteri)
- Group Analytic Music Therapy (Ahonen-Eerikäinen)
- Guided Imagery and Music: The Bonny Method and Beyond (Bruscia & Grocke)
- Music and Consciousness: The Evolution of Guided Imagery and Music (Bonny)
- Music and Your Mind: Listening with a New Consciousness (Bonny & Savary)

- Music Therapy: Group Vignettes (Borczon)
- Psychodynamic Music Therapy: Case Studies (Hadley)

ORFF-SCHULWERK

- Alike and Different: The Clinical and Educational Uses of Orff-Schulwerk – Second Edition (Bitcon)

PIANO

- Functional Piano for Music Therapists and Music Educators (Massicot)
- Improvising in Styles: A Workbook for Music Therapists, Educators, and Musicians (Lee & Houde)

PROFOUND MENTAL RETARDATION

- Age-Appropriate Activities for Adults with Profound Mental Retardation – Second Edition (Galerstein, Martin & Powe)

PSYCHODRAMA

- Acting Your Inner Music (Moreno)

PSYCHIATRY – MENTAL HEALTH

- Music Therapy in the Treatment of Adults with Mental Disorders: Theoretical Bases and Clinical Interventions (Unkefer & Thaut)
- Psychiatric Music Therapy in the Community: The Legacy of Florence Tyson (McGuire)
- Psychodynamic Music Therapy: Case Studies (Hadley)
- Resource-Oriented Music Therapy in Mental Health Care (Rolvsjord)

RACE

- Experience Race as a Music Therapist: Personal Narratives (Hadley)

RESEARCH

- A Guide to Writing and Presenting in Music Therapy (Aigen)
- Multiple Perspectives: A Guide to Qualitative Research in Music Therapy (Smeijsters)
- Music Therapy Research: Quantitative and Qualitative Perspectives – First Edition (1995) (Wheeler)
- Music Therapy Research – Second Edition (2005) (Wheeler)
- Playin' in the Band: A Qualitative study of Popular Music Styles as Clinical Improvisation (Aigen)
- Qualitative Inquiries in Music Therapy: A Monograph Series (Free Downloads Available Here)
- Qualitative Music Therapy Research: Beginning Dialogues (Langenberg, Frömmer & Aigen)

SUPERVISION

- Music Therapy Supervision (Forinash)

THEORY

- Culture-Centered Music Therapy (Stige)
- Defining Music Therapy – Second Edition (Bruscia)
- Emotional Processes in Music Therapy (Pellitteri)
- Music and Life in the Field of Play: An Anthology (Kenny)

- Music as Therapy: A Dialogal Perspective (Garred)
- Music-Centered Music Therapy (Aigen)
- Music Therapy and its Relationship to Current Treatment Theories (Ruud)
- Music Therapy: A Perspective from the Humanities (Ruud)
- Music Therapy: Improvisation, Communication, and Culture (Ruud)
- Music—The Therapeutic Edge: Readings from William W. Sears (Sears)
- The Music Within You (Katsh & Fishman)
- Readings on Music Therapy Theory (Bruscia)
- Resource-Oriented Music Therapy in Mental Health Care (Rolvsjord)
- The Rhythmic Language of Health and Disease (Rider)
- Sounding the Self: Analogy in Improvisational Music Therapy (Smeijsters)

VOICE

- Authentic Voices, Authentic Singing (Uhlig)
- Psychiatric Music Therapy in the Community: The Legacy of Florence Tyson (McGuire)